ANNUAL EDITIONS

Aging

Twentieth Edition

07/08

EDITOR

Harold Cox

Indiana State University

Harold Cox, professor of sociology at Indiana State University, has published several articles in the field of gerontology. He is the author of *Later Life: The Realities of Aging* (Prentice Hall, 2000). He is a member of the Gerontological Society of America and the American Sociological Association's Occupation and Professions Section and Youth Aging Section.

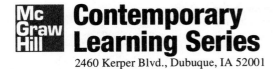
Contemporary Learning Series

2460 Kerper Blvd., Dubuque, IA 52001

Visit us on the Internet
http://www.mhcls.com

Credits

1. **The Phenomenon of Aging**
   Unit photo—IT Stock/PunchStock
2. **The Quality of Later Life**
   Unit photo—Bronwyn Kidd/Getty Images
3. **Societal Attitudes Toward Old Age**
   Unit photo—Donna Day/Getty Images
4. **Problems and Potentials of Aging**
   Unit photo—C. Lee/PhotoLink/Getty Images
5. **Retirement: American Dream or Dilemma**
   Unit photo—Steve Mason/Getty Images
6. **The Experience of Dying**
   Unit photo—Spike Mafford/Getty Images
7. **Living Environment in Later Life**
   Unit photo—Keith Brofsky/Getty Images
8. **Social Policies, Programs, and Services for Older Americans**
   Unit photo—Comstock Images/PictureQuest

Copyright

Cataloging in Publication Data
Main entry under title: Annual Editions: Aging. 2007/2008.
1. Aging—Periodicals. I. Cox, Harold, *comp.* II. Title: Aging.
ISBN-13: 978–0–07–339729–0   ISBN-10: 0–07–339729–6   658'.05   ISSN 2072–3808

Twentieth Edition

Cover image © Royalty free/Corbis and Photos.com
Printed in the United States of America   1234567890QPDQPD987   Printed on Recycled Paper

Editors/Advisory Board

Members of the Advisory Board are instrumental in the final selection of articles for each edition of ANNUAL EDITIONS. Their review of articles for content, level, currentness, and appropriateness provides critical direction to the editor and staff. We think that you will find their careful consideration well reflected in this volume.

EDITOR

Howard Cox
Indiana State University

ADVISORY BOARD

Barbara D. Ames
Michigan State University

Chalon E. Anderson
University of Central Oklahoma

Arthur E. Dell Orto
Boston University

Andrew W. Dobelstein
*University of North Carolina–
Chapel Hill*

Gayle Doll
Kansas State University

Phyllis Greenberg
St. Cloud State University

Lynne G. Hodgson
Quinnipiac University

Scott Hofer
Oregon State University

Christopher J. Johnson
University of Louisiana

Nancy J. King
St. Mary's College

Marcia Lasswell
California State Polytechnic University

Alinde J. Moore
Ashland University

Mark Novak
San Jose State University

Paul E. Panek
The Ohio State University–Newark

Sarah Pender
Folsom Lake College

Paul A. Roodin
SUNY College, Oswego

Rick J. Scheidt
Kansas State University

Shirley R. Simon
Loyola University

George F. Stine
Millersville University

Selwyn Super
University of Southern California

Dean VonDras
University Wisconsin–Green Bay

Caroline S. Westerhof
*Florida Metropolitan University–
Pinellas Campus*

Steve Wisensale
University of Connecticut

Staff

EDITORIAL STAFF

Larry Loeppke, Managing Editor
Jay Oberbroeckling, Developmental Editor
Jade Benedict, Developmental Editor
Nancy Meissner, Editorial Assistant

PERMISSIONS STAFF

Lenny J. Behnke, Permissions Coordinator
Lori Church, Permissions Coordinator
Shirley Lanners, Permissions Coordinator

TECHNOLOGY STAFF

Luke David, eContent Coordinator

MARKETING STAFF

Julie Keck, Senior Marketing Manager
Mary Klein, Marketing Communications Specialist
Alice Link, Marketing Coordinator
Tracie Kammerude, Senior Marketing Assistant

PRODUCTION STAFF

Beth Kundert, Production Manager
Trish Mish, Production Assistant
Kari Voss, Lead Typesetter
Jean Smith, Typesetter
Karen Spring, Typesetter
Sandy Wille, Typesetter
Tara McDermott, Designer
Maggie Lytle, Cover Graphics

Preface

In publishing ANNUAL EDITIONS we recognize the enormous role played by the magazines, newspapers, and journals of the public press in providing current, first-rate educational information in a broad spectrum of interest areas. Many of these articles are appropriate for students, researchers, and professionals seeking accurate, current material to help bridge the gap between principles and theories and the real world. These articles, however, become more useful for study when those of lasting value are carefully collected, organized, indexed, and reproduced in a low-cost format, which provides easy and permanent access when the material is needed. That is the role played by ANNUAL EDITIONS.

The decline of the crude birth rate in the United Sates and other industrialized nations combined with improving food supplies, sanitation, and medical technology has resulted in an ever increasing number and percentage of people remaining alive and healthy well into their retirement years. The result is a shifting age composition of the populations in these nations—a population composed of fewer people under age 20 and more people 65 and older. In 1990, approximately 3 million Americans were 65 years old and older, and they composed 4 percent of the population. In 2000, there were 36 million persons 65 years old and older, and they represented 13 percent of the total population. The most rapid increase in the number of older persons is expected between 2010 and 2030 when the "baby boom" generation reaches the age of 65. Demographers predict that by 2030 there will be 66 million older persons representing approximately 22 percent of the total population. The growing number of older people has made many of the problems of aging immediately visible to the average American. These problems have become widespread topics of concern for political leaders, government planners, and average citizens. Moreover, the aging of the population has become perceived as a phenomenon of the United States and the industrialized countries of Western Europe—it is also occurring in the underdeveloped countries of the world as well. An increasing percentage of the world's population is now defined as aged.

Today almost all middle-aged people expect to live to retirement age and beyond. Both the middle-aged and the elderly have pushed for solutions to the problems confronting older Americans. Everyone seems to agree that granting the elderly a secure and comfortable status is desirable. Voluntary associations, communities, and state and federal governments have committed themselves to improving the lives of older persons. Many programs for senior citizens, both public and private, have emerged in the last 15 years.

The change in the age composition of the population has not gone unnoticed by the media or the academic community. The number of articles appearing in the popular press and professional journals has increased dramatically over the last several years. While scientists have been concerned with the aging process for some time, in the last two decades there has been an expanding volume of research and writing on this subject. This growing interest has resulted in this twentieth edition of *Annual Editions: Aging 07/08.*

This volume is representative of the field of gerontology in that it is interdisciplinary in its approach, including articles from the biological sciences, medicine, nursing, psychology, sociology, and social work. The articles are taken from the popular press, government publications, and scientific journals. They represent a wide cross section of authors, perspectives, and issues related to the aging process. They were chosen because they address the most relevant and current problems in the field of aging, and present a variety of divergent views on the appropriate solutions to these problems. The topics covered include demographic trends, the aging process, longevity, social attitudes toward old age, problems and potentials of aging, retirement, death, living environments in later life, and social policies, programs, and services for older Americans. The articles are organized into an anthology that is useful for both the student and the teacher.

The goal of *Annual Editions: Aging 07/08* is to choose articles that are pertinent, well written, and helpful to those concerned with the field of gerontology. Comments, suggestions, or constructive criticism are welcomed to help improve future editions of this book. Please complete and return the postage-paid article rating form on the last page of this volume. Any anthology can be improved. This one will continue to be improved—annually.

Harold Cox
Editor

Contents

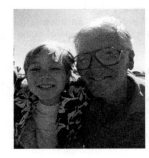

UNIT 1
The Phenomenon of Aging

The concepts in bold italics are developed in the article. For further expansion, please refer to the Topic Guide and the Index.

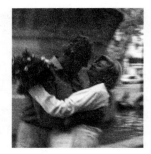

UNIT 2
The Quality of Later Life

UNIT 3
Societal Attitudes Toward Old Age

The concepts in bold italics are developed in the article. For further expansion, please refer to the Topic Guide and the Index.

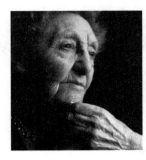

UNIT 4
Problems and Potentials of Aging

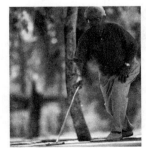

UNIT 5
Retirement: American Dream or Dilemma?

The concepts in bold italics are developed in the article. For further expansion, please refer to the Topic Guide and the Index.

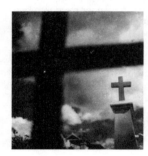

UNIT 6
The Experience of Dying

The concepts in bold italics are developed in the article. For further expansion, please refer to the Topic Guide and the Index.

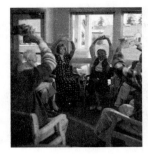

UNIT 7
Living Environment in Later Life

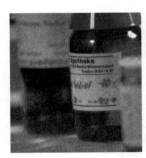

UNIT 8
Social Policies, Programs, and Services for Older Americans

The concepts in bold italics are developed in the article. For further expansion, please refer to the Topic Guide and the Index.

The concepts in bold italics are developed in the article. For further expansion, please refer to the Topic Guide and the Index.

Topic Guide

This topic guide suggests how the selections in this book relate to the subjects covered in your course. You may want to use the topics listed on these pages to search the Web more easily.

On the following pages a number of Web sites have been gathered specifically for this book. They are arranged to reflect the units of this *Annual Edition.* You can link to these sites by going to the student online support site at *http://www.mhcls.com/online/.*

ALL THE ARTICLES THAT RELATE TO EACH TOPIC ARE LISTED BELOW THE BOLD-FACED TERM.

Internet References

The following Internet sites have been carefully researched and selected to support the articles found in this reader. The easiest way to access these selected sites is to go to our student online support site at *http://www.mhcls.com/online/*.

AE: Aging 07/08

The following sites were available at the time of publication. Visit our Web site—we update our student online support site regularly to reflect any changes.

General Sources

Alliance for Aging Research
http://www.agingresearch.org/

The nation's leading non-profit organization dedicated to improving the health and independence of Americans as they age through public and private funding of medical research and geriatric education.

ElderCare Online
http://www.ec-online.net/

This site provides numerous links to eldercare resources. Information on health, living, aging, finance, and social issues can be found here.

FirstGov
http://www.firstgov.gov/

Whatever you want or need from the U.S. government, it's here on FirstGov.gov. You'll find a rich treasure of online information, services and resources.

UNIT 1: The Phenomenon of Aging

The Aging Research Centre
http://www.arclab.org/

The Aging Research Centre is dedicated to providing a service that allows researchers to find information that is related to the study of the aging process.

Centenarians
http://www.hcoa.org/centenarians/centenarians.htm

There are approximately 70,000 centenarians in the United States. This site provides resources and information for and about centenarians.

National Center for Health Statistics
http://www.cdc.gov/nchs/agingact.htm

NCHS is the Federal Government's principal vital and health statistics agency. NCHS is a part of the Centers for Disease Control and Prevention, U.S. Department of Health and Human Services.

UNIT 2: The Quality of Later Life

Aging with Dignity
http://www.agingwithdignity.org/

The non-profit Aging With Dignity was established to provide people with the practical information, advice and legal tools needed to help their loved ones get proper care.

The Gerontological Society of America
http://www.geron.org

The Gerontological Society of America promotes the scientific study of aging, and it fosters growth and diffusion of knowledge relating to problems of aging and of the sciences contributing to their understanding.

The National Council on the Aging
http://www.ncoa.org

The National Council on the Aging, Inc., is a center of leadership and nationwide expertise in the issues of aging. This private, nonprofit association is committed to enhancing the field of aging through leadership, service, education, and advocacy.

UNIT 3: Societal Attitudes Toward Old Age

Adult Development and Aging: Division 20 of the American Psychological Association
http://www.iog.wayne.edu/APADIV20/APADIV20.HTM

This group is dedicated to studying the psychology of adult development and aging.

American Society on Aging
http://www.asaging.org/index.cfm

The American Society on Aging is the largest and most dynamic network of professionals in the field of aging.

Canadian Psychological Association
http://www.cpa.ca/

This is the contents page of the Canadian Psychological Association. Material on aging and human development can be found at this site.

UNIT 4: Problems and Potentials of Aging

Alzheimer's Association
http://www.alz.org

The Alzheimer's Association is dedicated to researching the prevention, cures, and treatments of Alzheimer's disease and related disorders, and providing support and assistance to afflicted patients and their families.

A.P.T.A. Section on Geriatrics
http://geriatricspt.org

This is a component of the American Physical Therapy Association. At this site, information regarding consumer and health information for older adults can be found.

Caregiver's Handbook
http://www.acsu.buffalo.edu/~drstall/hndbk0.html

This site is an online handbook for caregivers. Topics include nutrition, medical aspects of caregiving, and liabilities of caregiving.

Caregiver Survival Resources
http://www.caregiver.com

Information on books, seminars, and information for caregivers can be found at this site.

AARP Health Information
http://www.aarp.org/bulletin

Information on a BMI calculator, the USDA food pyramid, healthy recipes and health related articles can be found at this site.

International Food Information Council

http://www.ific.org/

At this site, you can find information regarding nutritional needs for aging adults. The site focuses on information for educators and students, publications, and nutritional information.

University of California at Irvine: Institute for Brain Aging and Dementia

http://www.alz.uci.edu/

The Institute for Brain Aging and Dementia is dedicated to the study of Alzheimer's and the causes of mental disabilities for the elderly.

UNIT 5: Retirement: American Dream or Dilemma?

American Association of Retired People

http://www.aarp.org

The AARP is the nation's leading organization for people 50 and older. AARP serves their needs through information, education, advocacy, and community service.

Health and Retirement Study (HRS)

http://www.umich.edu/~hrswww/

The University of Michigan Health and Retirement Study surveys more than 22,000 Americans over the age of 50 every two years. Supported by the National Institute on Aging, the study paints an emerging portrait of an aging America; physical and mental health, insurance coverage, financial status, family support systems, labor market status, and retirement planning.

UNIT 6: The Experience of Dying

Agency for Health Care Policy and Research

http://www.ahcpr.gov

Information on the dying process in the context of U.S. health policy is provided here, along with a search mechanism. The agency is part of the Department of Health and Human Services.

Growth House, Inc.

http://www.growthhouse.org/

This award-winning web site is an international gateway to resources for life-threatening illness and end of life care.

Hospice Foundation of America

http://www.HospiceFoundation.org

On this page, you can learn about hospice care, how to select a hospice, and how to find a hospice near you.

Hospice HotLinks

http://www.hospiceweb.com/links.htm

Links with information about all aspects of hospice care can be found at this site.

UNIT 7: Living Environment in Later Life

American Association of Homes and Services for the Aging

http://www.aahsa.org

The American Association of Homes and Services for the Aging represents a not-for-profit organization dedicated to providing high-quality health care, housing, and services to the nation's elderly.

Center for Demographic Studies

http://cds.duke.edu

The Center for Demographic Studies is located in the heart of the Duke campus. The primary focus of their research is long-term care for elderly populations, specifically those 65 years of age and older.

Guide to Retirement Living Online

http://www.retirement-living.com

An online version of a free publication, this site provides information about nursing homes, continuous care communities, independent living, home health care, and adult day care centers.

The United States Department of Housing and Urban Development

http://www.hud.gov

News regarding housing for aging adults can be found at this site sponsored by the U.S. federal government.

UNIT 8: Social Policies, Programs, and Services for Older Americans

Administration on Aging

http://www.aoa.dhhs.gov

This site, housed on the Department of Health and Human Services Web site, provides information for older persons and their families. There is also information for educators and students regarding the elderly.

American Federation for Aging Research

http://www.afar.org/

Since 1981, the American Federation for Aging Research (AFAR) has helped scientists begin and further careers in aging research and geriatric medicine.

American Geriatrics Society

http://www.americangeriatrics.org

This organization addresses the needs of our rapidly aging population. At this site, you can find information on health care and other social issues facing the elderly.

Community Transportation Association of America

http://www.ctaa.org

C.T.A.A. is a nonprofit organization dedicated to mobility for all people, regardless of wealth, disability, age, or accessibility.

Consumer Reports State Inspection Surveys

http://www.ConsumerReports.org

To learn how to get state inspection surveys and to contact the ombudsman's office, click on "Personal Finance," then select "Assisted Living."

Medicare Consumer Information From the Health Care Finance Association

http://cms.hhs.gov/default.asp?fromhcfadotgov=true

This site is devoted to explaining Medicare and Medicaid costs to consumers.

National Institutes of Health

http://www.nih.gov

Information on health issues can be found at this government site. There is quite a bit of information relating to health issues and the aging population in the United States.

The United States Senate: Special Committee on Aging

http://www.senate.gov/~aging/

This committee, chaired by Senator Gordon Smith of Oregon, deals with the issues surrounding the elderly in America. At this site, you can download committee hearing information, news, and committee publications.

We highly recommend that you review our Web site for expanded information and our other product lines. We are continually updating and adding links to our Web site in order to offer you the most usable and useful information that will support and expand the value of your Annual Editions. You can reach us at: *http://www.mhcls.com/annualeditions/*.

UNIT 1
The Phenomenon of Aging

Unit Selections

1. **Elderly Americans**, Christine L. Himes
2. **The Economic Conundrum of an Aging Population**, Robert Ayres
3. **Living Longer**, Donna Jackson Nakazawa and Susan Crandall
4. **Puzzle of the Century**, Mary Duenwald
5. **The Demographic Drivers of Aging**, Kevin Kinsella and David R. Phillips
6. **Will You Live to Be 100?**, Thomas Perls and Margery Hutter Silver
7. **The 2005 White House Conference on Aging**, Maureen Shawn Kennedy

Key Points to Consider

- What factors contribute to the increasing life expectancy of the American people? What challenges do aging Americans face?

- Why are older Americans healthier than ever before?

- Will it ever be possible to slow down the aging process? Would this be desirable? Why or why not?

- What are the problems and advantages that society must consider in facing the increased aging population? Give examples.

Student Website

www.mhcls.com/online

Internet References

Further information regarding these websites may be found in this book's preface or online.

The Aging Research Centre
http://www.arclab.org/

Centenarians
http://www.hcoa.org/centenarians/centenarians.htm

National Center for Health Statistics
http://www.cdc.gov/nchs/agingact.htm

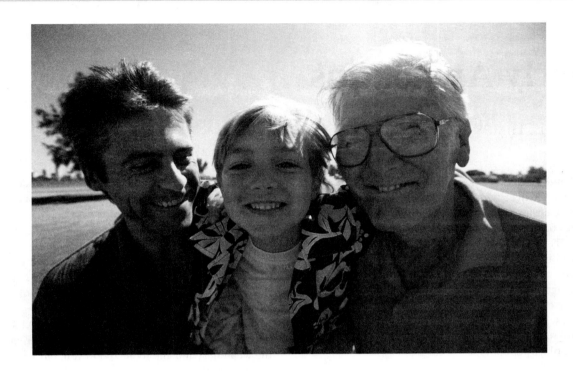

The process of aging is complex and includes biological, psychological, sociological, and behavioral changes. Biologically, the body gradually loses the ability to renew itself. Various body functions begin to slow down, and the vital senses become less acute. Psychologically, aging persons experience changing sensory processes; perception, motor skills, problem-solving ability, and drives and emotions are frequently altered. Sociologically, they must cope with the changing roles and definitions of self that society imposes on the individual. For instance, the role expectations and the status of grandparents is different from those of parents, and the roles of the retired are quite different from those of the employed. Being defined as "old" may be desirable or undesirable, depending on the particular culture and its values. Behaviorally, aging individuals may move slower and with less dexterity. Because they are assuming new roles and are viewed differently by others, their attitudes about themselves, their emotions, and, ultimately, their behavior can be expected to change.

Those studying the process of aging often use developmental theories of the life cycle—a sequence of predictable phases that begins with birth and ends with death—to explain individuals' behavior at various stages of their lives. An individual's age, therefore, is important because it provides clues about his or her behavior at a particular phase of the life cycle—be it childhood, adolescence, adulthood, middle age, or old age. There is, however, the greatest variation in terms of health and human development among older people than among any other age group. While every 3-year-old child can be predicted to have certain developmental experiences, there is a wide variation in the behavior of 65-year-old people. By age 65, we find that some people are in good health, employed, and performing important work

tasks. Others of this cohort are retired but in good health or are retired and in poor health. Still others have died prior to the age of 65. The articles in this section are written from biological, psychological, and sociological perspectives. These disciplines attempt to explain the effects of aging and the resulting choices in lifestyle, as well as the wider cultural implications of an older population.

In the article "Elderly Americans," Christine Himes delineates the increases in life expectancy and the aging of the American population that has occurred during the last century. Robert Ayres in "The Economic Conundrum of an Aging Population" examines the effect of a smaller labor pool and a larger older population on industrialized countries throughout the world. In "Living Longer," the authors discuss how the research findings in the areas of diet and exercise, if followed, could increase the individual's life expectancy by a number of years. Mary Duenwald in "Puzzle of the Century" tries to determine why so many Nova Scotians live to be 100 years or older. In "The Demographic Drivers of Aging," Kinsella and Phillips explain how a declining death rate, a declining crude birth rate, and an increase in life expectancy can lead to significant changes in the age composition of a population.

Thomas Perls and Margery Hutter Silver conducted a study at Harvard Medical School of long-living individuals. Following their research, they came up with a quiz that included dietary and lifestyle choices, as well as family histories to help the individual determine what his or her probabilities are of living to a very old age. "The 2005 White House Conference on Aging" passed a number of resolutions which are listed as a means of maintaining and improving current government senior service programs.

1

Elderly Americans

CHRISTINE L. HIMES

The United States is in the midst of a profound demographic change: the rapid aging of its population. The 2000 Census counted nearly 35 million people in the United States 65 years of age or older, about one of every eight Americans. By 2030, demographers estimate that one in five Americans will be age 65 or older, which is nearly four times the proportion of elderly 100 years earlier, in 1930. The effects of this older age profile will reverberate throughout the American economy and society in the next 50 years. Preparing for these changes involves more than the study of demographic trends; it also requires an understanding of the growing diversity within the older population.

The lives and well-being of older Americans attract increasing attention as the elderly share of the U.S. population rises: One-fifth will be 65 or older in 2030.

The aging of the U.S. population in the next 20 years is being propelled by one of the most powerful demographic forces in the United States in the last century: the "baby boom" cohort, born between 1946 and 1964. This group of 76 million children grabbed media attention as it moved toward adulthood—changing school systems, colleges, and the workplace. And, this same group of people will change the profile and expectations of old age in the United States over the next 30 years as it moves past age 65. The potential effects of the baby boom on the systems of old-age assistance already are being evaluated. This cohort's consumption patterns, demand for leisure, and use of health care, for example, will leave an indelible mark on U.S. society in the 21st century. Understanding their characteristics as they near older ages will help us anticipate baby-boomers' future needs and their effects on the population.

Until the last 50 years, most gains in life expectancy came as the result of improved child mortality. The survival of larger proportions of infants and children to adulthood radically increased average life expectancy in the United States and many other countries over the past century. Now, gains are coming at the end of life as greater proportions of 65-year-olds are living until age 85, and more 85-year-olds are living into their 90s. These changes raise a

multitude of questions: How will these years of added life be spent? Will increased longevity lead to a greater role for the elderly in our society? What are the limits of life expectancy?

Increasing life expectancy, especially accompanied by low fertility, changes the structure of families. Families are becoming more "vertical," with fewer members in each generation, but more generations alive at any one time. Historically, families have played a prominent role in the lives of elderly people. Is this likely to change?

As much as any stage of the life course, old age is a time of growth, diversity, and change. Elderly Americans are among the wealthiest and among the poorest in our nation. They come from a variety of racial and ethnic backgrounds. Some are employed full-time, while others require full-time care. While general health has improved, many elderly suffer from poor health.

The older population in the 21st century will come to later life with different experiences than did older Americans in the last century—more women will have been divorced, more will have worked in the labor force, more will be childless. How will these experiences shape their later years?

The answers to these questions are complex. In some cases, we are confident in our predictions of the future. But for many aspects of life for the elderly, we are entering new territory. This report explores the characteristics of the current older population and speculates how older Americans may differ in the future. It also looks at the impact of aging on the U.S. society and economy.

Increasing Numbers

The United States has seen its elderly population—defined at those age 65 or older—grow more than tenfold during the 20th century. There were just over 3 million Americans age 65 or older in 1900, and nearly 35 million in 2000.

At the dawn of the 20th century, three demographic trends—high fertility, declining infant and child mortality, and high rates of international immigration—were acting in concert in the United States and were keeping the population young. The age distribution of the U.S. population was heavily skewed toward younger ages in 1900, as illustrated by the broad base of the population age-sex pyramid for that year in Figure 1. The pyramid, which shows the proportion of each age and sex group in the population, also reveals that the elderly made up a tiny

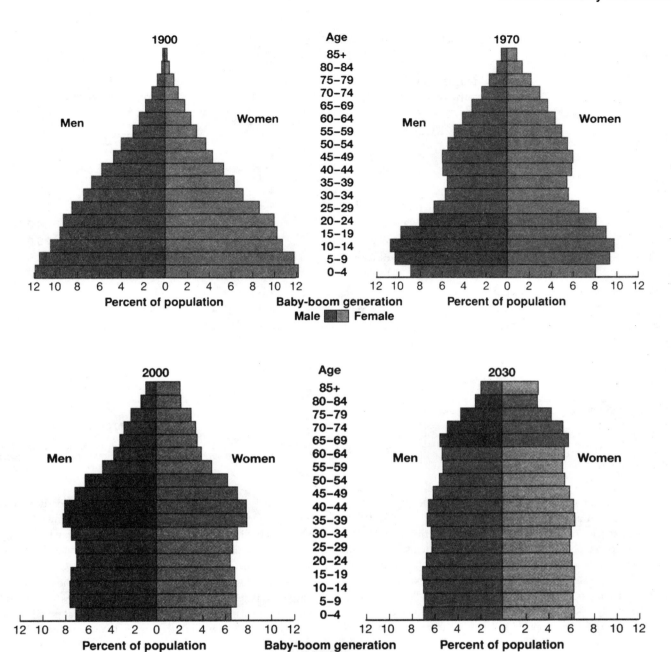

Figure 1 U.S. Population by Age and Sex, 1900, 1970, 2000, and 2030

Sources: U.S. Census Bureau Publications: *Historical Statistics of the United States: Colonial times to 1970* (1975); *Census 2000 Summary File* (SFI) (http://factfind-er.census.gov, accessed Sept. 5, 2001); and "Population Projections of the United States by Age, Sex, Race, Hispanic Origin, and Nativity: 1999 to 2100" (www.census.gov/population/projections/nation/summary/np-t4-a.txt, accessed Sept. 25, 2001).

Note: U.S. population in 1900 does not include Alaska or Hawaii. The baby-boom generation includes persons born between 1946 and 1964.

share of the U.S. population in 1900. Only 4 percent of Americans were age 65 of older, while more than one-half (54 percent) were under age 25.

But adult health improved and fertility fell during the first half of the century. The inflow of international immigrants slowed considerably after 1920. These trends caused an aging of the U.S. population, but they were interrupted after World War II by the baby boom. In the post-war years, Americans were marrying and starting families at younger ages and in greater percentages than they had during the Great Depression. The surge in births between 1946 and 1964 resulted from a decline in childlessness (more women had at least one child) combined with larger family sizes (more women had three or more children). The sustained increase in birth rates during their 19-year period fueled a rapid increase in the child population. By 1970, these baby boomers had moved into their teen and young adult years, creating a bulge in that year's age-sex pyramid shown in Figure 1.

Table 1 U.S. Total Population and Population Age 65 or Older, 1900–2060

| Year | Population (in thousands) | | Percent 65+ | Percent increase from preceding decade | |
	Total	Age 65+		Total	Age 65+
Actual					
1900	75,995	3,080	4.1		
1910	91,972	3,950	4.3	21.0	28.2
1920	105,711	4,933	4.7	14.9	24.9
1930	122,755	6,634	5.4	16.1	34.5
1940	131,669	9,019	6.8	7.2	36.0
1950	150,697	12,270	8.1	14.5	36.0
1960	179,323	16,560	9.2	19.0	35.0
1970	203,212	20,066	9.9	13.4	21.2
1980	226,546	25,549	11.3	11.5	27.3
1990	248,710	31,242	12.6	9.8	22.3
2000	281,422	34,992	12.4	13.2	12.0
Projections					
2020	324,927	53,733	16.5	8.4	35.3
2040	377,350	77,177	20.5	7.5	9.8
2060	432,011	89,840	20.8	7.0	9.6

Note: Data from 1900 to 1950 exclude Alaska and Hawaii. All data refer to the resident U.S. population.

Sources: U.S. Census Bureau publications: *Historical Statistics of the United States: Colonial Times to 1970* (1975); *1980 Census of Population: General Population Characteristics* (PC80-1-B1); *1990 Census of Populations: General Population Characteristics* (1990-CP1); *Census 2000 Demographic Profile*, (www.census.gov/Press-Release/www/2001/tables/dp_us_2000.xls, accessed Sept. 19, 2001); and *Population Projections of the United States by Age, Sex, Race, Hispanic Origin, and Nativity: 1999 to 2100* (www.census.gov/population/projections/nation/summary/np-t4-a.txt, accessed Sept. 25, 2001).

The baby boom was followed by a precipitous decline in fertility: the "baby bust." Young American women reaching adulthood in the late 1960s and 1970s were slower to marry and start families than their older counterparts, and they had fewer children when they did start families. U.S. fertility sank to an all-time low. The average age of the population started to climb as the large baby boom generation moved into adulthood, and was replaced by the much smaller baby-bust cohort. By 2000, the baby-boom bulge had moved up to the middle adult ages. The population's age structure at younger and older ages became more evenly distributed as fluctuations in fertility diminished and survival at the oldest ages increased. By 2030, the large baby-boom cohorts will be age 65 and older, and U.S. Census Bureau projections show that the American population will be relatively evenly distributed across age groups, as Figure 1 shows.

The radical shift in the U.S. population age structure over the last 100 years provides only one part of the story of the U.S. elderly population. Another remarkable aspect is the rapid growth in the number of elderly, and the increasing numbers of Americans at the oldest ages, above ages 85 or 90. The most rapid growth in the 65-or-older age group occurred between the 1920s and the 1950s (see Table 1). During each of these decades, the older population increased by at least 34 percent, reaching 16.6 million in 1960. The percentage increase slowed after 1960, and between 1990 and 2000, the population age 65 or older increased by just 12 percent. Since the growth of the older population largely reflects past patterns of fertility, and U.S. fertility rates plummeted in the 1930s, the first decade of the 21st

century will also see relatively slow growth of the elderly population. Fewer people will be turning 65 and entering the ranks of "the elderly." Not until the first of the baby-boom generation reaches age 65 between 2010 and 2020 will we see the same rates of increase as those experienced in the mid-20th century.

In the 1940s and 1950s, the rapid growth at the top of the pyramid was matched by growth in the younger ages—the total U.S. population was growing rapidly, and the general profile was still fairly young. That was not the case in the second half of the 20th century, as the share of the population age 65 or older increased to around 12 percent. The elderly share will increase much faster in the first half of the 21st century. This growth in the percentage age 65 or older constitutes population aging.

Many policymakers and health care providers are more concerned about the sheer size of the aging baby-boom generation than the baby boom's share of the total population. The oldest members of this group will reach age 65 in 2011, and by 2029, the youngest baby boomers will have reached age 65. This large group will continue to move into old age at a time of slow growth among younger age groups. The Census Bureau projects that 54 million Americans will be age 65 or older in 2020; by 2060, the number is projected to approach 90 million. The size of this group, and the general aging of the population, are important in planning for the future. Older Americans increasingly are healthy and active and able to take on new roles. At the same time, increasing numbers of older people will need assistance with housing, health care, and other services.

The Oldest-Old

The older population is also aging as more people are surviving into their 80s and 90s. In the 2000 Census, nearly one-half of Americans age 65 or older were above age 74, compared with less than one-third in 1950; one in eight were age 85 or older in 2000, compared with one in 20 in 1950 (see Figure 2).

As the baby boomers enter their late 60s and early 70s around 2020, the U.S. elderly population will be younger: The percentage ages 65 to 74 will rise to 58 percent, as shown in Figure 2. By 2040, however, just 44 percent will be 65 to 74, and 56 percent of all elderly will be age 75 or older.

Those age 85 or older, the "oldest-old," are the fastest growing segment of the elderly population. While those 85 or older made up only about 1.5 percent of the total U.S. population in 2000, they constituted about 12 percent of all elderly. More than 4 million people in the United States were 85 or older in the 2000 Census, and by 2050, a projected 19 million will be age 85 or older. These oldest-old will make up nearly 5 percent of the total population, and more than 20 percent of all elderly Americans. This group is of special interest to planners because those 85 or older are more likely to require health services.

Gender Gap

Women outnumber men at every age among the elderly. In 2000, there were an estimated three women for every two men age 65 or older, and the sex ratio is even more skewed among the oldest-old.

The preponderance of women among the elderly reflects the higher death rates for men than women at every age. There are approximately 105 male babies born for every 100 female babies, but higher male death rates cause the sex ratio to decline

as age increases, and around age 35, females outnumber males in the United States. At age 85 and older, the ratio is 41 men per 100 women.[1]

Changes in the leading causes and average ages of death affect a population's sex ratio. In 1900, the average sex ratio for the U.S. total population was 104 men for every 100 women. But during the early 1900s, improvements in health care during and after pregnancy lowered maternal mortality, and a greater proportion of women survived to older ages. Adult male mortality improved much more slowly; death rates for adult men plateaued during the 1960s.

In recent years, however, male mortality improved faster than female mortality, primarily because of a marked decline in deaths from heart disease. The gender gap at the older ages has narrowed, and it is expected to narrow further. The U.S. Census Bureau projects the sex ratio for those age 65 or older to rise to 79 men for every 100 women by 2050. A sex ratio of 62 is anticipated for those age 85 or older.

Most elderly women today will outlive their spouses and face the challenges of later life alone: Older women who are widowed or divorced are less likely than older men to remarry. Older women are more likely than older men to be poor, to live alone, to enter nursing homes, and to depend on people other than their spouses for care. Many of the difficulties of growing older are compounded by past discrimination that disadvantaged women in the workplace and now threatens their economic security.

As the sex differential in mortality diminishes, these differences may lessen, but changes in marriage and work patterns, family structures, and fertility may mean that a greater proportion of older women will not have children or a living spouse. High divorce rates and declining rates of marriage, for instance, mean that many older women will not have spousal benefits available to them through pensions or Social Security.

Ethnic Diversity

The U.S. elderly population is becoming more racially and ethnically diverse, although not as rapidly as is the total U.S. population. In 2000, about 84 percent of the elderly population were non-Hispanic white, compared with 69 percent of the total U.S. population. By 2050, the proportion of elderly who are non-Hispanic white is projected to drop to 64 percent as the growing minority populations move into old age (see Figure 3). Although Hispanics made up only about 5 percent of the elderly population in 2000, 16 percent of the elderly population of 2050 is likely to be Hispanic. Similarly, blacks accounted for 8 percent of the elderly population in 2000, but are expected to make up 12 percent of elderly Americans in 2050.

The major racial and ethnic groups are aging at different rates, depending upon fertility, mortality, and immigration among these groups. Immigration has a growing influence on the age structure of racial and ethnic minority groups. Although most immigrants tend to be in their young adult ages, when people are most likely and willing to assume the risks of moving to a new country, U.S.

Percent of 65+ population

■ Age 65–74   ■ Age 75–84   ■ Age 85+

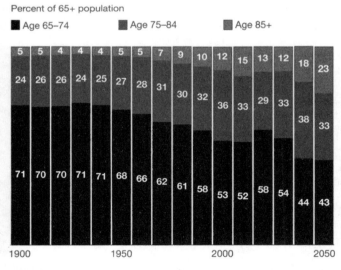

Figure 2 Age Distribution of Older Americans, 1900–2000, and Projection to 2050

Sources: U.S. Census Bureau publications: *Historical Statistics of the United States: Colonial Times to 1970* (1975); *1980 Census of Population: General Population Characteristics* (PC80-1-B1); *1990 Census of Populations: General Population Characteristics* (1990-CP1); *Census 2000 Demographic Profile*, (www.census.gov/2001/tables/dp_us_2000.xls, accessed Sept. 19, 2001); and "Projections of the Resident Population by Age, Sex, Race, Hispanic Origin, 1990 to 2100" (www.census.gov/population/www/projections/natdet-D1A.html, accessed July 6, 2001).

Percent of population age 65+

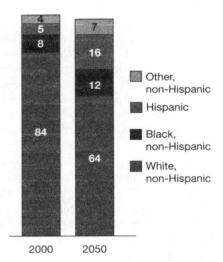

Other, non-Hispanic

Hispanic

Black, non-Hispanic

White, non-Hispanic

2000   2050

Figure 3 Elderly Americans by Race and Ethnicity, 2000 and 2050

Sources: U.S. Census Bureau, *Census 2000 Demographic Profile* (2001); and U.S. Census Bureau, "Projections of the Resident Population by Age, Sex, Race and Hispanic Origin, 1999-2100" (www.census.gov/population/www/projections/natdet-D1A.html, accessed Sept. 19, 2001).

Note: The 2000 figures refer to residents who identified with one race. About 2% of Americans identified with more than one race in the 2000 census.

immigration policy also favors the entry of parents and other family members of these young immigrants. The number of immigrants age 65 or older is rapidly increasing as more foreign-born elderly move to the United States from Latin America, Asia, or Africa to join their children.[2] These older immigrants, plus the aging of immigrants who entered as young adults, are altering the ethnic makeup of elderly Americans.

References

1. U.S. Census Bureau, *Population Projections of the United States by Age, Sex, Race, Hispanic Origin, and Nativity: 1999 to 2100* (2000), accessed online at: www.census.gov/population/projections/nation/summary/np-t3-a.txt, on Sept. 19, 2001.
2. Janet M. Wilmoth, Gordon F. DeJong, and Christine L. Himes, "Immigrant and Non-Immigrant Living Arrangements in Later Life," *International Journal of Sociology and Social Policy* 17 (1997): 57–82.

The Economic Conundrum of an Aging Population

ROBERT AYRES

In a large part of the world, old age is an incentive to have many children. That may seem puzzling to Europeans or Americans, for whom old age can be a welcome escape from the burdens of buying kids' clothes or paying for college tuition. Retired people in affluent countries usually have savings or pensions, as well as government-provided retirement income. But in poor countries, where hundreds of millions of people have no such income after they stop working, adult male children are the equivalent of social security. For this reason, there are strong cultural imperatives for children to provide support for their elderly parents, in preference (if a choice is necessary) to their own young. The result is a combination of too many children and too little care for those children—a potent formula for yet another generation of poorly educated and impoverished young people, including more young men whose frustrations make them prime prospects for militias and terrorists, and young women who have few prospects other than to have more children. It's a self-perpetuating cycle, which ironically becomes harder to break as life expectancies increase and the number of old people in poor countries continues to increase.

Aging Populations Have Fewer Children, But...

The incentives for having fewer children in rich industrialized countries are the mirror image of the reasons for having large families in poor countries. In poor countries, most people live on subsistence farms where child labor is valuable. In rich countries, most people live in cities where children are required by law to go to school. Children are an expensive luxury for people who live in cities and who have jobs outside the home. They must be housed, fed, and schooled. They add nothing to family income. If the mother has a job, she must find (and pay for) a baby-sitter or nanny to look after young children. Urban teenagers are often neglected by working parents, and too many of them—lacking adult guidance—engage in high-risk or costly behavior, from profligate consumption of video games or TV shows exhibiting extreme violence, to unsafe sex, drug-taking, or even crime. If unemployed, children may be an economic burden on parents into their thirties. In Italy, especially, unmarried children have be-

come notoriously inclined to continue to live with their aging parents and enjoy mama's cooking. For that reason, among others, Italy now has one of the lowest birth rates in the world. Some Italians would like to see that trend reversed.

The shift to a stable population will increase the "dependency ratio" of old to young. While that may stem environmental decline, it could bring economic hardship to the countries that first achieve it. The only real chance of escaping this dilemma is to eliminate the huge economic inequities that now prevail in the world.

Last fall, *The Economist* magazine published a story, "Work Longer, Have More Babies." The illustration showed a horrified young woman—presumably in shock over the news that she is expected to stop having fun and start reproducing, for the good of western society. The underlying message, of course, was that as the populations of rich countries get older, with smaller percentages of them of child-bearing age—and as fewer of them care to bear the expense of having kids in any case—the populations of those countries will shrink and their cultures will risk being overrun by others, whose populations are rapidly expanding.

It is true that all of the industrialized countries, including the United States, are aging. The number of old people supported by social security, compared to the number of younger employed people paying into the retirement system, is growing. This "dependency ratio"—the number of people over 65 as a percentage of the number in the 20–24 age group—is a good indicator of the fundamental demographic problem. This ratio is now just over 20 percent for the United States, about 27 percent for the Euro zone, and 28 percent for Japan. However, by 2050, according to the World Bank, the dependency ratio will be close to 46 percent for the United States, 60 percent for Europe, and 70 percent for Japan.

The number of workers supporting each German pensioner today, via the main government "pay-as-you-go" (PAYG) system, is about three. By 2030, if current trends continue, the number of active workers per pensioner will be only 1.5. If each of the active workers earned 100 Euros before the transfer, he (or she) would get to keep 60, and the retiree would also get 60 Euros (1.5 X 100 = 2.5 X 60 = 150). The other costs of government would be taken (via taxation) out of the 60 Euros of income each person has. Costs of government, net of pensions, are at least 25 percent of GDP for industrialized countries, so taxes would take at least 15 Euros from each worker and retiree. The original 100 Euros is therefore down to 45, or less. From that, the future worker must think about saving for his own future retirement when the overstressed PAYG system collapses, as many people now expect.

A Demographic Dilemma

To an environmentalist, an aging population might seem a good thing—proof that birthrates have fallen and that overall population will stabilize or decline. But a small aging population like that of Italy, in a world of huge younger populations like those of China or Brazil, may not be sustainable. First, there's that pressure from those who don't want their traditional culture (of Italy, or Spain, or France) to be overrun, and who want to encourage their young families to have more children. But even if that weren't a factor, there'd be the economic pressure on a country with a high dependency ratio to alleviate the imbalance, by delaying retirements or reducing retirement benefits. There's also the kind of pressure created by the Bush administration in the United States, to allow active workers to divert part of their social security taxes into privately controlled savings or investment accounts. It's a tempting idea because share prices have increased in value faster than government bonds (in which social security funds are invested), but it would take money away from the PAYG funds available to support current retirees, thus imposing either a very large near-term tax burden or additional government debt to make up the difference.

All things considered, an aging population of non-workers will necessitate an increased tax burden or increased public sector debt, or both. In the past, a few countries have lived with taxes in the 50-percent range, especially in wartime, but not happily. However, this is no longer plausible. In a globalized world with no restrictions on capital flows, where nations compete for investment and where multinational firms can—and do—move money around at the touch of a button, high taxes are a major barrier to investment. In the world of 2030, the United States will be somewhat better off than Europe or Japan, thanks to its lower dependency ratio. On the other hand, China and India will have much lower dependency ratios than the United States, in addition to having lower wages. Even if they had to pay much higher wages, as they must do eventually, those countries would, and will, continue to absorb most of the capital available for investment, including whatever savings the workers of the (formerly) rich countries can manage to divert from current needs.

When environmentalists began to worry about population in the 1970s, the idea that having a *declining* population could spell trouble for a country might have seemed unimaginable. After all,

wasn't that the ultimate goal? But in a globalized economy, a declining national population means a nation with a high percentage of elderly, non-working people will compete against nations of young, productive (often low-wage) people—and lose. The change of perspective since the 1970s can be attributed to three factors.

- First, *retirement ages have gotten younger*, putting greater burdens on the social security system. According to the European Commission, the average age of retirement in Western Europe was 65 in 1960, but is 60 today. Civil servants and some unionized workers, such as truck drivers, are able to retire considerably earlier. In the United States, the average age of retirement was 66 in 1960, but is down to under 63 today. Moreover, when firms "downsize," which happens with alarming frequency these days, they often do so by offering early retirement schemes to older workers without replacing them with younger ones. This cuts payroll costs and shifts some or all of the burden to the government. Employees who were previously paying into the social security system are suddenly withdrawing funds from the system.

- Meanwhile, *birth rates in the industrialized countries have declined*, just as environmentalists hoped they would—but with some unforeseen consequences. In 1950, the average overall birth rate in the European union was still above replacement (2 children per woman), at 2.7. Today it is 1.5 and falling. Similar rates are now observed in Japan, China, and Russia. In the United States, the birth rate is just above 2, in part because many of the country's Latino immigrants still prefer large families. If current trends continue, the working-age population of Europe will fall by 18 percent (40 million people) by 2050, while the corresponding U.S. group will increase by a similar amount. In that period the average age of the German population will increase to 54, while the average American will still be only 35. This discrepancy is very disturbing to most European economists, and politicians, who are concerned about economic competition with the United States, not to mention China and India.

- Finally, *life expectancies have been increasing* since the beginning of the 18th century, and especially fast since the early 19th century. When Thomas Malthus warned of explosive population growth, in 1798, the average life expectancy was probably no more than 35. When Otto von Bismarck introduced the first state pension in Germany in 1889, the average life expectancy was 48, whereas the retirement age was set at 70. No wonder the German PAYG system was fiscally sound when it was introduced. There were a lot of active workers and very few retirees. The ratio was probably more than 100 to 1. Now, of course, the life expectancy of Europeans, Japanese, and Americans alike is around 77 (slightly more for women, slightly less for men) and still rising.

An older population requires more health and other services, and produces less wealth, than a younger population. At least that is the conventional wisdom. What is certain is that existing pension plans and social security programs are in deep trouble, even in the United States, and more so in Europe and Japan.

What Would an Aging Society Be Like?

Imagine a society ruled by the old. College professors, army generals, CEOs, doctors, judges, and legislators would hang on to their jobs into their seventies or eighties, or even longer. Promotion in big corporations, civil service, colleges and universities, and the military officer corps would slow almost to a halt, as vacancies due to retirement become rare. Even poorly paid jobs like teaching children in primary or secondary schools, or nursing, or processing forms in government agencies, would most likely require advanced degrees. Computers already do much of the work formerly done by clerks and middle managers. Computers are learning to talk to each other. The need for human interfaces will continue to decline.

Highly skilled construction, repair, and maintenance jobs, such as heavy machine operation, auto repair, plumbing, masonry, plastering, plumbing, electrical work, and electronics repair, would continue to be important and well-paid. However, many such jobs tend to be passed on from father to son. Union membership would be essentially closed to outsiders. Without an expanding economy to absorb them, young people on the lower rungs of the education ladder would be chronically unemployed—or forced to take jobs that most people are unwilling to do, such as collecting and separating trash or cleaning fish.

It is unlikely that there would be enough such jobs for all. But unemployment, especially among the young, is socially destabilizing. Moreover, it discriminates against ethnic minorities of all kinds. It is not at all unlikely that half or more of the present U.S. prison population—disproportionately black and Hispanic, and the largest in the industrialized world—would never have got into trouble with the law if there had been enough decent job opportunities for the less privileged.

Of course there is nothing new about this situation. It has been with us for a long time. The children of the rich are less likely to steal or commit crimes for money, since they don't need to. If they are caught driving while drunk, or accused of date rape, they will be defended by high-priced lawyers or released on a convenient technicality to avert the expense of a trial without an assured outcome, or worse, the loss of a wealthy campaign contributor. When the rich commit financial crimes that cause vast losses for customers or shareholders, they can afford to hire even more expensive lawyers skilled in the black arts of confusion, obstruction, obfuscation, and delay. Very few millionaire malefactors are convicted, still fewer punished. In the future, as the rich get richer—and older people become more demographically dominant—this sort of inequity will almost surely get worse before it gets better.

One way it's likely to get worse is in access to medical services. The rich can afford services that the poor can only dream of. No matter what the Christian and/or Islamic fundamentalists and their moral police think, and no matter whether it is legal in the United States and other major Christian or Islamic countries, cloning of stem cells from human embryos for therapeutic purposes is on the way. Clinics will soon—probably within a decade—be available in China, Russia, the Ukraine, Armenia, or other countries, where custom-grown livers, kidneys, hearts, lungs, or even legs and arms can be had for a suitably high price. The technology is already well along in development. Demand will surely follow. The more effective the gene therapies and stem cell technologies become, the longer their lucky recipients will live—and block the promotion prospects for younger people.

Given these trends, there is growing risk that the aging society of a mature industrial nation will be an increasingly inequitable society, ruled by the rich (and the old) for their own benefit and perpetuation in power. It will be controlled by means of hired guardians who will perform the same duties as today's police and military, but with added civil powers. Having high unemployment or underemployment, and no real power, the rest of our urban society will inevitably revert to a form of existence analogous to that of the Romans who were kept satisfied and entertained by bread and circuses. Its bread will be junk food and its circuses will be our 200 TV channels and omnipresent movieplexes, as well as our sports stadiums and NASCAR race tracks. But just as Rome was overrun, this self-indulgent senior culture (more toys for 65-year-old boys, with fewer actual children) could well be overrun by needier and more aggressive outsiders.

In a society thus dominated by the old, the young are doubly disadvantaged—by their subordinate positions in the major institutions of society and by their reduced capacity to pay the costs of social security. But the real killer is the fact that these overburdened young Europeans, Americans, or Japanese will be competing with nations that have both cheaper wages *and* lower dependency ratios—countries that will not only get the lion's share of investment but also will have to spend less of it on supporting their elders. To a policymaker in Brussels, Washington, or Tokyo, the advent of stable population will look worrisome indeed—unless the inequities between the enviable "old" and hungry or resentful "young" countries are bridged.

Supporting the Old Without Lots More Young?

The standard economist's formula for dealing with overpopulation is economic growth. The reasoning behind this formula is uncomfortable for environmentalists, but there is an inescapable logic: people with higher incomes, in countries that have social security for the elderly, want and need fewer babies; they do not need children to provide security. So, there's an enormous dilemma. Economic growth drives consumption, and waste, which is the reason population is a problem in the first place. But economic growth is also what's necessary to raise incomes to the point where population stabilizes.

It's here where the politics of economic development and the population stabilization that can follow become complicated. Environmentalists are not alone in their uneasiness about the full-throttle economic growth that increases incomes but also increases consumption of nonrenewable resources, degrades the environment, and may undermine social stability. They find some of their concerns echoed by their most fanatical adversaries—fundamental Islamists who regard

9

Western modernization as decadent, but who have notoriously suppressed women's empowerment. The discomfort is made all the more excruciating by the fact that the anti-capitalist Muslims have become de facto bedfellows with some of *their* ideological enemies, the pro-capitalist Christian conservatives, in their mutual hatred of the "sexual revolution" of the past quarter-century. Experts on population virtually all agree that female empowerment, starting with education, is a necessary condition for reducing birthrates.

What's needed, to raise incomes and empower women while *also* mitigating concerns about profligate consumption, is an engine to drive economic growth without the kind of consumption that depends on the exploitation of remaining stocks of natural resources. How would this engine differ from the one that now drives global GDP yet leaves hundreds of millions of people in poverty and dependence on children—and vulnerable to social unrest?

To begin with, it would probably be a more "dematerialized" economy, in which economic productivity is not so rigidly tied to the extraction of ever more oil, minerals, wood, and other physical resources from the Earth as it is now. Aside from the costs of the ecological disruption and pollution that such industries impose, past experience shows that logging, mining, and drilling concessions tend to benefit mainly the very few (and often very corrupt) who have the power to make such deals. The natural wealth has never been widely distributed beyond this elite group. Governments in countries like Nigeria or Indonesia, which still have important natural resource stocks of oil or timber, also have vast populations of poor people for whom having children is a source of income. For this reason alone, it is essential that the global community address the inequity problem—and the closely related problem of corruption—far more quickly and seriously than it has. The rich Western countries have a big stake in the equitable development of the rest of the world, because equitable growth is the only effective tool for ameliorating international terrorism and its close cousin, uncontrollable immigration.

In the short run, though, *controlled* immigration is probably one of the most promising answers to the conundrum raised at the beginning of this article—the lack of enough new young workers (because of declining birthrates) to replace the retiring workers. Immigrants are demonstrably hardworking and willing to do the jobs our own pampered children scorn. Immigrants (being predominantly young adults) even tend to pay more in taxes than they get back in social services. They are a bargain, economically speaking. They also have fewer children than their age group in their home countries, as well as contributing enormously to the economic development of their home countries by sending back significant amounts of their earnings to parents or siblings.

That's only a short-term, partial solution, however. In the larger picture, the rich countries need to provide far more development aid, and to provide it with much tighter—and smarter—strings, to prevent misuse. Investment by the private sector can and will be the dominant source of capital, but that investment should not be going into exploitation of increasingly scarce natural resources. International lending agencies should stop encouraging this sort of investment, and in fact they should create barriers to discourage or prevent it. By the same token, international development agencies should concentrate much greater efforts on education and on creating the institutions needed to assure the rule of law.

As long as there are large economic disparities between nations, there will be unstoppable pressures both to have more children in the poor countries and to endure uncontrolled immigration of the poor into richer countries. When incomes are more equitable worldwide, the problem of smaller working populations supporting their elders will continue to be a problem as birthrates decline, *but* with all nations then sharing common constraints, the present incentives to have more babies and/or migrate to richer countries will disappear. Instead of being shackled by the destabilizing effects of poor people having large families to produce free labor and/or illegally migrating into rich countries in search of jobs, all governments can then focus on finding ways to build economic productivity through an increasingly non-extractive economy, enough to allow people everywhere to support their elders while living comfortably in their home countries.

ROBERT AYRES is professor emeritus of management and environment at the European business school INSEAD and King Gustav XVIth professor of environmental science in Sweden.

Living Longer: Diet

In the search for the fountain of youth, researchers keep coming back to one fact: what you eat has a tremendous impact not only on your health but on your longevity. Here's why every bite you take counts

DONNA JACKSON NAKAZAWA

It's hard to get through your first cup of morning coffee without reading a headline about food. Eat blueberries! Inhale kale! Such antioxidant-rich foods will clear your arteries and help prevent the buildup of Alzheimer's plaque in your brain. Add in a cup of green tea in the morning and swish down an ounce or two of dark chocolate with a glass of red wine in the evening and you will be nicely tanked up on healthy fuel for the day.

Or will you? Almost every day, it seems, new studies emerge on the antiaging properties of various foods. One day, soy is good; the next, we find out soy's health benefits may have been oversold. To add to the confusion, this year *The Journal of the American Medical Association (JAMA)* published a study that found caloric restriction—eating about 25 percent less than normal—could extend your life.

So which headlines should we believe? And why should we believe them? The answers lie in research that shows exactly how various foods work at the cellular level. In particular, antioxidant-rich fruits and vegetables are emerging as powerful medicine in the fight against cellular aging.

Here's how it works. In the normal process of metabolism, cells produce unstable oxygen molecules—called free radicals—that damage cells. Worse still, the older we get, the more free radicals we produce. Recent studies suggest that the havoc free radicals wreak "plays a central role in virtually every age-related disease, including cardiovascular diseases such as stroke and atherosclerosis, Parkinson's disease, Alzheimer's, and type 2 diabetes," says Mark Mattson, Ph.D., chief of the Laboratory of Neurosciences at the National Institute on Aging at the National Institutes of Health.

It sounds pretty grim, but in this battle there are, thankfully, superheroes. Enter the vibrant world of antioxidants—substances that bind with free radicals and inhibit them from damaging cells. They are abundant in the most colorful fruits and vegetables, including spinach, broccoli, spirulina (blue-green algae), red apples, cranberries, blueberries, cherries, and grapes, as well as in chocolate and red wine. When you hear doctors say that eating five helpings of fruits and vegetables a day is good for you, antioxidants are the main reason. In the past five years an impressive

body of research has emerged showing how antioxidants may protect the body and brain against the ravages of aging.

Paula Bickford, Ph.D., a researcher at the University of South Florida Center of Excellence for Aging and Brain Repair, is particularly interested in the role of antioxidants in brain health. The brain is a good place to study the benefits of antioxidants, says Bickford, because it has one of the highest percentages of fats of any organ in the body, and it is in our fats that free radicals inflict much of their damage. As we age, "communications between neurons become damaged, kind of like what happened to the Tin Man in *The Wizard of Oz*," she explains. "Oxidative damage caused the Tin Man to grow rusty—until Dorothy came along and oiled him." Similarly, antioxidants help to "regrease the lines of communication" in the cells in our brain, says Bickford.

To measure how the communication between cells was affected when groups of rats ate different diets, Bickford and her colleagues placed electrodes in the brains of 20-month-old rats—the equivalent of 60-year-old humans. She then fed one group of rats a diet supplemented with spirulina, another with apples, and a third with cucumbers, which lack the antioxidant qualities of spirulina and apples. Bickford and her colleagues were surprised by the robustness with which "both the spirulina and apple groups demonstrated improved neuron function in the brain, a suppression of inflammatory substances in the brain, and a decrease in oxidative damage." By contrast, there was no improvement in rats fed a diet containing cucumbers. Bickford, who calls the findings "dramatic," reproduced her results in another study, in which rats fed a spinach-rich diet had a reversal in the loss of learning ability that occurs with age.

Most recently, Bickford examined whether eating a diet high in antioxidant-rich spinach and blueberries makes a difference in lab animals suffering from stroke and Parkinson's. "We've seen very positive effects with both of these diseases, as well," she says. "We believe that antioxidants can help people either to delay the onset or to slow the progression of a range of diseases that we tend to get as we age."

Tempting though it may be now to go out and gorge on anti-oxidant-rich dark chocolate, resist the urge. The hottest discovery in the search to find the fountain of youth through the foods we eat is to—gulp!—eat a lot less of them. A 2006 article in *JAMA* caused a stir by announcing that in both men and women, caloric restriction—as spartan as 890 calories a day—resulted in a decrease in fasting insulin levels and body temperature, two biomarkers of longevity. Why? Because restricting calories also helps to eliminate those nefarious free radicals. Mattson explains: "When you overeat and more energy comes into the cells than you burn off by being active, you are going to have more excess free radicals roaming around." Still, he advises, don't panic over the idea of having to subsist on 890 calories a day. Mattson, who calls such a diet "starvation," believes we can all gain the benefits of healthy eating with a lot less pain.

Richard Miller, M.D., Ph.D., professor of pathology and geriatric medicine at the University of Michigan, agrees. He has spent the last 20 years studying the ways in which dietary and genetic changes can slow the aging process. The research has shown that mice, rats, and monkeys that have undergone severe caloric restriction demonstrate all kinds of mental and physical benefits such as better mental function, less joint disease, and even fewer cases of cataracts. But it's unrealistic to try to replicate that in humans. "To copy what's happening in the lab, a man weighing 200 pounds would have to decrease his caloric intake by 40 percent for life, which would put him at about 120 pounds," Miller explains. "That's just not tenable."

Instead, Mattson and Miller advocate a more moderate approach. According to the Centers for Disease Control and Prevention, the average man in the United States consumes about 2,475 calories a day. That's roughly 500 more, on average, than he really needs. Likewise, the average American woman consumes 1,833 calories, yet probably needs only about 1,600. One way to ratchet down your caloric consumption would be to follow this simple equation: men should aim for about 500 calories at both breakfast and lunch, while women should strive for about 300 at each meal. Both sexes can then shoot for 1,000 calories at dinner.

Bickford, who prefers to think of caloric restriction as caloric selection, underscores the importance of getting as much of your caloric intake as you can not only from antioxidant-rich fruits and vegetables but also from nuts and flaxseed, which are loaded with vitamin E and omega-3 and omega-6 fatty acids. In fact, Bickford takes a page out of her own lab studies and starts her day with an antioxidant smoothie. You can try it at home by blending together one cup of frozen blueberries with half a tablespoon of spirulina (available in any health food store), half a cup of nonfat plain yogurt, one teaspoon of ground flaxseed,

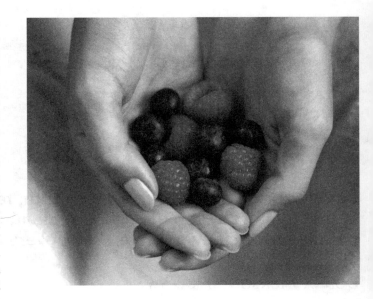

one tablespoon of almond butter or a half-handful of almonds, and a dash of soy milk. Consider what's in that blender as a gas tank full of high-antioxidant fuel for the day.

Of course, one can't help but ask: what's the fun of living to 102 if you're subsisting on spirulina shakes? Not to worry. If you splurge on a stack of pancakes with eggs, bacon, and sausage—packing in 2,000 calories before 10 a.m.—you can always take heart in new data about to emerge from Mattson's lab, which show that periodic fasting—skipping a meal here and there—can also help to eliminate free radicals quite beautifully. "From an evolutionary standpoint we just aren't used to constant access to food," he explains. "Our bodies are used to going days without eating anything. Yet all of a sudden, we are taking in calories all day long."

In other words, we have gone from thousands of years of intermittently restricting our calories and eating a high-antioxidant diet to, in the past century, constantly eating a low-antioxidant diet. And that means more free radicals and more disease. So indulge in the pancakes or the cheese steak, but not both. Then skip a couple of meals and make your next one an all-out antioxidant feast. It may be counter to the don't-skip-meals philosophy our mothers all taught us; yet as it turns out, Mother Nature just might know better.

DONNA JACKSON NAKAZAWA is a health writer whose next book, a medical mystery about what's behind rising rates of autoimmune disease, will be published by Touchstone/Simon & Schuster in 2007.

Living Longer: Exercise

Regular physical activity has been shown to reduce your risk of heart attack, stroke, Alzheimer's, and some cancers. Now we're finding it also may add years to your life. That's powerful medicine indeed

SUSAN CRANDELL

There are no guarantees in life and even fewer in death. But if you wish to prolong the former and delay the latter, scientists can now pretty much promise that regular exercise will help. "So many of what we thought were symptoms of aging are actually symptoms of disuse," says Pamela Peeke, M.D., a University of Maryland researcher and author of *Body for Life for Women* (Rodale, 2005). "This is a monster statement." It means that your health is not just a throw of the genetic dice but a factor that is largely under your control. "Our bodies are built for obsolescence after 50," Peeke says. "Up to 50 you can get away with not exercising; after that, you start paying the price."

The most dramatic declines due to aging are in muscle strength. "Unless you do resistance exercise—strength training with weights or elastic bands—you lose six pounds of muscle a decade," says Wayne Westcott, Ph.D., the highly respected fitness research director at the South Shore YMCA in Quincy, Massachusetts. That change in body composition not only saps our strength; it also lowers our metabolism and exposes us to greater risk of age-related disease. In fact, the loss of muscle (and accompanying increase in body fat) puts extra strain on the heart, alters sugar metabolism (increasing the risk for diabetes), and can tip the balance of healthy lipids in the blood, leading to heart attack and stroke.

Building muscle is much easier than you might think. Strength training just 20 minutes a day, two or three times a week, for 10 to 12 weeks can rebuild three pounds of muscle and increase your metabolism by 7 percent. Do you really need a boost in metabolism? Yes, if you want to feel more energetic, more alert, more vital and alive. Plus, the added muscle has a halo effect on many systems of the body, reducing blood pressure, improving your ability to use glucose from the blood by 25 percent, increasing bone mass by 1 to 3 percent, and improving gastrointestinal efficiency by 55 percent. "It's like going from a four-cylinder engine to a six," Westcott says.

If that's not enough to get your attention, consider this: a regular exercise program (30 minutes of physical activity at least three days a week) can reduce your risk of dying in the next eight years by 40 percent, improve brain function, cut your risk of Alzheimer's disease by up to 60 percent, and blunt the symptoms of depression. This is powerful medicine, given that 80 percent of the population over 65 suffers from at least one chronic condition, and half have two or more, according to a report from the Census Bureau and the National Institute on Aging.

What is it about physical activity that makes it such a panacea? As scientists learn more about how the aging process works, they're finding that exercise—both aerobic exercise and strength training—has a tremendous impact on every cell in the body, reducing inflammation, increasing blood flow, and even reversing the natural declines in oxygen efficiency and muscle mass that come with aging.

Westcott points to a study his organization conducted at a nursing home in Orange City, Florida. Nineteen men and women with an average age of 89, most of whom used wheelchairs, did just ten minutes of strength training a week. "After 14 weeks almost everybody was out of their wheelchairs," Westcott says. "One woman moved back into independent living." The results were published in *Mature Fitness*.

Another inspiring study, published last spring in the *Journal of the American College of Cardiology*, reported that people in their 60s and 70s who walked or jogged, biked, and stretched for 90 minutes three times a week for six months increased their exercise efficiency—their ability to exercise harder without expending more energy—by a whopping 30 percent. But here's the shocker: a comparison group of people in their 20s and 30s showed an efficiency increase of just 2 percent. The results caught even study author Wayne C. Levy, M.D., an associate professor of cardiology at the University of Washington in Seattle, by surprise. "I hadn't anticipated that the older people would improve more than the group in their 20s and 30s," he says.

The explanation, Levy believes, may involve improvement in the function of the mitochondria—spherical or rod-shaped structures in our cells that take glucose, protein, and fat from the food we eat and turn them into energy. In fact, scientists believe that most of the dramatic benefits we get from exercise can be traced to this improvement in the mitochondria. "Mitochondrial function naturally declines with age," explains Kevin Short, Ph.D., who studies mitochondria and exercise at the Mayo Clinic in Rochester, Minnesota. But exercise, he found, can reverse that decline.

When Short and his colleagues put 65 healthy nonexercisers ranging in age from 21 to 87 on a bicycle training program three days a week, they found that everyone's maximum aerobic capacity had increased by about 10 percent after four months. When they studied thigh-muscle samples, they found out why: the mitochondria were pumping out more adenosine triphosphate (ATP), the fuel muscles use to move.

Now, if mightier mitochondria aren't enough to get you on your exercise bike each morning, this might be: it appears physical activity may also combat oxidative damage (see "Browning apples: oxidation at work". "During exercise there's a tremendous burst of oxidative agents that are injurious to tissue," says Abraham Aviv, M.D., director of the Center of Human Development and Aging at the University of Medicine and Dentistry of New Jersey.

The theory is that although you take in more oxygen while exercising, regular exercise slows your resting heart rate, thereby decreasing the amount of oxygen you need overall and reducing the rate at which you create harmful free radicals.

Finally, to all these substantial benefits of exercise add one more: Professor Tim Spector, director of the TwinsUK registry at St. Thomas' Hospital in London, is conducting experiments to determine whether exercise slows down the rate at which our telomeres shrink. (Telomeres are DNA sequences, located on the ends of chromosomes, that shorten as we age—see "Telomeres: your body's biological clock". Although the results have not yet been published, preliminary findings suggest that in exercising and sedentary twin pairs, the twin who exercises has much longer telomeres "even when you adjust for differences in weight and smoking," says Spector.

In short, the evidence is clear: daily physical activity can transform your life. And it's never too late to start. "I started strength-training my father when he was 82," recalls Westcott. "He's six feet tall, but he was emaciated by the stress of my mother's death and weighed only 124 pounds. In a year and a half, he added 24 pounds of muscle. At 97, he's stronger than people half his age."

SUSAN CRANDELL is the author of *Thinking About Tomorrow: Reinventing Yourself at Midlife,* to be published by Warner Books in January 2007.

Reprinted from *AARP The Magazine,* September/October 2006, pp. 78, 80, 82; 84, 86-87. Copyright © 2006 by Donna Jackson Nakazawa and Susan Crandell. Reprinted by permission of American Association for Retired Persons (AARP) and the authors. www.aarpmagazine.org 1-888-687-2227.

Puzzle of the Century

Is it the fresh air, the seafood, or genes? Why do so many hardy 100-year-olds live in, yes, Nova Scotia?

Maybe it's that her face is so smooth and pink or the way she aims her green eyes right into yours, talking fast and crisply articulating each word. Her gestures are as nimble as a hatmaker's. You would be tempted to say Betty Cooper isn't a day over 70. She's 101. "If I couldn't read, I'd go crazy," she says, lifting the magazine on her lap. "I like historical novels—you know, Henry VIII and Anne Boleyn and all that kind of stuff. I get a big batch from the Books for Shut-ins every three weeks, and I read them all."

Betty wears bifocals, and it's no small thing to see as clearly as she does after watching a century go by. Though her hearing is not what it used to be, a hearing aid makes up for that. Complications from a knee operation more than 30 years ago keep her from walking easily. But she continues to live in her own apartment, in Halifax, Nova Scotia, with assistance from women who drop by to cook meals, run errands and help her get around.

Cooper's health and independence confound the notion that living a very long life entails more pain and suffering than it's worth. "I do have a problem remembering," she allows. "I go to say someone's name and it escapes me. Then five minutes later, I remember it." Of course, lots of people half her age have that complaint.

MARY DUENWALD

Betty Cooper is a diamond-quality centenarian, whose body and brain appear to be made of a special material that has scarcely worn down. But just being a Nova Scotian may have something to do with it. At least that's the suspicion of medical researchers who plan to study Cooper and others in Nova Scotia to learn more about the reasons for their very long—and hardy—lives. In parts of Nova Scotia, centenarians are up to 3 times more common than they are in the United States as a whole, and up to 16 times more common than they are in the world population.

Why? Nova Scotians have their own theories. "We're by the sea, and we get a lot of fresh air," says Grace Mead, 98, of Halifax. "I've always been one for fresh air."

"I was a very careful young girl," says Hildred Shupe, 102, of Lunenburg. "I never went around with men."

"I mind my own business," says Cora Romans, 100, of Halifax.

"The Lord just expanded my life, I guess," says Elizabeth Slauenwhite, 99, of Lunenburg. "I'm in His hands, and He looked after me."

Delima Rose d'Entremont, a tiny, brown-eyed woman of 103, of Yarmouth, says the piano helped keep her going. "I won two medals in music when I was younger, and I taught piano all my life," she says, sitting straight in her wheelchair and mimicking herself at the keys. She occasionally performs for friends at her nursing home, Villa St. Joseph-du-Lac.

Cooper grew up on a farm in Indian Harbor Lake, on the province's eastern shore, and remembers meals that few followers of today's nonfat regimens would dare contemplate. "I ate the right stuff when I was growing up," she explains. "Lots of buttermilk and curds. And cream—in moderation. And when I think of the homemade bread and butter, and the toast with cups of cocoa," she says, trailing off in a high-calorie rhapsody. Then she adds: "I never smoked. And I never drank to excess. But I don't know if that made the difference."

In some ways, Nova Scotia is an unlikely longevity hot spot; a healthful lifestyle is hardly the provincial norm. Physicians say that despite abundances of brisk sea air, fresh fish and lobster and locally grown vegetables and fruits, Nova Scotians as a group do not take exceptionally good care of themselves. "The traditional diet is not that nutritious," says Dr. Chris MacKnight, a geriatrician at Dalhousie University in Halifax who is studying the centenarians. "It's a lot of fried food." Studies show that obesity and smoking levels are high and exercise levels low. Also, the two historically most important industries—fishing and logging—are dangerous, and extract a toll. "In fact," Mac Knight says, "we have one of the lowest *average* life expectancies in all of Canada."

"Nova Scotians had something up their sleeve" that enabled so many of them to reach such an advanced age, says a U.S.-based longevity expert. "Someone had to look into it."

Yet the province's cluster of centenarians has begged for a scientific explanation ever since it came to light several years ago. Dr. Thomas Perls, who conducts research on centenarians at the Boston Medical Center, noticed that people in his study often spoke of very old relatives in Nova Scotia. (To be sure, the two regions have historically close ties; a century ago, young Nova Scotians sought their fortunes in what they called "the Boston States.") At a gerontology meeting, Perls talked to one of MacKnight's Dalhousie colleagues, who reported seeing a centenarian's obituary in a Halifax newspaper nearly every week. "That was amazing," Perls recalls. "Down here, I see obituaries for centenarians maybe once every five or six weeks." Perls says he became convinced that "Nova Scotians had something up their sleeve" that enabled them to reach such advanced ages. "Someone had to look into it."

MacKnight and researcher Margaret Miedzyblocki began by analyzing Canadian census data. They found that the province has about 21 centenarians per 100,000 people (the United States has about 18; the world, 3). More important, MacKnight and Miedzyblocki narrowed the quest to two areas along the southwestern coast where 100-year-olds were extraordinarily common, with up to 50 centenarians per 100,000 people. One concentration is in Yarmouth, a town of 8,000, and the other is in Lunenburg, a town of 2,600.

To the researchers, the notable feature was not that Yarmouth and Lunenburg were started by people from different countries. Rather, the key was what the two towns have in common: each is a world of its own, populated to a significant degree by descendants of original settlers. And as the researchers learned, longevity tends to run in families. Elroy Shand, a 96-year-old in Yarmouth, says he has a 94-year-old aunt and had two uncles who lived into their 90s. Delima Rose d'Entremont's mother died at 95. Betty Cooper's father died at 98. Says MacKnight: "It's very possible that the 100-year-olds in Nova Scotia have some genetic factor that has protected them—even from all the bad effects of the local environment."

O nly a three-hour ferry ride from Bar Harbor, Maine, Nova Scotia extends like a long foot into the Atlantic, connected to New Brunswick by a thin ankle. Almost all the stormy weather that roars up the Eastern Seaboard crashes into Nova Scotia. In winter, powerful northeasters batter the province with snow and freezing rain. The windswept shoreline, the vast expanse of ocean beyond, and frequent low hovering clouds make the place feel remote.

Unlike most Nova Scotians, whose ancestors were English, Irish and Scottish, Lunenburg residents largely trace their heritage to Germany. In the mid-1700s, the province's British government moved to counteract the threat posed by French settlers, the Acadians, who practiced Catholicism and resisted British rule. The provincial government enticed Protestants in southwestern Germany to immigrate to Nova Scotia by offering them tax-free land grants, surmising they would not sympathize with either the unruly Acadians or the American revolutionaries in the colonies to the south.

Settling predominantly along the south shore of Nova Scotia, the Germans eventually gave up on farming because the soil is so rocky. They turned to fishing and shipbuilding. For generations, they kept mostly to themselves, marrying within the community and hewing to tradition. Lunenburg has so retained its original shipbuilding, seafaring character that the United Nations has named it a World Heritage Site.

Grace Levy, of Lunenburg, is a petite 95-year-old woman with blue eyes, shining white hair and impossibly smooth skin. She has two sisters, both of whom are still living at ages 82 and 89, and five brothers, four of whom drowned in separate fishing accidents. She left school at age 13 to do housework for other families in Lunenburg. The hardships seem not to have dampened her spirit—or health. "My Dad said you've gotta work," she recalls. "He was a kind of a hard taskmaster. He didn't mind using a piece of rope on our back if we did the least little thing. But Mom was so good and kind."

Grace married a man from nearby Tancook. Although the two were not blood relatives, their ancestries so overlapped they had the same last name. "My name has always been Levy," she says with a smile that flashes white teeth. "I had a brother named Harvey Levy and I married a Harvey Levy."

The town of Yarmouth was settled by New Englanders, but areas just to the south and north were settled by the French, whose plight is dramatized in Henry Wadsworth Longfellow's epic poem *Evangeline*. It tells the story of lovers from Nova Scotia's northern "forest primeval" who were separated during the brutal Acadian expulsion of 1755, when the English governor, fed up with the French peasants' refusal to swear allegiance to Britain, banished them to the American colonies and Louisiana. Later, large numbers of Acadians returned to Nova Scotia and settled the coastline from Yarmouth north to Digby.

After their rough treatment by the English, the Acadians were not inclined to mix with the rest of the province. Today, many people in the Yarmouth area still speak French and display the blue, white and red Acadian flag. Local radio stations play Acadian dance music, a country-French sound not unlike Louisiana zydeco.

"The Yarmouth area would have been settled by only 20 or 30 families," MacKnight says. "Many of the people who live there now are their descendants." The question is, he says, did one of the original ancestors bring a gene or genes that predisposed them to extreme longevity, which have been passed down through the generations?

In Boston, Perls and his colleagues, who have been studying centenarianism for almost a decade, gathered promising evidence to support the notion of a genetic basis for extreme longevity: a woman with a centenarian sibling is at least eight times more likely to live 100 years than a woman without such a sibling; likewise, a man with a centenarian sibling is 17 times more likely to reach 100 than a man without one. "Without the appropriate genetic variations, I think it's extremely difficult to get to 100," Perls says. "Taking better care of yourself might add a decade, but what matters is what you're packin' in your chassis."

Additional evidence comes from recent studies on DNA. Drs. Louis M. Kunkel and Annibale A. Puca of Children's

Hospital in Boston—molecular geneticists working with Perls—examined DNA from 137 sets of centenarian siblings. Human beings have 23 pairs of chromosomes (the spindly structures holding DNA strands), and the researchers discovered that many of the centenarians had similarities in their DNA along the same stretch of chromosome No. 4. To Perls and colleagues, that suggested that a gene or group of genes located there contributed to the centenarians' longevity. The researchers are so determined to find one or more such genes that they formed a biotechnology company in 2001 to track them down: Centagenetix, in Cambridge, Massachusetts.

Scientists suspect there may be a handful of age-defying genes, and the competition to pinpoint and understand them is heated. Medical researchers and drug company scientists reason that if they can figure out exactly what those genes do, they may be able to develop drugs or other treatments to enhance or mimic their action. To skeptics, that might sound like the same old futile quest for a fountain of youth. But proponents of the research are buoyed by a little-appreciated fact of life for many of the super old: they're healthier than you might think.

That, too, has been borne out in Nova Scotia. "I'm forgetful, I can't help it," says 96-year-old Doris Smith of Lunenburg. "But I've never had an ache nor a pain."

"I can't remember being sick, not a real sickness," Hildred Shupe says. "But my legs are beginning to get kind of wobbly now. I don't expect to live to be 200."

Alice Strike, who served in the Royal Air Corps in World War I and lives in a veteran's healthcare facility in Halifax, doesn't recall ever being in a hospital before. She is 106.

Scientists suspect there may be a few age-defying genes and hope to develop drugs that mimic their action. To skeptics, that sounds like a futile quest for the fountain of youth.

Centenarians often are healthier and livelier than many people in their 70s or 80s, according to research by Perls. He says that 40 percent of centenarians avoid chronic illnesses until they're 85 or older, and another 20 percent until they're over 100. "We used to think that the older you were the sicker you were," Perls says. "The fact is, the older you are, the healthier you've been."

He speculates that longevity-enabling genes may work via several possible mechanisms, such as protecting against chronic diseases and slowing down the aging process. Then again, those processes may amount to much the same thing. "If you slow down the rate of aging, you naturally decrease susceptibility to illnesses like Alzheimer's, stroke, heart disease and various cancers," he says.

Clues to how such genes might operate come from a centenarian study being conducted by Dr. Nir Barzilai, a gerontologist and endocrinologist at Albert Einstein College of Medicine in the Bronx. Barzilai has found that his research subjects—more than 200 Ashkenazi Jewish centenarians and their children—have abnormally high blood levels of high-density lipoprotein, or HDL, a.k.a. the "good" cholesterol. The average woman has an HDL level of 55, he says, whereas the grown children of his centenarians have levels up to 140.

He believes that a gene or genes are responsible for the extremely high HDL levels, which may have helped the very old people in his studies maintain their sharp minds and clear memories. He says their high HDL levels, which are presumably controlled by genes, might protect them from heart disease; HDL clears fat from coronary arteries, among other things.

Other researchers say that longevity-enabling genes might protect people in much the same manner as caloric restriction, the only treatment or dietary strategy shown experimentally to extend life. Studies with laboratory rats have found that those fed an extremely low-calorie diet live at least 33 percent longer than rats that eat their fill. The restricted animals also seem to avoid ailments connected with aging, such as diabetes, hypertension, cataracts and cancer. Another possibility is that longevity-enabling genes limit the activities of free radicals—unpaired electrons known to corrode human tissue. Medical researchers have suggested that free radicals spur atherosclerosis and Alzheimer's disease, for instance. "Free radicals are a key mechanism in aging," Perls says. "I wouldn't be surprised if something to do with free-radical damage pops up in our genetic studies."

If MacKnight receives funding to pursue the research, he and his associates plan to interview Nova Scotian centenarians about their histories as well as examine them and draw blood samples for genetic analysis. He hopes to work with Perls to compare the Nova Scotians' genetic material to that from Perls' New England subjects, with an eye for similarities or differences that might betray the presence of longevity-enabling genes.

Like all students of the extremely old, MacKnight is interested in their habits and practices. "We're trying to look at frailty," MacKnight says, "or, what makes some 100-year-old people seem like they're 60 and some seem like they're 150. What are the differences between those who live in their own homes and cook their own breakfast and those who are blind and deaf and mostly demented and bed-bound? And can we develop some kind of intervention for people in their 50s and 60s to keep them from becoming frail?"

Not all centenarians—not even all of those in Nova Scotia—seem as young as Betty Cooper. And though it could be that the difference between the frail and the strong is determined largely by genes, researchers say it is also true that some people who reach 100 in fine shape have been especially prudent. Among centenarians, smoking and obesity are rare. Other qualities that are common to many centenarians include staying mentally engaged, having a measure of financial security (though not necessarily wealth) and remaining involved with loved ones. And though healthy nonagenarians and centenarians often say they've led physically active lives—"I did a lot of hard labor," says 90-year-old

Arthur Hebb, of Lunenburg County, who eagerly reads the newspaper every day—Perls and other researchers haven't definitively answered that question.

Nor do researchers fully understand all the centenarian data, such as why the great majority are women. In the United States, women older than 100 outnumber men by more than four to one. But men at 100 are more likely than women the same age to be in good health and clearheaded. Perls and his colleague Margery Hutter Silver, a neuropsychologist, have found that about 70 percent of centenarian women show signs of dementia, compared with only 30 percent of the men. A surprisingly high proportion of the women—14 percent—have never married. In contrast, almost all centenarian men are, or have been, married.

Centenarians tend to be healthier than you might think: 40 percent avoid chronic illnesses until they're 85 or older; 20 percent postpone age-related debilities until they're 100.

Whether they've survived so long because they're resilient, or they're resilient because they've survived so long, centenarians are often possessed of exceptional psychological strength. "They're gregarious and full of good humor," Perls says. "Their families and friends genuinely like to be with them, because they're basically very happy, optimistic people." A genial attitude makes it easier for people to handle stress, he adds: "It isn't that centenarians have never suffered any traumatic experiences. They've been through wars, they've seen most of their friends die, even some of their own children. But they get through."

Paradoxically, that centenarians have lived such long and eventful lives makes it all the more difficult to pinpoint any one advantage they may have shared. No matter how much researchers learn about longevity-enabling genes, no matter how well they discern the biological protections that centenarians have in common, the very old will always be an exceptionally diverse group. Each one will have a story to tell—as unique as it is long.

"I started fishing when I was 14," says Shand, of Yarmouth. "Then I built fishing boats for 35 years." He uses a wheelchair because a stroke 18 years ago left him with some disability in his right leg. He is broad-chested, robust—and sharp. "I don't think hard work ever hurt anybody."

"We had a lot of meat and a lot of fish and fowl," says Elizabeth Slauenwhite, 99, of Lunenburg. There were also "vegetables and fruit," she adds. "And sweets galore."

MARY DUENWALD, former executive editor of *Harper's Bazaar*, writes about health.

The Demographic Drivers of Aging

Kevin Kinsella and David R. Phillips

When asked "Why do populations age?," most people intuitively think of changes in longevity. We know that life expectancy has been rising in most countries throughout the world, so it seems reasonable that population aging is an outcome of people living longer. Yet, the most prominent historical factor in population aging has been declining fertility. If we think of population aging as an increase in the percent of people age 65 or older, we realize that, over time, a decline in the number of babies will mean fewer young people and proportionally more people at older ages.

Fertility—The Primary Driver

The decrease in fertility in industrialized nations during the last century has pushed the average number of children per woman in almost all more developed countries below the population replacement level of 2.1 children. Sustained low fertility since the late 1970s has reduced the size of successive birth cohorts and increased the proportion of older people in these countries' populations. Fertility decline in the less developed world has been more recent and more rapid; most regions have seen large reductions in fertility rates during the last 30 years. Although the aggregate total fertility rate (TFR, the average number of children per woman given current birth rates) remains in excess of 4.5 children per woman in Africa and many countries of the Middle East, overall levels in Asia and Latin America decreased by about 50 percent (from 6 to 3 children per woman) between 1965 and 1995. The TFR in many less developed countries is now at or below replacement level—notably in the world's most populous country, China. By 2000, a majority of the world's population lived in countries with near- or below- replacement fertility. The UN projects that, by 2050, three of every four of today's less developed countries will have below-replacement fertility.

At very old ages, the rate of increase in mortality tends to slow.

Populations with high fertility tend to have low proportions of older people and vice versa. The term "demographic transition" is used to describe a gradual process of change from high rates of fertility and mortality to low rates of fertility and mortality. The process is characterized first by declines in infant and childhood mortality, as infectious and parasitic diseases are controlled through expansion of public health services and facilities and disease eradication programs. This improvement in mortality occurs while fertility is still high, resulting in large birth cohorts and an expanding proportion of children relative to adults. Other things being equal, the initial decline in mortality generates a younger population age structure.

Increasing Importance of Mortality

In countries where infant mortality rates are relatively high but declining, most of the improvement in life expectancy at birth results from helping infants survive the high-risk early years of life. Reductions in maternal mortality also contribute to increased life expectancy at birth. As a nation's infant, childhood, and maternal mortality reach low levels, longevity gains at older ages become more prominent contributors to increased life expectancy. Most countries today are experiencing a rise in life expectancy at older ages, which contributes to rising life expectancy at birth. For example, the average Japanese woman reaching age 65 in 2000 could expect to live more than 22 additional years, and the average man more than 17 years. Japanese life expectancy at age 65 for both sexes combined increased 44 percent from 1970 to 2000, while life expectancy at birth increased only 9 percent. Comparative figures for the United States are 19 percent and 9 percent, respectively.

The speed at which death rates at advanced ages decline will play a major role in determining future numbers of older, and especially of very old, populations. The remaining life expectancy of 80-year-old women in England and Wales is about 50 percent higher today than it was in 1950. Hence, the number of female octogenarians is about 50 percent higher than it would have been had oldest-old mortality remained at 1950 levels. In absolute terms, there are more than 500,000 British women age 80 or older alive today who otherwise would have died if death rates for the oldest-old had not improved.

Until the mid-1990s, conventional demographic wisdom held that the human death rate increases with age in an exponential manner. Newer research has documented that, at very old ages, the rate of increase in the mortality rate tends to slow down. A study of 28 countries with reliable data for 1950 to 1990 found not only a decline in mortality rates at ages 80 and older, but also a tendency toward greater decline in more recent years. Other work has confirmed this tendency, and one study in the United States suggests that the age at which mortality deceleration occurs is rising.

There are at least two potential explanations of this deceleration of mortality at the oldest ages. The "heterogeneity" hypothesis, an extension of the notion of "survival of the fittest," posits that the deceleration in old-age mortality is a result of frailer older people dying at younger ages, thus creating a very old population with exceptionally healthy attributes resulting from genetic endowment and/or lifestyle. A second, "individual-risk" hypothesis, suggests that the rate of aging may slow down at very old ages, and/or that certain genes that are detrimental to survival may be suppressed. The observed deceleration in mortality, combined with the fact that human mortality at older ages has declined substantially, has led to the questioning of many of the theoretical tenets of aging. Important insights are being garnered from "biodemographic" research that attempts to crossfertilize the biologic and demographic perspectives of aging and senescence. A clearer picture of the causes of mortality deceleration at very old ages may emerge from the study of evolutionary biology and aging in nonhuman species. But recognition of this slowdown in old-age mortality—at a time when numbers of the very old are growing rapidly—has important policy implications.

Changes in Life Expectancy

The dramatic increases in life expectancy that began in the mid-1800s often are thought to be the result of medical breakthroughs. In fact, the major impact of improvements in medicine and sanitation did not occur until the late 19th century. Prior innovations in industrial and agricultural production and distribution, which improved nutrition for large numbers of people, were more powerful forces in mortality reductions. A growing multidisciplinary research consensus attributes the gain in human longevity since the 1800s to the interplay of advancements in medicine and sanitation against a backdrop of new modes of familial, social, economic, and political organization. Life expectancy at birth in Japan approached 82 years in 2003, the highest level among the world's major countries. Life expectancy is at least 79 years in several other developed nations, including Australia, Canada, Italy, Iceland, Sweden, and Switzerland. Average life expectancy in the United States and most other developed countries ranged between 76 and 78 years.

Throughout the less developed world, there are extreme variations in life expectancy at birth. Some nations have levels equal to or higher than those in many European nations, whereas life expectancy at birth in numerous African countries is less than 45 years. The average person born in a more developed country can now expect to outlive his or her counterpart in the less developed world by 14 years.

In some nations, life expectancy more than doubled during the 20th century (see Table). Increases in life expectancy were more rapid in the first half than in the second half of the century. Between 1900 and 1950, many Western nations added 20 or more years to their average life expectancy. Reliable estimates of life expectancy for less developed countries prior to 1950 are scarce, but changes in life expectancy in these countries have been fairly uniform since then. Practically all nations have shown continued improvement, with some exceptions in Latin America and more recently in Af-rica, the latter due to the impact of the HIV/AIDS epidemic. The most dramatic gains have occurred in East Asia, where average life expectancy at birth for the region increased from less than 45 years in 1950 to more than 72 years today.

An increasing gender differential in life expectancy was a hallmark of mortality patterns in more developed countries in the 20th century, reflecting the generally lower mortality of females than males in every age group and for most causes of death. In Europe in 1900, women typically outlived men by two or three years. Today, the average gap between the sexes is approximately seven years, and may be as high as 12 years in parts of the former Soviet Union. Gender differentials tend to be smaller (between three and six years) in less developed countries, and are reversed in a few South Asian and Middle Eastern societies in which such cultural factors as low female social status and a preference for male rather than female offspring affect female life expectancy.

Changing Age Structure

Populations begin to age when fertility declines and adult mortality rates improve. Successive birth cohorts eventually become smaller, although the trend may be interrupted by "baby-boom echoes" as women of prior large birth cohorts reach childbearing age. International migration usually does not play a major role in the aging process, but can be important in smaller populations. Some Caribbean nations, for example, have experienced a combination of emigration of working-age adults, immigration of retirees from other countries, and return migration of older former emigrants; all three factors contribute to population aging. Many observers expect international migration to assume a more prominent role in the aging process, particularly in "older" countries where persistently low fertility has led to stable or even declining population size.

Most if not all countries once had a youthful age structure similar to that of less developed countries as a whole in 1950, with a large percentage of the entire population under age 15. Given the comparatively high rates of fertility that prevailed in most less developed countries from 1950 through the early 1970s, the pyramidal shape of the age and sex profile of less developed countries had not changed greatly by 1990. However, the effects of fertility and mortality decline can be seen in the projected age-sex pyramid for 2030, which loses its strictly triangular shape as the size of younger five-year cohorts stabilizes and the older portion of the total population increases.

The picture in more developed countries has been and will be quite different. In 1950, there was relatively little variation in the size of five-year groups between the ages of 5 and 24. The beginning of the post-World War II baby boom can be seen in the 0-to-4 age group. By 1990, the baby-boom cohorts were ages 25 to 44, and younger cohorts were successively smaller. If projected fertility rates are reasonably accurate through 2030, the aggregate pyramid will start to invert, with more weight on the top than on the bottom, and the size of the oldest-old population (especially women) will increase substantially.

Table   Life Expectancy at Birth in Years, Selected Countries, 1900, 1950, and 2003

Region/country	Circa 1900		Circa 1950		Circa 2003	
	Male	**Female**	**Male**	**Female**	**Male**	**Female**
More developed countries						
Western Europe						
Austria	38	40	63	68	75	81
France	45	49	64	70	75	83
Sweden	53	55	70	73	78	83
United Kingdom	46	50	67	72	76	81
Southern and eastern Europe						
Hungary	37	38	62	66	68	76
Italy	43	43	64	68	76	82
Spain	34	36	62	66	76	83
Other						
Australia	53	57	67	72	76	82
Japan	43	44	60	63	78	85
United States	48	51	66	72	74	80
Less developed countries						
Africa						
Egypt	—	—	41	44	67	71
Ghana	—	—	40	44	57	59
Mali	—	—	31	34	48	49
South Africa	—	—	44	46	45	51
Uganda	—	—	39	42	45	47
Asia						
China	—	—	39	42	69	73
India	—	—	39	38	63	65
Kazakhstan	—	—	52	62	61	72
South Korea	—	—	46	49	72	79
Syria	—	—	45	47	71	73
Latin America						
Argentina	—	—	60	65	71	78
Bolivia	—	—	39	43	62	66
Brazil	—	—	49	53	64	73
Costa Rica	—	—	56	59	76	81
Mexico	—	—	49	52	70	76

— Not available.
Note: Average number of years a person born in those years could expect to live.

Source: UN Population Division, *World Population Prospects: The 2002 Revision* (2003); and G. Siampos, *Statistical Journal of the United Nations Economic Commission for Europe* 7, no. 1 (1990): 13–25.

Will You Live to Be 100?

After completing a study of 150 centenarians, Harvard Medical School researchers Thomas Perls, M.D., and Margery Hutter Silver, Ed.D., developed a quiz to help you calculate your estimated life expectancy.

Longevity Quiz

	Score
1 Do you smoke or chew tobacco, or are you around a lot of secondhand smoke? Yes (–20) No (0)	
2 Do you cook your fish, poultry, or meat until it is charred? Yes (–2) No (0)	
3 Do you avoid butter, cream, pastries, and other saturated fats as well as fried foods (eg., French Fries)? Yes (+3) No (–7)	
4 Do you minimize meat in your diet, preferably making a point to eat plenty of fruits, vegetables, and bran instead? Yes (+5) No (–4)	
5 Do you consume more than two drinks of beer, wine, and/or liquor a day? (A standard drink is one 12-ounce bottle of beer, one wine cooler, one five-ounce glass of wine, or one and a half ounces of 80-proof distilled spirits.) Yes (–10) No (0)	
6 Do you drink beer, wine, and/or liquor in moderate amounts (one or two drinks/day)? Yes (+3) No (0)	
7 Do air pollution warnings occur where you live? Yes (–4) No (+1)	
8 **a** Do you drink more than 16 ounces of coffee a day? Yes (–3) No (0) **b** Do you drink tea daily? Yes (+3) No (0)	
9 Do you take an aspirin a day? Yes (+4) No (0)	
10 Do you floss your teeth every day? Yes (+2) No (–4)	
11 Do you have a bowel movement less than once every two days? Yes (–4) No (0)	
12 Have you had a stroke or heart attack? Yes (–10) No (0)	
13 Do you try to get a sun tan? Yes (–4) No (+3)	
14 Are you more than 20 pounds overweight? Yes (–10) No (0)	
15 Do you live near enough to other family members (other than your spouse and dependent children) that you can and want to drop by spontaneously? Yes (+5) No (–4)	
16 Which statement is applicable to you? **a** "Stress eats away at me. I can't seem to shake it off." Yes (–7) **b** "I can shed stress." This might be by praying, exercising, meditating, finding humor in everyday life, or other means. Yes (+7)	
17 Did both of your parents either die before age 75 of nonaccidental causes or require daily assistance by the time they reached age 75? Yes (–10) No (0) Don't know (0)	
18 Did more than one of the following relatives live to at least age 90 in excellent health: parents, aunts/uncles, grandparents? Yes (+24) No (0) Don't know (0)	
19 **a** Are you a couch potato (do no regular aerobic or resistance exercise)? Yes (–7) **b** Do you exercise at least three times a week? Yes (+7)	
20 Do you take vitamin E (400–800 IU) and selenium (100–200 mcg) every day? Yes (+5) No (–3)	

Score

STEP 1: Add the negative and positive scores together. Example: –45 plus +30 = –15. Divide the preceding score by 5 (–15 divided by 5 = –3).

STEP 2: Add the negative or positive number to age 84 if you are a man or age 88 if you are a woman (example: –3 + 88 = 85) to get your estimated life span.

The Science Behind The Quiz

Question 1 Cigarette smoke contains toxins that directly damage DNA, causing cancer and other diseases and accelerating aging.

Question 2 Charring food changes its proteins and amino acids into heterocyclic amines, which are potent mutagens that can alter your DNA.

Questions 3, 4 A high-fat diet, and especially a high-fat, high-protein diet, may increase your risk of cancer of the breast, uterus, prostate, colon, pancreas, and kidney. A diet rich in fruits and vegetables may lower the risk of heart disease and cancer.

Questions 5, 6 Excessive alcohol consumption can damage the liver and other organs, leading to accelerated aging and increased susceptibility to disease. Moderate consumption may lower the risk of heart disease.

Question 7 Certain air pollutants may cause cancer; many also contain oxidants that accelerate aging.

Question 8 Too much coffee predisposes the stomach to ulcers and chronic inflammation, which in turn raise the risk of heart disease. High coffee consumption may also indicate and exacerbate stress. Tea, on the other hand, is noted for its significant antioxidant content.

Question 9 Taking 81 milligrams of aspirin a day (the amount in one baby aspirin) has been shown to decrease the risk of heart disease, possibly because of its anticlotting effects.

Question 10 Research now shows that chronic gum disease can lead to the release of bacteria into the bloodstream, contributing to heart disease.

Question 11 Scientists believe that having at least one bowel movement every 20 hours decreases the incidence of colon cancer.

Question 12 A previous history of stroke and heart attack makes you more susceptible to future attacks.

Question 13 The ultraviolet rays in sunlight directly damage DNA, causing wrinkles and increasing the risk of skin cancer.

Question 14 Being obese increases the risk of various cancers, heart disease, and diabetes. The more overweight you are, the higher your risk of disease and death.

Questions 15, 16 People who do not belong to cohesive families have fewer coping resources and therefore have increased levels of social and psychological stress. Stress is associated with heart disease and some cancers.

Questions 17, 18 Studies show that genetics plays a significant role in the ability to reach extreme old age.

Question 19 Exercise leads to more efficient energy production in the cells and overall, less oxygen radical formation. Oxygen (or free) radicals are highly reactive molecules or atoms that damage cells and DNA, ultimately leading to aging.

Question 20 Vitamin E is a powerful antioxidant and has been shown to retard the progression of Alzheimer's, heart disease, and stroke. Selenium may prevent some types of cancer.

Adapted from *Living to 100: Lessons in Living to Your Maximum Potential at Any Age* (Basic Books, 1999) by Thomas Perls, M.D., and Margery Hutter Silver, Ed.D., with John F. Lauerman.

The 2005 White House Conference on Aging

Real policymaking—or rubber stamping?

MAUREEN SHAWN KENNEDY

Baby boomers, the 78 million Americans born between 1946 and 1964, are coming of age—retirement age, that is—and will soon be eligible for Social Security and Medicare.

As of January 1 of this year, the first official boomers began turning 60, and the cumulative effects of the exodus of this large group out of the workforce and into a world of free time—and greater need for social support and health programs—are worrying many government, health care, financial, and social organizations. These concerns, as well as the sobering national outlook for program funding, were the focus of the 2005 White House Conference on Aging (WHCoA), December 12–14 in Washington, DC (www.whcoa.gov).

As it has roughly every 10 years since 1961, the WHCoA brings together delegates from around the nation to "vote on resolutions that are intended to set the national aging policy agenda for the future." Of the 1,199 delegates selected, 440 were appointed by governors, Congress, the National Congress of American Indians, and other organizations; 759 "at large" delegates were selected by the WHCoA Policy Committee.

This 17-member bipartisan committee—appointed by the president and Congress—developed 73 resolutions based on input from 130,000 people at events held throughout the year. These resolutions cover a variety of issues, from creating a national strategy for prosecuting elder abuse to making workplaces "senior friendly" to improving access to care in rural communities and assuring an adequate supply of health care providers knowledgeable about aging.

The delegates voted on which 50 of the 73 resolutions the committee will send to the White House and Congress for consideration—hopefully to emerge as legislated and funded programs or policies addressing the resolutions.

The Bush administration doesn't value input, complained many delegates, who pointed out that this is the first WHCoA at which delegates weren't allowed to introduce or amend resolutions, a process that every other WHCoA has used. Tony Fransetta, president of the Florida Alliance for Retired Americans (a 192,000-member senior-advocacy group) said, "What they are

Other Highlights

For the first time ever at a White House Conference on Aging, there were exhibits, including booths displaying new technologies for monitoring activity, falls, medications, and health parameters, as well as robotics and products that enhance independent mobility.

Ken Dychtwald, who has been writing about aging since 1998, helped launch an ad campaign for volunteerism aimed at baby boomers, saying that retiring boomers are moving from a "quest for success" to a "quest for significance." The campaign slogan is "Lead. Inspire. Change the world. Again." (For more information, go to wwwv.getinvolved.gov.)

doing is wrong. They lined up speakers philosophically attuned with White House policies, and we can only address resolutions they picked. What's the point?"

Twenty-three percent of the delegates agreed with him, signing a petition asking for the process to be reinstated. It was not.

Others were less concerned, saying that there was plenty of input prior to the conference. Policy committee member Tom Gallagher, speaking at a press conference, agreed, saying that the group could spend the time developing specific recommendations on implementing the resolutions, "rather than waste time wordsmithing resolutions."

It was hard, though, to dismiss the glaring absence of the traditional convener of the meeting—the U.S. president. For the first time in the WHCoA's history, the sitting president failed to address the delegates. Several delegates said the gesture gave them little confidence that the work of this conference would be seriously considered.

The presentation that generated the most discussion was given by David Walker, comptroller general of the United States and head of the Government Accountability Office, who painted a bleak picture of the national financial situation and declared current fiscal policy "unsustainable" unless drastic steps are taken to address the growing deficit and anticipated increases in the costs of Medicare, Medicaid, and Social Security.

The Top 10
Resolutions from the 2005 White House Conference on Aging.

1. Reauthorize the Older Americans Act within the first six months after the 2005 WHCoA.

2. Develop a coordinated, comprehensive long-term care strategy by supporting public and private sector initiatives that address financing, choice, quality, service delivery, and the paid and unpaid workforce.

3. Ensure that older Americans have transportation options to retain their mobility and independence.

4. Strengthen and improve the Medicaid program for seniors.

5. Strengthen and improve the Medicare program.

6. Support geriatric education and training for all health care professionals, paraprofessionals, health profession students, and direct care workers.

7. Promote innovative models of noninstitutional long-term care.

8. Improve recognition, assessment, and treatment of mental illness and depression among older Americans.

9. Attain adequate numbers of health care personnel in all professions who are skilled, culturally competent, and specialized in geriatrics.

10. Improve state and local health care delivery systems to meet the needs of seniors in the 21st century.

He offered several strategies for reforming retirement benefits and health care, pointing out that "half of the federally supported programs cannot demonstrate that they are making a difference in outcomes." He was especially critical of "companies [that aren't] delivering on their promises [to retiring workers] and federal law that allows them to evade those promises." (To view slides from Walker's presentation, go to www.gao.gov/cghome/whitehousewalker1205/index.html.)

Jennie Chin Hansen is a senior fellow at the Center for the Health Professions at the University of San Francisco and was for 25 years the executive director of On Lok, a highly regarded community health organization for older adults in the Bay Area. She is also a board member at the American Association of Retired Persons (AARP) and one of two nurses appointed to the Medicare Payment Advisory Commission (Sheila Burke is the other). Hansen was a delegate to the 1995 WHCoA and agrees that the process has in the past been more democratic and involved more input from delegates. "The mike wasn't shut off until everyone was finished," she says. For her, the important issues are funding, implementation, and accountability. "We need to look at all the rules and regulations and remove the ones that have become barriers to care. The big questions are Where will we be in five years? and What did this WHCoA and Congress accomplish?"

MAUREEN SHAWN KENNEDY, MA, RN, news director

UNIT 2
The Quality of Later Life

Unit Selections

Key Points to Consider

- What are the stable unchanging factors in women's sexuality as they age?

- What country is identified as taking the best care of its older citizens? Why?

- Are cohabitants found to be better or worse off than married or unmarried persons?

- What are the critical factors that Lou Ann Walker identifies as contributing to a long healthy life?

Student Website
www.mhcls.com/online

Internet References
Further information regarding these websites may be found in this book's preface or online.

Aging with Dignity
   http://www.agingwithdignity.org/
The Gerontological Society of America
   http://www.geron.org
The National Council on the Aging
   http://www.ncoa.org

Although it is true that one ages from the moment of conception to the moment of death, children are usually considered to be "growing and developing" while adults are often thought of as "aging." Having accepted this assumption, most biologists concerned with the problems of aging focus their attention on what happens to individuals after they reach maturity. Moreover, most of the biological and medical research dealing with the aging process focuses on the later part of the mature adult's life cycle. A commonly used definition of senescence is "the changes that occur generally in the post-reproductive period and that result in decreased survival capacity on the part of the individual organism" (B. L. Shrehler, Time, Cells and Aging, New York: Academic Press, 1977).

As a person ages, physiological changes take place. The skin loses its elasticity, becomes more pigmented, and bruises more easily. Joints stiffen, and the bone structure becomes less firm. Muscles lose their strength. The respiratory system becomes less efficient. The individual's metabolism changes, resulting in different dietary demands. Bowel and bladder movements are more difficult to regulate. Visual acuity diminishes, hearing declines, and the entire system is less able to resist environmental stresses and strains.

Increases in life expectancy have resulted largely from decreased mortality rates among younger people, rather than from increased longevity after age 65. In 1900, the average life expectancy at birth was 47.3 years; in 2000, it was 76.9 years. Thus, in the last century the average life expectancy rose by 29.6 years. However, those who now live to the age of 65 do not have an appreciably different life expectancy than did their 1900 cohorts. In 1900, 65-year-olds could expect to live approximately 11.9 years longer, while in 2000 they could expect to live approximately 17.9 years longer, an increase of 6 years. Although more people survive to age 65 today, the chances of being afflicted by one of the major killers of older persons is still about as great for this generation as it was for their grandparents.

While medical science has had considerable success in controlling the acute diseases of the young—such as measles, chicken pox, and scarlet fever—it has not been as successful in controlling the chronic conditions of old age, such as heart disease, cancer, and emphysema. Organ transplants, greater knowledge of the immune system, and undiscovered medical technologies will probably increase the life expectancy for the 65-and-over population, resulting in longer life for the next generation.

Although people 65 years of age today are living only slightly longer than 65-year-olds did in 1900, the quality of their later years has greatly improved. Economically, Social Security and a multitude of private retirement programs have given most older persons a more secure retirement. Physically, many people re-

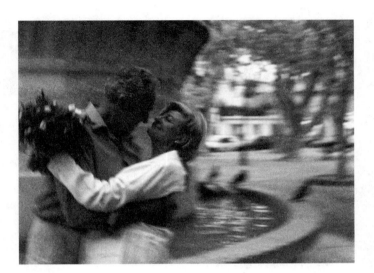

main active, mobile, and independent throughout their retirement years. Socially, most older persons are married, involved in community activities, and leading productive lives.

While they may experience some chronic ailments, most are able to live in their own homes, direct their own lives, and involve themselves in activities they enjoy. The articles in this section examine health, psychological, social, and spiritual factors that affect the quality of aging. All of us are faced with the process of aging, and by putting a strong emphasis on health, both mental and physical, a long, satisfying life is much more attainable.

In "Women's Sexuality As They Age: The More Things Change, The More They Stay the Same," the authors attempt to determine the effect of the women's menstrual status and aging on their sexuality.

Mike Edwards in "As Good As It Gets" points out the advantages that older persons living in the Netherlands have over other countries throughout the world in terms of the number and quality of retirement and government services they are provided.

In "Cohabitation Among Older Adults: A National Portrait," the authors point out that cohabitants, in later life, are considerably less well off than married or unmarried persons. Lou Ann Walker, in "We Can Control How We Age," gives specific recommendations for what the individual can do to improve his or her chances of aging well.

Women's Sexuality as They Age: The More Things Change, the More They Stay the Same

PATRICIA BARTHALOW KOCH, PH.D.
Associate Professor, Biobehavioral Health & Women's Studies

PHYLLIS KERNOFF MANSFIELD, PH.D.
Professor, Women's Studies & Health Education
Pennsylvania State University State College, PA

With the aging of the baby boomers and the development and hugely successful marketing of Viagra® to treat erectile dysfunction, attention from sexologists, pharmaceutical companies, and the public has become focused on the sexuality of aging women.[1]

Some of the burning questions that are currently being pursued are: Does women's sexual functioning (sexual desire, arousal, orgasm, activity, and/or satisfaction) decrease with age and/or menopausal status? And what can be done to enhance aging women's sexual functioning?

As researchers try to provide answers for women, pharmaceutical companies, and other interested parties, what is becoming crystal clear is that we (the scientific community, health care professionals, and society at large) don't understand women's sexuality as they age because we don't understand women's sexuality. Therefore, we may not even be pursuing the right questions. For example, are specific elements of sexual "functioning" the most important aspects of women's sexuality or do we need to shift our focus?

Models of Female Sexuality: The Importance of Context

Much of the information accumulated about women's sexuality has been generated from theories, research methodologies, and interpretation of data based on male models of sexuality, sexual functioning, and scientific inquiry.

As explained by Ray Rosen, Ph.D., at a recent conference on "Emerging Concepts in Women's Health," sexology has pursued a path of treating male and female functioning as similar, as evidenced by Masters and Johnson's development of the human sexual response cycle.[2]

What has resulted is a lack of appreciation for and documentation of the unique aspects of women's sexual functioning and expression. There is a growing chorus of sexologists acknowledging that women's sexuality, including their sexual response, merits different models than those developed for men.[3]

As Leonore Tiefer, Ph.D., has advocated, what is needed is a model of women's sexuality that is more "psychologically-minded, individually variable, interpersonally oriented, and socio-culturally sophisticated."[4] Such models are beginning to emerge.[5]

The new models of female sexual response have been developed from quantitative and qualitative research findings and clinical practice assessments that more accurately reflect women's actual experiences than previous male-centered models.

A key component of these models is the importance of context to women's sexual expression. Context has been defined as "the whole situation, background, or environment relevant to some happening."[6] For example, unlike men whose sexual desire often is independent of context, women's sexual desire is often a responsive reaction to the context (her partner's sexual arousal, expressions of love and intimacy) rather than a spontaneous event.[7] Jordan identified the central dynamic of female adolescent sexuality as the relational context.[8] She described young women's sexual desire as actually being "desire for the experience of joining toward and joining in something that thereby becomes greater than the separate selves."[9]

So throughout women's development and the transitions in their lives (adolescence, pregnancy, parenthood, menopause) context is a key factor in their sexual expression. Thus, the more things change (their bodies, their relationships, their circumstances), the more they stay the same (the importance of context to their sexual expression).

Insights From the Midlife Women's Health Survey

Applying the new models of women's sexuality that emphasize the importance of context helps us to better understand women's sexuality as they age. Findings from the Midlife Women's Health Survey (MWHS), a longitudinal study of the menopausal transition that is part of the broader Tremin Trust Research Program on Women's Health, support these new models.[10]

The Tremin Trust is a longitudinal, intergenerational study focusing on menstrual health that first enrolled 2,350 university women in 1934 and a second cohort of 1,600 young women between 1961 and 1963. (See the Tremin Trust Web site at www.pop.psu.edu/tremin/). In 1990, an additional 347 mid-life women were enrolled in order to better study various aspects of the menopausal transition, including sexual changes.

All the participants complete a daily menstrual calendar, recording detailed information about their menstrual health. They also complete a yearly comprehensive survey, assessing biopsychosocial information about their health and aging, life experiences, and sexuality, among other factors. These surveys collect both quantitative and qualitative data. Throughout the years, some of the women have been called upon to participate in special qualitative studies in which they have been interviewed. One hundred of the perimenopausal women who are not taking hormone replacement therapy have also supplied daily morning urine specimens so that hormonal analysis could be conducted.

The Tremin Trust participants are incredibly dedicated to the project. For example, they keep daily records throughout their lives (for some almost 70 years) and enlist participation from their daughters, granddaughters, and great-granddaughters. The study's potential for providing a greater understanding of women's sexuality throughout their lives, and the factors that affect sexual changes, is unparalleled. The greatest limitation is the lack of diversity among the participants, since over 90 percent are well-educated white women. However, data collection has been conducted with additional samples of African-American and Alaskan women as well as lesbians. More diverse cohorts may be enlisted in the future.

Analysis of the sexuality data is ongoing, with more data being collected each year. Interesting findings have emerged regarding midlife women's sexuality (ages 35 through 55 years of age) as they progress through menopausal transition. The average age of menopause is 51, with perimenopause beginning as early as the late thirties. In an open-ended question asking what they enjoyed most about their sexuality, more than two-thirds of the women referred to aspects of their relationships with their partners.[11] Most of these responses described some aspect of intimacy, including love, closeness, sharing, companionship, affection, and caring, as described below. About 15 percent of the women noted feeling comfortable and secure in their relationship, emphasizing feelings of mutual trust and honesty.

It is the most healthy relationship I've ever been in. Sex in the context of a respectful, caring, non-exploitative relationship is very wonderful.

Wow! The sexual experience is another heightened way we share the humor that comes from shared experiences such as canoeing, fine music, backyard work, scuba trips. It makes the "union" a joyous and complete one!

Many of the lesbian participants felt that the intimacy they shared in their relationships was even greater than what they had experienced or observed in male-female relationships.

Many straight women in 20-to-25-year marriages are distant and emotionally separate from their husbands. I think this is a time when lesbian women and their partners really come into their own—their best time together. There's much greater emotional intimacy with less emphasis on sex. It's very nurturing and increases the bond between us.

Another very important contextual feature that at least one in ten women enjoyed about their sexuality was a newly-found sexual freedom they experienced as they aged, either from their children leaving home or from being with a new partner.

Freedom and ability to be spontaneous with our sexual desires due to the "empty nest."

The freedom to have sex at his apartment. The growing intimacy and closeness that goes along with sex itself. The sexual playfulness and frivolity that threads itself through regular daily activities (teasing, sexual nuances, private jokes, and touches).

Approximately 20 percent of the women discussed some particular aspect to their sexual interactions, with mutual sexual satisfaction, continuing sexual interest, desire, and attraction, and lessened inhibitions and increased experimentation mentioned most often.

We seem to enjoy sex more and more as the years go by. The orgasms seem even better. We both respond well to each other sexually since we feel safe in our loving monogamous relationship.

One-third of these discussions emphasized that touching, kissing, hugging, and cuddling were the most important aspects of the sexual interactions.

You may not consider it sexual, but sleeping together in a queen-sized bed in the last year and a half. While the kids were growing up, we had twin beds. We enjoy the cuddling this provides daily.

Qualities exhibited by their sexual partners, who are most often the women's husbands, have been found to significantly impact the women's sexual responding.[12] Specifically, the more love, affection, passion, assertiveness, interest, and equality expressed by the sexual partners, the higher the women's sexual desire, arousal, frequency, and enjoyment. Women also expressed appreciation for a non-demanding partner who was responsive to their needs.

> My partner is very accepting about how I feel and what I like and what I don't like even though it changes often. I also appreciate that he doesn't expect me to have an orgasm every time we make love.

Sexual Changes As Women Age

Each year the women report many changes in their sexual responding. Some women have reported enjoying sex more (8.7 percent), easier arousal (8.7 percent), desiring sexual relations more (7 percent), easier orgasm (6.7 percent), and engaging in sexual relations more often (4.7 percent).[13] The women attribute their improved sexuality most often to changes in life circumstances (new partner, more freedom with children leaving home), improved emotional well-being, more positive feelings toward partner, and improved appearance.[14]

However, two to three times more women have reported declines in their sexual responding, including: desiring sexual relations less (23.1 percent), engaging in sexual relations less often (20.7 percent), desiring more non-genital touching (19.7 percent), more difficult arousal (19.1 percent), enjoying sexual relations less (15.4 percent), more difficult orgasm (14 percent), and more pain (10 percent).

Women are much more likely to attribute declining sexual response to physical changes of menopause than to other factors.[15] Analysis of the health data has found a statistically significant relationship between having vaginal dryness and decreased sexual desire and enjoyment.[16] However, no statistically significant relationship between menopausal status and decreased sexual desire, enjoyment, or more difficulty with orgasm was found. On the other hand, sexual desire and enjoyment were significantly related to marital status, with decreases associated with being married. The woman's age was also significantly related to her sexual enjoyment, with enjoyment decreasing as the woman became older. Further, a significant relationship has been found between poor body image and decreased sexual satisfaction.[17]

Other studies among general populations of aging women have failed to find clear associations between menopausal status and declines in sexual functioning.[18] Similar to the MWHS findings, they found psychosocial factors to be more important determinants of sexual responding among midlife (perimenopausal and menopausal) women than menopausal status.[19] The factors include sexual attitudes and knowledge; previous sexual behavior and enjoyment; length and quality of relationship; physical and mental health; body image and self-esteem; stress; and partner availability, health, and sexual functioning.

Sexual Satisfaction and the Importance of Sex For Women

Even with many aging women in the MWHS identifying declines in their sexual desire, frequency, or functioning, about three-quarters of them reported overall sexual satisfaction (71 percent), including being physically and emotionally satisfied (72 percent).

> Even though sex is less frequent and it takes much longer to feel turned on, it is still very satisfying.
>
> I have been a very fortunate person. The man I married I still love dearly. We both respect each other and try to keep each other happy. We don't have sex as much as we used to but we kiss and hug and hold each other a lot.

The importance of sexual expression varied in the midlife women's lives and was affected by the circumstances in which they found themselves (married, divorced, widowed, in a same-sex relationship). Once again, women evaluated the importance of sexuality in the overall context of their lives. Some women who had lost their sexual partners to death or divorce reported missing a sexual relationship, mostly because of the lack of intimacy.

> I find being a widow at a young age to be very lonely. I find that I miss the desire to have a sexual closeness with a man. I also feel very sad and confused as my husband was the only man I have ever been with. Having lost him, I fear beginning a new relationship.
>
> I have been alone for 18 years after a 14 year marriage and three children. I miss regular sex, but *most* of all I miss touching, cuddling, body-to-body contact, not the sex act.

Yet many women without partners had decided that having sexual relations was not worth the price if the overall relationship was not fulfilling.

> I am single by choice (heterosexual) and have never wanted children. I am finding it difficult to meet men as I get older and my relationships are further apart. My sexual response is still very strong, but I am not willing to compromise what I want in a relationship just for sex. My attitude is that if that doesn't happen, I am doing fine, and am happy with my life.
>
> I find myself wishing for a "partner" but only if he's a real friend. My celibacy is comfortable at the moment. It has become apparent to me that our culture has taught most females to sacrifice themselves to their partner's desires and not to defend themselves. I hope I don't fall in that trap again. I find that I satisfy my physical sexual desires better than my husband ever did.

On the other hand, sexual interaction is very important to many of the aging women.

Half of Americans Over 60 Have Sexual Relations at Least Once a Month

Nearly half of all Americans over the age of 60 have sexual relations at least once a month, and 40 percent would like to have it more often. In addition, many seniors say their sex lives are more emotionally satisfying now than when they were in their forties.

These findings were part of the latest Roper-Starch Inc. survey of 1,300 men and women over the age of 60 conducted by the National Council on the Aging.

"This study underscores the enduring importance of sex among older men and women—even among those who report infrequent sexual activity," said Neal Cutler, director of survey research for the Council. "When older people are not sexually active, it is usually because they lack a partner or because they have a medical condition."

As most people might expect, the survey found that sexual relations taper off with age, with 71 percent of men and 51 percent of women in their sixties having sex once a month or more and 27 percent of men and 18 percent of women in their eighties saying they do. Cutler said women had sex less often in part because women are more likely to be widowed.

Thirty-nine percent of people said they were happy with the amount of sexual relations they currently have—even if it is none—while another 39 percent said they would like to make love more often. Only four percent of the people surveyed said they would like to have sexual relations less frequently. The people who had sex at least once a month said it was important to their relationship.

The survey also found that 74 percent of men and 70 percent of women find their sex lives more emotionally satisfying now that they are older than when they were in their forties. As to whether it is physically better, 43 percent say it is just as good as or better than in their youth, while 43 percent say sex is less satisfying.

"When it comes to knowledge about sex, older people are not necessarily wiser than their children. A third of the respondents believed it was natural to lose interest in sex as they got older," said Cutler.

I am 58 and as horny as ever.... The sex urge is still with me, not much different from my earlier years. Maybe I am too physically active and healthy! I can't seem to get it into my head that I am approaching a different time of life.... There is little or no speaking about a situation like mine in books or media. Yet women my age say the same thing: "Where are the men? Men want only younger women. The 'good men' are married or in relationships.".... My request to you is—listen to the voice of the horny women. When we hear each other and gain our dignity, solutions will come!

Conclusion

Results from the MWHS, some of which have been shared in this article, illustrate that women experience their sexuality as complex and holistic. Thus, it is doubtful that a particular drug or other substance or device that could improve physical functioning (increase libido or vasocongestion) would be the "magic bullet" to transform women's sexuality as they age. In order to understand and enhance women's sexuality throughout their lives, we must listen to their voices, learn from their experiences, and appreciate the importance of context to their sexual expression.

References

1. R. Basson, J. Berman, et al., "Report on the International Consensus Development Conference on Female Sexual Dysfunction: Definitions and Classifications," *Journal of Urology,* vol. 163, pp. 888–93; J. Hitt, "The Second Sexual Revolution," *The New York Times Magazine,* February 20, 2000, pp. 34–41, 50, 62, 64, 68–69; J. Leland, "The Science of Women and Sex," *Newsweek,* May 29, 2000, pp. 48–54; P. K. Mansfield, P. B. Koch,

and A. M. Voda, "Qualities Midlife Women Desire in Their Sexual Relationships and Their Changing Sexual Response," *Psychology of Women Quarterly,* vol. 22, pp. 285–303.
2. R. Rosen, *Major Issues in Contemporary Research in Women's Sexuality.* (Roundtable discussion at the Women's Health Research Symposium, Baltimore, MD.)
3. R. Basson, "The Female Sexual Response: A Different Model," *Journal of Sex and Marital Therapy,* vol. 26, pp. 51–65. S. R. Leiblum, "Definition and Classification of Female Sexual Disorders," *International Journal of Impotence Research,* vol. 10, pp. S102–S106; R. Rosen, *Major Issues in Contemporary Research in Women's Sexuality.*
4. L. Tiefer, "Historical, Scientific, Clinical and Feminist Criticisms of the Human Sexual Response Cycle," *Annual Review of Sex Research,* vol. 2, p. 2.
5. R. Basson, "The Female Sexual Response: A Different Model," pp. 51–65; L. Tiefer, "A New View of Women's Sexual Problems: Why New? Why Now?," *The Journal of Sex Research,* vol. 38, no. 2, pp. 89–96.
6. *Webster's New World Dictionary of the American Language: College Edition* (New York: The World Publishing Company, 2000).
7. R. Basson, "The Female Sexual Response: A Different Model," pp. 51–65.
8. J. Jordan, *Clarity in Connection: Empathic Knowing, Desire and Sexuality,* work in progress (Wellesley, MA: Stone Center Working Papers Series, 1987).
9. J. Jordan, *Clarity in Connection: Empathic Knowing, Desire and Sexuality.*
10. A. M. Voda and P. K. Mansfield, *The Tremin Trust and the Midlife Women's Health Survey: Two Longitudinal Studies of Women's Health and Menopause.* (Paper presented at the Society for Menstrual Cycle Research Conference, Montreal, June 1995.); A. M. Voda, J. M. Morgan, et al., "The Tremin Trust Research Program" in N. F. Taylor and D. Taylor, editors, *Menstrual Health and Illness* (New York: Hemisphere Press, 1991), pp. 5–19.
11. *Midlife Women's Health Survey,* 1992, unpublished data.

12. P. K. Mansfield, P. B. Koch, et al., "Qualities Midlife Women Desire in Their Sexual Relationships and Their Changing Sexual Response," *Psychology of Women Quarterly,* vol. 22, pp. 285–303.
13. Ibid.
14. P. K. Mansfield, P. B. Koch, et al., "Midlife Women's Attributions for Their Sexual Response Changes," *Health Care for Women International,* vol. 21, pp. 543–59.
15. Ibid.
16. P. K. Mansfield, A. Voda, et al., "Predictors of Sexual Response Changes in Heterosexual Midlife Women," *Health Values,* vol. 19, no. 1, pp. 10–20.
17. D. A. Thurau, *The Relationship between Body Image and Sexuality among Menopausal Women.* (Unpublished master's thesis, Pennsylvania State University, 1996).
18. N. E. Avis, M. A. Stellato, et al., "Is There an Association between Menopause Status and Sexual Functioning?," *Menopause,* vol. 7, no. 5, pp. 297–309; K. Hawton, D. Gaith, et al., "Sexual Function in a Community Sample of Middle-aged Women with Partners: Effects of Age, Marital, Socioeconomic, Psychiatric, Gynecological, and Menopausal Factors, *Archives of Sexual Behavior,* vol. 23, no. 4, pp. 375–95.
19. N. E. Avis, M. A. Stellato, et al., "Is There an Association between Menopause Status and Sexual Functioning?," pp. 297–309; I. Fooken, "Sexuality in the Later Years—The Impact of Health and Body-Image in a Sample of Older Women," *Patient Education and Counseling,* vol. 23, pp. 227–33; K. Hawton, D. Gaith, et al., "Sexual Function in a Community Sample of Middle-aged Women with Partners: Effects of Age, Marital, Socioeconomic, Psychiatric, Gynecological, and Menopausal Factors," *Archives of Sexual Behavior,* vol. 23, no. 4, pp. 375–95; B. K. Johnson, "A Correlational Framework for Understanding Sexuality in Women Age 50 and Older," *Health Care for Women International,* vol. 19, pp. 553–64.

(**DR. MANSFIELD** is director of the Tremin Trust Research Program on Women's Health. **DR. KOCH** is assistant director. Dr. Koch is also adjunct professor of human sexuality at Widener University in West Chester, PA.)

—Editor

As Good As It Gets

What country takes the best care of its older citizens? The Netherlands rates tops in our exclusive survey of 16 nations. But no place is perfect

Mike Edwards

Every week, Anna Sophia Fischer greets a clutch of tourists in the medieval central square of Utrecht and, with a spring in her step, guides them on a stroll among 14th-century Dutch monasteries and houses. She knows every arch, garden, and alley and, at 75, goes about her daily business by bicycle, as do the swarms of people around her. "You have to go by bike if you live in town," she says. (Could this be one reason that the Dutch live longer than we do—an average 78.6 years, compared with 77.3 in the U.S.?) A retired physician, Fischer is living her dream. "I wanted to do something different," she says. "I'm not rich, but I can do the things I want to do."

Wim van Essen, 69, is a former teacher, tall, vigorous, an ardent hiker, a fanatical chess player—and a one-man pep squad for the Dutch way of retirement. "You see how we live," he says, inviting a guest into his brick home in the leafy city of Amersfoort. There's a fireplace in the living room, a wildflower garden out back. Extra bedrooms upstairs await visiting grandchildren. On a coffee table are photos of Van Essen trekking in the Austrian Alps with his wife, Lamberta Jacoba Maria, nicknamed Bep. (Every year, the two of them take a major trip, partly subsidized by the government.) The couple receive government and work pensions and various perks. All told, it's a wonderful life, based on what Van Essen calls "a beautiful pension," which, when everything is added up, comes to about $45,000 a year.

In a world that is rapidly aging, the Netherlands, perhaps more than any other country, has created a society in which people have the luxury of growing old well, according to a survey conducted by AARP THE MAGAZINE. We weighed 17 criteria (see the PDF chart "And the Winner is...") in selected industrialized nations that approximate as closely as possible the lifestyle of most AARP members. We focused on key quality-of-life issues such as health care, work, education, taxes, and social programs.

But if you're already thinking of packing your bags, stop right there. The purpose of this report is not to encourage American retirees to immigrate to the Netherlands or to some of the other top scorers in our study. Most nations aren't keen to share their pensions and health care benefits with noncitizens just off a plane. Rather, our goal is to shed light on what retirees enjoy elsewhere in the world as a reference point for our own country's policies.

In the Netherlands, all citizens receive the full old-age pension at 65 if they've lived in the country for a minimum of 50 years between ages 15 and 64. Unlike our Social Security, however, the pension doesn't require a work history. The full amount per month is nearly $1,000 for singles and nearly $1,400 for couples, married or not. The old-age pension is in addition to an occupational, or employer-provided, pension based on payments over the years by worker and employer. And every pensioner gets a "holiday allowance" of about $700, thoughtfully paid in May, just in time for spring.

Pension generosity is a major reason that, by international measurements, only 6.4 percent of the elderly fall in the bottom quarter of income distribution, as compared with the U.S. percentage of 20.7. Although the U.S. has a far larger per capita income than the Netherlands—$26,448 a year versus $17,080—it scores poorly in two other comparisons: First, all Dutch citizens have government insurance for medical conditions and nursing-home care; 45 million Americans have no health insurance at all. Second, prescription drugs are available to all Dutch citizens, with few if any copayments; Americans get drugs in many different ways and those without insurance pay top dollar. Even when Medicare drug coverage begins in 2006, most enrollees will still face substantial out-of-pocket costs.

"The European attitude is, we're all in this together and sooner or later we're all going to become older and need some help. The U.S. attitude is, we're all rugged individualists and we're going to take care of ourselves, not others."

How do the Dutch do it? How do their euros stretch further than our dollars? The key factor is lower costs. Although medicine isn't completely socialized—physicians and pharmacists, for example, aren't state employees—the government regulates almost all health expenses. That helps explain why, in the view of Professor Gerard F. Anderson of the Johns Hopkins Bloomberg School of Public Health, "in the U.S. we pay a lot more than anybody else for pretty much the same stuff." In analyzing health

And the Winner Is . . . The Netherlands, which scored highest on key quality-of-life issues important to older people and society in general.

On a scale of 1 to 5 FIVE IS TOPS	Netherlands	Australia	Sweden	Finland	Switzerland	Norway	Denmark	Japan	France	Canada	Ireland	Spain	United States	United Kingdom	Germany	Italy
Mandatory Retirement	1	5	1	1	1	1	1	1	1	1	1	1	5	1	1	1
Age-Discrimination Laws	5	5	4	5	1	1	1	1	3	5	5	5	5	1	1	3
Unemployment Rate	5	4	4	2	5	5	4	5	2	3	5	1	4	5	2	2
College Education	4	3	2	2	2	5	4	3	1	3	2	2	5	3	1	1
Per Capita Income	3	3	2	2	3	5	3	2	2	3	4	1	5	3	2	2
Total Tax Burden	3	5	1	2	5	2	1	5	2	4	5	4	5	3	4	2
Home Care	3	5	2	3	2	4	5	2	2	4	1	1	2	1	2	1
Retirement Age for Full Benefits	3	3	3	3	3	1	1	3	5	3	3	3	1	3	3	3
Public Pension Replacement Rate	4	1	4	3	3	2	3	2	4	1	1	5	2	1	1	4
Employers Pension Coverage	5	5	5	5	5	3	5	3	5	2	3	1	3	3	3	1
Economic Inequality	4	2	5	5	4	5	4	3	4	3	3	3	1	2	4	2
Economic Inequality for the Elderly	5	1	5	5	4	3	5	5	4	5	3	4	2	3	5	4
Public Spending on Social Programs	3	2	5	4	3	4	5	1	3	2	1	3	1	3	5	4
Total Health Costs	4	4	4	5	3	4	4	5	4	4	5	5	1	5	3	5
Universal Health Care	5	5	5	5	5	5	5	5	5	5	5	5	4	5	5	5
Universal Rx	5	5	5	5	5	5	5	5	5	4	5	5	3	5	5	5
Life Expectancy at Birth	2	4	4	2	4	3	1	5	3	3	1	3	1	2	2	3
TOTAL	64	62	61	59	58	58	57	56	55	55	53	52	50	49	49	48

Understanding the Chart . . .

Mandatory Retirement Australia and the United States are the only countries on the list above that prohibit companies from making their employees retire at a certain age.

Age-Discrimination Laws The EU expects to have laws by 2006, but experts are skeptical that all countries will make the deadline.

Unemployment Rate In 2003, the Netherlands averaged lowest (3.8%); Spain, the highest (11.3%). The U.S. had 6%.

College Education The U.S. and Norway both get an A on this one: 28% of adults age 25–64 have a college degree.

Per Capita Income Compared with the countries above, the U.S. has the highest average standard of living; Norway is next.

Total Tax Burden Sweden collects the most taxes (51.4% of GDP).

Home Care In Australia and Denmark, more than 20% of those 65 and over receive home help—from medical care to tidying up. (In the Netherlands, its 12.8%; in the U.S., less than 10%.)

Retirement Age for Full Benefits Most grant benefits at 65. France is lowest—at 60—with citizens strongly protesting change; Denmark is 67.

Public Pension Replacement Rate Spains retirement benefit as a percentage of an average workers earnings is highest, at 88%. Spain also has a high tax burden and the lowest income.

Employers Pension Coverage About 50% of U.S. workers have pension coverage at work. In some countries—Finland and Australia—employer pensions are required by law.

Economic Inequality Using an international definition, this is the percent of those whose income is in the lower quarter.

Economic Inequality for the Elderly In the U.S., the elderly fare slightly better than the general population.

Public Spending on Social Programs Income-support programs, such as social security and welfare, vary widely. Scandinavian countries traditionally offer the most.

Total Health Costs Americans spend the most (14.6% of GDP); Finland and Ireland, the least (7.3%).

Universal Health Care The U.S. is odd man out: 45 million—41%—have no health insurance, though most seniors have Medicare.

Universal Rx Canada has limitations and some gaps at the provincial level; 88% have coverage. The U.S. scores lowest, but changes in Medicare represent progress for the elderly.

Life Expectancy at Birth In the U.S., babies born in 2004 can expect to live to 77.3; in the Netherlands, to 78.6. Japan is highest at 81.9.

For more details on these criteria, go to www.aarpmagazine.org.

Finland
Model Home

Drop a few coins into a slot machine in a local casino in Finland and you contribute to the care and comfort of retirees. Legal gambling in Finland is the exclusive province of the Slot Machine Association, a government-controlled nonprofit that pumps more than $50 million a year into the welfare of the country's 65-plus population (800,000 out of a total of 5.2 million).

Slot machine profits, for example, helped build the four-story Saga Senior Center, a complex of 138 units in Helsinki with cheerful apartments that are emphatically uninstitutional and that allow older people to have their own space and their own life. "It's the classiest senior home in Finland," says Leif Sonkin, a housing expert. "It's really like a spa." Indeed. Sunshine pours through the glass roof of the atrium, nourishing a lush semitropical garden. The swimming pool is indoor-outdoor and heated in winter. In the basement are saunas, essentials of Finnish life, and a well-equipped gym. (Pay no attention to its thick steel doors; the government requires bomb shelters in all buildings, a holdover from Cold War days.)

"The Saga center isn't a place for rich people," says administrator Mariana Boneva. A small apartment rents for about $600 a month. Most retirees can afford that, but "if they need it to live here, people can get a government housing subsidy," she adds.

Saga is one of three residences owned by the nonprofit Ruissalo Foundation. Although municipalities are charged by law with caring for older people, nonprofits have taken a major role; they operate more than half of Finland's "service housing" homes for the elderly. This shared responsibility is an extension of the egalitarian streak that started permeating policy in the 1950s, when Finland, along with Sweden, Norway, and Denmark, embraced an unabashedly liberal form of tax-supported welfare.

Finland's taxes are formidable. "I cannot say we love taxes," says Erikki Vaatanen, who lives with her husband, Orvokki, in the Wilhelmiina House, a new senior center. "But we know that schools, hospitals, and highways would go down if we didn't pay." Still, Vaatanen recently faced a drawback. After waiting a year for surgery for an arthritic wrist, she applied again, only to be told: "Little lady, you must wait two years more." So she went to a private physican for treatment and paid herself. —M.E.

systems in the Netherlands and other industrialized nations, Anderson found that drugs, hospitals, and physicians' services were from 30 to 50 percent more expensive in the U.S., "and their health status is as good or better than ours."

Another factor is attitude. A strong feeling of "social solidarity," as Anderson sees it, makes Europeans inclined to be generous to older people, more willing to support them. "Their attitude is, we're in this together and sooner or later we're going to become older and we'll need some help," he says. "The U.S. attitude is, we're all rugged individualists and we're going to take care of ourselves, not others."

The Netherlands demonstrates its attitude toward older citizens (2 million are over 65) by showering them with numerous friendly perks, in addition to the big-ticket items such as pensions and health care. One example: seven days of free travel a year on the efficient rail system. "I go as far as possible," says Joris Korst, a 65-year-old civil servant in Nieuwegein. That's never very far in the Netherlands, which is only a third the size of Pennsylvania, but the destinations can be exhilarating—like the windswept beaches that Korst strolls in the West Frisian Islands. Museums, movies, concerts, campgrounds, and holiday bungalows are discounted, too. All this and a country that's worldly, prosperous, tolerant, steeped in art, and graced by canals, windmills, and tulip fields. What's not to like?

Health Care

The Dutch are accustomed to paying minuscule copayments for expensive treatment.

Dutch health insurance took care of teacher Van Essen when he needed a heart pacemaker. "He never saw a bill," his wife, Bep, recalls. Neither did civil servant Korst, who remembers that there were no charges when his wife, Trees, had cancer surgery followed by 32 chemotherapy treatments. "The whole country paid," he says, referring to the state-regulated insurance. In the U.S., those 32 treatments alone could have cost $30,000 or more, depending on the type and number of drugs used. Medicare might cover 80 percent, but the patient still could owe thousands.

Compare Trees's experience with that of Harold Powers, 79, and his wife, Ozelle, 82, retired educators in Tennessee. Powers paid about $200 of the bill for his bypass heart surgery because Medicare picked up 80 percent of the tab and his private Medigap insurance (which costs extra) paid most of the rest. But, in addition, he and Ozelle spend about $3,000 a year for medicines, and Medicare won't cover any of that until 2006. Van Essen, on the other hand, pays nothing for the medicine he takes to prevent migraines. In 2003, however, the Dutch health ministry proposed that everyone make a copayment of $1.75 for each prescription—but backed down when the people protested.

There is also a government limit on the amount a hospital may bill an insurance company for a pacemaker—Van Essen's was $5,750, plus the expense of the procedure. In the U.S., a pacemaker can cost as much as a car—$15,000 to $20,000, just for the device. The whole procedure can zoom up to $50,000. In the Netherlands, government pressure on hospitals, doctors, and manufacturers helps to keep costs down.

These kinds of controls are not always painless. Just this past year, the Dutch government hit a nerve when it decided to boost the $6-per-hour cost of home care by 250 percent. Half a million citizens, most of them beyond the age of 65, have been receiving subsidized home visits by health professionals or workers who clean and tidy up (like most developed countries, the Netherlands wants to help people maintain their independence and avoid going into nursing homes as long as possible). However, at the increased rate of about $15 an hour, despite government subsidies, home care is rapidly climbing out of sight for many low-income retirees. This increase takes effect, moreover, at an awkward time when the country has a nursing-home waiting list of some 50,000.

Still, all things considered, the Dutch like their health care. In a Harvard School of Public Health survey (taken before the increase in home-care costs), 70 percent said they were satisfied with the system. The same study rated the satisfaction level in the U.S. at 40

Sweden
Shrinking Benefits

In a suburb of Stockholm, care for Aina Karlsson, 85, arrives twice a day, seven days a week. In the morning a *vårdbiträde* (care assistant) helps her bathe and dress; in the evening she helps her get ready for bed. Once a month she cleans the apartment that Aina shares with her husband, Einar. And twice a week she takes Aina to a gymnasium for exercise.

Life expectancy in Sweden is 80.4, one of the highest in Europe. Good care could be one reason. Aina has been receiving *hemhjälp* (home help) assistance since she suffered a stroke four years ago. Cost to the Karlssons: $159 a month. "Not very much," says Einar, a retired union official. To the municipal government, which provides Aina's care, the real cost is about five times greater. And if the Karlssons couldn't afford even $159, the government would provide a subsidy. "That's why Swedish taxes are so high," Einar says cheerfully, noting that income taxes shrink his own pension of $4,400 a month by a third.

Sweden is democratic, capitalistic, high-tech, and industrialized, well known for Ikea and Volvo. It is also well known as a prime example of a welfare state. Social spending, which includes payments such as pensions and welfare, equals 28.5 percent of GDP. In the U.S. it's 16.4 percent.

The income tax rate tops out at a breathtaking 58.2 percent, and there's a 25 percent VAT tax on most purchases. "Of course, many people say taxes are too high," remarks Nils-Erik Hogstedt, a home-care manager. "But the complaint isn't against the elderly. The great majority favor the care." Adds Pernilla Berggren, the manager of a retirement home: "People in Sweden are used to the community doing everything. You grow up expecting society to help take care of Mom."

Tens of thousands use *hemhjälp*, which enables people to remain in their own homes. "Sometimes we visit just once a month to clean," says Chatrin Engbo, head of a Stockholm district care office. "But if needed, we may go several times a day and at night."

This sounds nice—but expensive. To contain costs, the government recently sanctioned sharp cuts in home care by the municipalities, a move that upset many. "Home care used to include visits just to sit and have coffee two or three times a week, or just to take someone for a walk," says Berggren. "We do the essentials, but we can't afford those social moments anymore.

Reductions are also in the pipeline for the pension system, but for now a worker on the job for 30 years is customarily rewarded with a pension that replaces about 60 percent of his pay. (In the U.S. the Social Security replacement rate ranges from about 30 to 60 percent.)

The government's worry about future solvency began in the 1990s. The percentage of 65-plussers, almost one in five of the 8.9 million Swedes, is one of Europe's highest. As with U.S. Social Security, pension payments made by active workers support retirees. With low birth rates and the increase of pensioners, experts estimate that by 2035 the system will be seriously out of balance, with about two workers supporting each older person. (By then, America will be in the same boat.)

Looking ahead, the parliament recently approved drastic, complicated revisions. Out the window went the defined-benefit pension—a set amount based on salary and years of service—replaced by a system based on contributions by worker and employer. The benefit will be indexed to wage growth, with a built-in expectancy that the rate will grow 1.6 percent annually. If wages don't grow that much, the benefit drops. The plan phases in fully in 2019, with the retirement of those born in 1954.

There's yet another new wrinkle: mandated private investments. Besides paying into the pension's main part (employee and employer contribute a total of 16 percent of the worker's wages), all workers are required to put an additional 2.5 percent into their choice of investments—an idea that has become popular among world pension experts. A voluntary form of this setup is favored by President George W. Bush.

Swedes were optimistic in 2000, when this change took effect, even though many were confused by the hundreds of funds, Swedish and foreign, competing for their kronor. The timing proved terrible. The return averaged 3.5 percent in 2001, and then *katastrof!* Or so said a civil servant who saw a thousand dollars vanish from her stock account as markets toppled worldwide. More than 2 million Swedes lost 30 to 40 percent of their mandated investments. (By July 2004, the average fund had recovered nearly 19 percent.)

One likely outcome of the radically revised system: to earn higher pension benefits more Swedes will work beyond the typical retirement age of 60. Says Barbro Westerholm, president of the Swedish Association of Senior Citizens: "I've recommended to my children that they plan to work until they are 70."

percent. And this even when the U.S. spends far more on health care than any other nation in the world—an average of $5,440 per person, with a large share of that going toward retirees.

Canada, by the way, doesn't score much better. Just 46 percent say they are satisfied. Although Canadians receive low-cost prescription drugs, thanks to government controls, health services are underfunded and waiting periods for treatment are long (see the sidebar "O Canada!").

Waiting. That seems to be the tradeoff. Someone who needs open-heart surgery in the Netherlands might have to sit around for 14 weeks before a time slot and hospital space become available. Hip surgery? You're maybe looking at an average wait of eight weeks. Like much of Europe and also Canada, the Netherlands is short of hospital beds and medical staff. Dutch officials say no one has to wait for emergency attention, and some patients are being sent to Germany and Belgium for faster treat-

O Canada!

The pain in her back was terrible, recalls Diane Tupper, who lives in a Vancouver suburb. When she finally got a consultation with a neurosurgeon—after waiting eight months—he said he could fix her spine. Then he delivered the bad news: "Our surgery waiting time is a year and a half to two years."

If Tupper, a 63-year-old lawyer, could hold out, her surgery would be free under Canada's universal-care system. But if she hopped over the border to St. Joseph Hospital in Bellingham, Washington, she could be in the operating room in days. The cost would be about $47,000. "I'm not a well-off person," Tupper says, "but I felt I didn't have any choice." Tupper took out two lines of credit, borrowed $14,500 from a friend, and went to Bellingham.

To many Americans, Canada may look like health care's promised land. Care for all 32.5 million citizens is paid for from taxes. Drugs are typically 30 to 50 percent cheaper than in the U.S.—which is why more than a million statesiders now get prescriptions filled in Canada.

But recently, Canada's system has fallen behind, hobbled by budget cuts, regulations, and shortages of physicians, nurses, and sophisticated equipment such as MRI machines. A recent survey put the backlog of unperformed procedures at 876,584. The waiting time for a hip replacement in Tupper's province, British Columbia, is nearly a year, even longer for a knee replacement.

Filling that gap are U.S. border cities such as Buffalo, New York, and Great Falls, Montana. Minot, North Dakota, attracts people needing CT scans and MRIs, for which they'd wait months in Saskatchewan. Randy Schwan of Trinity Health in Minot says Canadians are amazed to find that "a doctor says we've got to get a test, and the same day someone wheels them down the hall for that test." At the globally famous Mayo Clinic in Rochester, Minnesota, Canadians are the largest foreign-patient constituency.

Some provinces cover care outside of Canada under special circumstances. To trim the waiting list of cancer patients needing radiation treatment, Ontario picked up the bill for 1,650 people who went to the U.S. in 2000 and 2001.

So, get to a Canadian hospital's emergency room after a heart attack and you'll be treated promptly—with no worry about cost. But the system, once the nation's pride, has become, as one official says, "functionally obsolete." —*M.E.*

ment. Still, the delays underscore a major difference between Dutch and U.S. care. Says one not-so-happy Dutch resident: "I don't care what they say. If you need open-heart surgery here, you can die before you get it."

"In America we love responsiveness," says Anderson, the Johns Hopkins expert. "We're the best on responsiveness." But ready access to care, he adds, is one of the reasons Americans pay more than people do in other countries. Anderson is one of a number of health specialists and economists who have been pointing out the built-in inefficiencies of U.S. care. Some critics argue that the huge number of health-insurance providers—HMOs, PPOs, Medicare, Medicaid, and all the rest—consumes far more in overhead than

would one or two providers and that their many forms and complicated rules drive up hospital administrative costs. Others point to the huge sums spent advertising and marketing drugs and hospitals.

In Sweden, with its low birth rate and increasing number of pensioners, experts estimate that by 2035 the system will be seriously out of balance, with only about two workers supporting each older person.

Taxes

The Dutch in particular pay quite a lot to take care of one another. The personal income tax rate in the Netherlands isn't Europe's highest, but it's well up there, with a top rate of 52 percent on any income over $60,000. (The top U.S. rate has been going down during the presidency of George W. Bush and now stands at 35 percent. A family of four with an income of about $60,000 would be in the 25 percent tax bracket.)

Almost half of Dutch taxes go to the universal pension fund, known as the AOW, which provides the basic pension that everyone receives at age 65. The AOW takes a salary bite of 17.9 percent. Most Dutch workers have an employer-provided pension based on payments by worker and employer—that's another salary bite of 6 or 7 percent.

Then comes a bigger bite: a 12.05 percent contribution to help pay for basic state health insurance, known as the AWBZ, which, like the basic pension, is universal. Besides paying for care for grave illnesses and a place in a nursing home (after a wait), it also covers part (but less now) of the cost of home care. Most workers also have government-regulated insurance with private or nonprofit companies for lesser medical expenses and medicines. Employers usually pay most of this cost; the worker's share is only about 1.7 percent of income.

On top of that formidable raft of outlays, there's also a stiff value-added tax (VAT tax) of 19 percent on most things you buy. There's a 12 percent tax on food. And a whopping tax of as much as 40 percent on new cars (plus roughly $6 for a gallon of gas). Yet costs like these haven't stopped Wilhelmina and Cornelius van der Hoop, both retired teachers, from driving all around Europe towing a trailer.

The couple has a combined pension of about $41,000 after all deductions. "We have no reason to complain," Wilhelmina says. "All those taxes help other people."

In fact, polls show that the majority of Dutch citizens don't object to the large salary deduction that sustains the AOW. "The general attitude in the Netherlands—if you ask the man in the street—is that people who have worked their entire lives should be protected from poverty," says pension expert Maarten Lindeboom, an economist at the Free University of Amsterdam.

Dutch citizens with higher-than-average incomes usually invest in a private pension plan or annuities. That's what retired physician-turned-tour guide Anna Sophia Fischer did years ago. These investments put her annual income in the $60,000 range, where the taxman ordinarily takes a large bite. But thanks to reductions granted to people over 65, her tax is only about 30 percent of her income. As a physician, Fischer was well acquainted with the fabled liberality of the health system. "If you want a sex-change operation, the government will pay for it," she says. "I do think that goes a bit too far." A recent innovation: marijuana available by prescription for pain.

A noticeable difference in most of Europe's treatment of older people is the absence of laws that forbid discrimination and age-based mandatory retirement. In the U.S., mandatory retirement has been illegal for most occupations since 1986. Says one Dutch pension expert: "Here it is automatic that at 65 the job is over." The European Union has mandated that its 25 member states introduce laws against age discrimination by 2006, but the word is that loopholes will permit mandatory retirement to continue. Laurie McCann, senior attorney with AARP Foundation Litigation, concludes that the EU is a long way from either "talking the talk" or "walking the walk" when it comes to eliminating age discrimination.

Today some 14 percent of Americans 65 and older—about 4.8 million people in all—are still on the job; that's one of the highest rates in the industrialized world. Most European workers retire at age 60 or so, taking advantage of pension generosity.

The need for a ban on mandatory retirement hasn't seemed all that urgent. Frits Velker, a foreman at a Dutch plumbing and sheet-metal company, was 59 when the company was sold. "I looked around and saw so many other people who had retired early," he says. So Velker did too. His company pension is about $27,000, and when he turns 65 he and wife Gerrie will receive about $14,000 a year from the AOW, the state pension fund. In general, a worker in the Netherlands can expect a total pension equaling about 70 percent of his salary if he worked for 40 years. Thanks to cost-of-living adjustments, former teacher Van Essen's pension is slightly higher—72 percent of his salary—even though his teaching career stopped after 38 years.

Such generous retirement benefits are under siege all across Europe (and Japan). Cutbacks and proposed cutbacks in care and pensions provoked angry strikes last year in France, Italy, Germany, and Austria. Even in Sweden, shining star of the Scandinavian welfare-state constellation, benefits have shrunk. With increasing concern, governments are facing challenging demographics: swelling ranks of longer-living older citizens and thinning ranks of workers able—and willing—to pay for benefits.

MIKE EDWARDS, a writer and editor for *National Geographic* magazine for 34 years, has received national awards for articles on Chernobyl and pollution in the former U.S.S.R. Also contributing to this article was **SOPHIE KORCZYK,** an economist and consultant based in Alexandria, Virginia.

Cohabitation Among Older Adults: A National Portrait

SUSAN L. BROWN, GARY R. LEE, AND JENNIFER ROEBUCK BULANDA
Department of Sociology and Center for Family and Demographic Research, Bowling Green State University, Ohio

The prevalence of heterosexual cohabitation in the United States has increased enormously in recent decades. The number of cohabiting couples grew by a factor of 10 between 1970 and 2000, from about 500,000 to around 5 million (U.S. Census Bureau, 2001). Today, even though only about 45% of all cohabiting unions eventuate in marriage, more than half of all marriages are preceded. by cohabitation (Bumpass & Lu, 2000; Smock, 2000).

Most of the public attention surrounding cohabitation, as well as most of the research, has focused on younger adults, who usually cohabit as either a prelude or an alternative to first marriage (Smock, 2000). However, cohabitation is actually more common among the formerly married than the never married (Bumpass & Lu, 2000). According to the 2000 Census, of the roughly 10 million individuals currently cohabiting, more than 1 million are older than age 30. It is clear that the rising incidence of cohabitation crosses the age spectrum. Yet with few exceptions (Brown, Bulanda, & Lee, 2005; Chevan, 1996; De Jong Gierveld, 2004; Hatch, 1995; King & Scott, 2005), the research literature has ignored the cohabitation experiences of older adults (Cooney & Dunne, 2001). Research on the living arrangements of older persons (e.g., Angel, Angel, McClellan, & Markides, 1996; Wilmoth, 1998, 2001) has not considered cohabitation.

The objective of this study was to use Census 2000 data and national data from the 1998 Health and Retirement Study to describe the characteristics of cohabitors aged 51 and older and to show how these individuals compare with their contemporaries of different union statuses. As will be shown in the Results section, nearly all older cohabitors have prior marital experience; that is, they are divorced or widowed. Consequently, we will emphasize comparisons across the previously married: cohabitors, remarrieds, and unpartnereds. In other words, to explore the significance of union type, we will investigate how those who are formally remarried differ from those who are cohabiting in informal unions. This research contributes to an understanding of the antecedents and consequences of cohabitation in the later stages of the life cycle, issues that will become increasingly important to gerontologists as the number of older cohabitors continues to rise.

Background

Several demographic processes are responsible for the increase in cohabitation among middle-aged and older persons. A major cause is simple cohort replacement. Substantial increases in cohabitation among younger adults first occurred in the baby boom cohorts. These people are now aging into their later middle-age years, meaning that an increasing share of older adults is likely to be favorably disposed towards cohabitation (De Jong Gierveld, 2004). Moreover, divorce rates have been relatively high among these cohorts, and remarriage rates have decreased (Allen, Blieszner, & Roberto, 2000; Cooney & Dunne, 2001), yielding more adults who are unmarried and available for partnering. Cohabitation is also more common among Blacks and Hispanics than among non-Hispanic Whites (Raley, 1996; Wherry & Finegold, 2004), and these groups are increasing as a proportion of the older population. In consequence, a smaller fraction of the older population will be married in coming decades, and a higher proportion is likely to be cohabiting. Because the older population is growing, this will produce an even greater increase in the number of older co-habitors. There were just more than 25 million Americans aged 55 and older in 1950; by 2000 this number had increased to nearly 60 million (U.S. Census Bureau, 2002). Although growth in this age group has been modest over the past decade, it is expected to accelerate between 2010 and 2020 as baby boomers age into this group. Indeed, Chevan's (1996) estimates of cohabitation among persons aged 60 and older indicate that whereas fewer than 10,000 were cohabiting in 1960, more than 400,000 were cohabiting by 1990. Brown and colleagues (2005) report that more than 1.2 million persons aged 50 and older were cohabiting in 2000; we calculate that more than 500,000 of these were aged 60 and older.

Like the demographic trends, Americans' attitudes and values regarding cohabitation are changing. Research shows a dramatically increased tolerance of unmarried cohabitation among both younger and older persons (Thornton & Young-DeMarco, 2001), a trend that appears to comprise both cohort and period effects. Well over a decade ago, Bulcroft and Bulcroft (1991) reported that unmarried adults older than age 60 were as interested in cohabiting as in remarrying. These trends point to an increasing diversity of living arrangements among the older population that includes, notably, cohabitation (Cooney & Dunne, 2001).

From a theoretical standpoint, cohabitation likely has a unique meaning and plays a different role in the life course of older adults than it does in that of younger adults (Chevan, 1996; Hatch, 1995; King & Scott, 2005). Research on dating and remarriage among older adults suggests that theories developed to explain these behaviors among young and middle-aged adults are inadequate as they ignore the significance of life-course stage in structuring opportunities and outcomes (e.g., Bulcroft & Bulcroft, 1991; Bulcroft, Bulcroft, Hatch, & Borgatta, 1989). Similarly, the motivations for cohabitation among the older population are likely to differ from those of young adults.

Several researchers assert that older adults, particularly women, are not especially interested in remarriage (Bulcroft & Bulcroft, 1991; Bulcroft et al., 1989; Chevan, 1996; Hatch, 1995; Talbott, 1998). Chevan (1996) maintains that the disincentives for remarriage are greater among older adults, who are especially likely to have economic resources whose value may be undermined by remarriage. For instance, provisions governing social security and pension receipt typically depend on one's marital status. Also, adult offspring may encourage their parents to cohabit rather than to remarry in order to protect their estates (i.e., the offspring's inheritances).

In summary, there are important demographic and theoretical reasons for investigating the composition of the older adult cohabiting population and for assessing how this group compares with other union statuses. Despite the growth of the older population, which is increasingly composed of unmarrieds who may enter into cohabitation, research on this topic is scarce and dated. For instance, Chevan's (1996) study of cohabitors older than age 60 relied on decennial census data from 1960–1990, and Hatch's (1995) research on older cohabitors used census data from 1980. Not only were these analyses conducted at a time when cohabitation was much less common, but both studies were also undermined by significant data constraints, including the availability of only indirect measures of cohabitation and a very narrow set of sociodemographic correlates to explore. Until 1990, cohabitation had to be inferred from census data; respondents were not directly asked whether they were currently involved in an intimate, heterosexual, coresidential relationship (Casper & Cohen, 2000). Moreover, Chevan's analyses compared cohabitors only to other unmarrieds; marrieds were excluded. A few recent analyses have incorporated cohabitation into studies of mental health (Brown et al., 2005) and repartnering following marital dissolution in The Netherlands (De Jong Gierveld, 2004) among older adults, but these studies do not describe the older adult cohabiting population and how it compares with other union statuses.

The Present Study

The present study updates and extends the limited prior work in this area by drawing on two data sources. We will construct a detailed portrait of older cohabitors, providing explicit compar-

isons to those in other union statuses (i.e., marriage, remarriage, separation or divorce, widowhood, and the never-married state). By examining older adults' characteristics across these union statuses, we will document the composition of the older adult cohabiting population and the extent to which these older adults are similar to (and different from) those in other union statuses. We will investigate multiple features of older adults' lives according to union status, emphasizing factors that were shown in prior research to be related to union status among older adults: (a) demographic characteristics, (b) economic resources, (c) physical health, and (d) social relationships.

Demographic characteristics.— Union status is associated with individual demographic characteristics, including gender, age, and race. Union formation and dissolution processes differ for men and women, particularly among the older population. This is largely an artifact of the skewed sex ratio: Unmarried women outnumber unmarried men by a ratio of 2.5:1 among the 55 and older population (U.S. Census Bureau, 2002: Table 48). This imbalance is exacerbated by gender-specific mate selection strategies, whereby men tend to partner with younger women whereas women often partner with older men. These dynamics indicate that older men will be more likely to form and maintain unions than women. Indeed, older cohabitors are also disproportionately men. Men compose only about 25% of the elderly unmarried population but account for nearly 60% of cohabitors older than age 60 (Chevan, 1996). Among older unmarrieds, age is negatively associated with cohabitation (Chevan, 1996; De Jong Gierveld, 2004). In the general population, cohabitation is especially common among African Americans and Hispanics (Raley, 1996). As the older population becomes more racially and ethnically diverse with the changing composition of the American population and the lengthening life expectancies of non-Whites, there is no reason not to expect that African Americans and Hispanics will continue to be more likely than Whites to cohabit. Among older persons, Blacks are more likely to reside in cohabiting unions than Whites, but Hispanics do not differ from Whites (Chevan, 1996; Hatch, 1995).

Economic resources.— Among younger persons (especially men), economic stability is associated with marriage versus cohabitation (Clarkberg, 1999; Oppenheimer, 2003; Smock, Manning, & Porter, 2005; Xie, Raymo, Goyette, & Thornton, 2003). Cohabitation is particularly common among those with lower levels of education, although its popularity has increased among individuals of all educational strata. Among older persons, the association between education and cohabitation is unclear. Hatch (1995) documents a negative relationship between education and cohabitation, but Chevan (1996) finds no significant association. In the present study, we tested whether education was negatively related to cohabitation among older adults, as it is for younger adults. Chevan's analysis of cohabitation among older unmarried adults shows that poverty is positively related to cohabitation. Nonetheless, he also finds that labor force participation is positively associated with cohabitation among men, perhaps because it serves as a proxy for health and social integration. Or, economically active men may be more attractive partners. In contrast, Hatch's analysis of 1980 Census data indicates that cohabiting older men are less likely to be working and earn smaller incomes than either married or single older men. Women exhibit a distinct pattern; cohabitors have higher levels of employment than marrieds or singles. Older cohabiting women report higher earnings than single women but lower earnings than married women. Additional economic factors associated with cohabitation among older adults include renting (vs owning) a home and receipt of entitlement income (Hatch, 1995).

Physical health.— Despite being younger, on average, than marrieds, cohabitors report poorer physical health (Brown et al., 2005). Relative to marriage, cohabitation may be selective of individuals in worse health. Those in poor health may be less attractive as potential spouses, leaving these less healthy individuals at risk of a cohabiting union, which typically requires a weaker commitment from a partner. Among older men, poor health is positively related to cohabitation versus being single (Hatch, 1995), perhaps because older men in ill health are seeking support. This finding is consistent with Talbott's (1998) assertion that older women are reluctant to assume the burden of caregiving that may follow from remarriage at older ages, particularly when men's traditional familial obligation of economic provision ends in old age. Existing studies of caregiving, even those focused on ethnic minorities among whom cohabitation is more common, essentially ignore cohabitation (e.g., Pinquart & Sorenson, 2005).

Social relationships.— There are competing hypotheses regarding the association between social relationships and cohabitation among older adults (Hatch, 1995; Talbott, 1998). The compensatory hypothesis suggests that those individuals who do not receive adequate support from friends and family members will be especially motivated to form a union to achieve support through an intimate partner. Alternatively, the complementary hypothesis states that those individuals who enjoy the highest levels of social interaction with friends and family will be most interested in—and effective at—forming an intimate partnership, which these individuals view as offering unique, non-overlapping forms of support. Widows with close friends are more interested than those without close friends in forming a new partnership, supporting the complementary approach to social relationships (Talbott, 1998). Additional support for this hypothesis comes from a study of dating among older unmarrieds that documents a positive relationship between organizational participation and dating (Bulcroft & Bulcroft, 1991). To the extent that social relationships enhance individual well-being and promote social integration, we expected that they would be positively associated with cohabitation. Religious commitment and affliiation are negatively associated with cohabitation not only because some religions frown upon living together outside of formal marriage, but also because religious persons tend to espouse more traditional, conservative family attitudes that are disapproving of cohabitation (Clarkberg, Stolzenberg, & Waite, 1995; Thornton, Axinn, & Hill, 1992). One study of repartnering among older adults conceptualized the absence of religious af-

filiation as an indicator of individualism, which was positively associated with forming a cohabiting union (De Jong Gierveld, 2004). Older adults' relationships with their children may influence their own relationship trajectories. Close relationships with children may weaken an older adult's interest in forming a cohabiting (or marital) union. Or, children may pressure parents to avoid the legal complexities that would accompany remarriage and may suggest cohabitation as an alternative (Bulcroft & Bulcroft, 1991; Chevan, 1996; Hatch, 1995). Indeed, Hatch contends that children actively discourage their widowed mothers from remarrying, and De Jong Gierveld posits that the parent-child relationship weakens following repartnering. Widowed older women with children are less likely than their childless counterparts to remarry, but children are not associated with older men's remarriage patterns (Wu, 1995).

In summary, we expect cohabitors, remarrieds, and those who were previously married but are now unpartnered (i.e., the divorced and widowed) to differ in terms of demographic characteristics, economic resources, physical health, and social relationships. Additionally, these union status differences are likely to be distinct for men and women. We extend prior work on remarriage following divorce or widowhood by including cohabitation as a competing risk.

Methods

We used two sources of data. Initially, we drew on the Census 2000 Public-Use Microdata Samples 5% sample to document the prevalence of cohabitation among older adults by age and union status. This basic census information provided a point of comparison for our findings from the main source of data we employed: the 1998 Health and Retirement Study (HRS; Health and Retirement Study, 1998). Designed to examine health and retirement decision making as well as how older adults and their families respond to declining health in later life, the HRS is a nationally representative sample comprising 21,384 noninstitutionalized persons born in 1947 and earlier. Thus, at the time of the 1998 interview, respondents were as young as 51 years old.

Of the 21,384 HRS respondents, 33 were eliminated from our sample because we were unable to determine their current marital status. Another 21 respondents were eliminated because they reported being in same-sex partnerships (although substantively of interest, the small number of cases prohibits meaningful analysis of this group). Finally, an additional 681 respondents were excluded because they did not have a sample weight (typically because they were institutionalized). We also limited our sample to individuals aged 51 and older, which resulted in the loss of an additional 922 respondents (i.e., younger spouses or partners of primary respondents), for a final sample size of 19,727.

Measures

Union status.— HRS respondents reported their union status at the time of interview. Approximately 2.2% of the sample was cohabiting, yielding 437 cohabitors for analysis. About 48.7% of the respondents (*n = 9,617*) were in first marriages, 19.8% (*n = 3,899*) were widowed, 16.5% (n = 3,255) were in remarriages, 9.9% (n = 1,948) were separated or divorced, and the remaining 2.9% (n = 571) had never married.

Demographic characteristics.— Gender was a dichotomous variable (1 = women). Race/ethnicity was composed of four dummy variables: non-Hispanic White (reference), nonHispanic Black, Hispanic, and non-Hispanic other race. Age was coded in years. Previously widowed (a dummy variable coded 1 for those whose marriage ended through death of the spouse and 0 for those whose marriage ended in divorce) was controlled for in the analyses that were restricted to the previously married.

Economic resources.— Several indicators of respondents' economic resources were included. Education was coded in years, ranging from 0 (no formal education) to 17 (post-college; i.e., more than 17 years of education). Household income was a constructed measure in the HRS data set that incorporated bracketed income responses using sophisticated imputation techniques. It was logged to minimize the effects of skewness. A dichotomous measure indicated whether the respondent owned his/her home (1 = yes). Employment status was dummy coded full-time employment (reference), part-time employment, unemployed, and not working. Retirement status indicated whether the respondent was retired (1 = yes). This measure was distinct from the employment status variable because some respondents were technically retired but working in a different job. We also included measures to tap receipt of Social Security and a pension (1 = yes). Health insurance coverage is gauged by four mutually exclusive dummy variables: private insurance (reference), Medicare, other insurance (e.g., Medicaid), and no insurance.

Physical health.— The activity of daily living (ADL) measure is a scale composed of the responses to 11 items asking the respondent whether, because of health problems, he or she has any difficulty with various ADLs (e.g., walking several blocks, sitting for about two hours, picking up a dime from a table). For each question, answers of *yes* are coded 1 and answers of *no* are coded 0. Responses are then added together to form the scale. Alcohol measured whether and how much the respondent drank. Those who indicated that they did not drink or have never drunk alcohol (more than 50% of the sample) were coded 1; those who responded that they drank alcohol but less than once a week were coded 2; those who responded that they drank alcohol at least once a week but not daily were coded 3; and those who reported drinking alcohol every day were coded 4.

Social relationships.— Social relationships were gauged by several measures. Neighborhood friends was coded 1 if the respondent reported having good friends living in the neighborhood and 0 otherwise. Relatives in the neighborhood was coded 1 if the respondent reported at least one relative residing in their neighborhood and 0 otherwise. (The term *neighborhood* is not explicitly defined by the HRS.) Religiosity is a measure of the reported significance of religion in the respondent's life, ranging from 1 = not too important to 3 = very important. Children is coded 1 if the respondent reported having at least one living biological child and 0 otherwise.

Analytic Strategy

We began by establishing the size and marital status distribution of the older adult cohabiting population using the Census 2000 data. These data provide a benchmark against which to compare the figures we obtained from the 1998 HRS. Next, we employed the HRS to compare older adults across six union statuses in terms of several sets of characteristics that are related to union status, including demographic characteristics, economic resources, physical health, and social relationships. Because roughly 90% of HRS cohabitors were previously married (i.e., had been divorced or widowed), the most appropriate comparison group for ascertaining the significance of union type was not individuals in marriages but rather those in remarriages. Previously published literature (e.g., Bulcroft et al., 1989; Burch 1990; Talbott 1998) has examined middle-aged and older adults' decisions to remarry following divorce or the death of a spouse, and we extended this line of inquiry by treating cohabitation and remarriage as competing risks. Thus, our final set of analyses was restricted to those who were previously married. Detailed comparisons by union type (i.e., cohabitation vs remarriage) were examined separately for women and men. We estimated multinomial logistic regression models of the competing risks of being in either a cohabiting union or remarriage (vs being unpartnered; i.e., being divorced or widowed) separately for women and men. Our objective is to describe the population of older cohabitors, so we are less concerned about causal order here; the set of independent variables likely includes both antecedents and consequences of union type. This analysis shows most clearly how older, previously married persons who cohabit differ from those who are remarried or unpartnered. These are critical comparisons because it is unclear whether cohabitation is better conceptualized as an alternative to marriage or to remaining unpartnered among older persons who have experienced divorce or widowhood. The complex sample design of the HRS means that the sample is not self-weighting. Thus, standard errors need to be adjusted to correct for design effects. Both descriptive and multivariate analyses were conducted in Stata (StataCorp LP, College Station, TX) using the survey procedure to correct for the complex sample design.

Results

According to Census 2000 data, 1,088,428 persons aged 51 and older are currently cohabiting (< 2% of this age group; see Table 1). Age is negatively associated with cohabitation; most of these cohabitors (n = 676,782) are between the ages of 51 and 59. Among those who are at risk of cohabiting (i.e., the unmarried), 4% are involved in cohabiting relationships. For unmarrieds aged 51–59, the number of cohabitors is nearly 9%. A majority of older cohabitors are divorced or separated (71 %), followed by widowed (18%), and never married (11%).

HRS data show slightly higher percentages of older adults cohabiting. Among respondents aged 51 and older, 2% (n = 437) are currently cohabiting. As in the census data, younger persons are more likely to cohabit. Among the unmarried,

Table 1 Older Cohabitors by Age and Marital Status

Population	2000 Census N	%	1998 HRS N	%
Total population				
≥ 51	1,088,428	1.49	437	1.97
51–59	676,782	2.50	193	3.00
60–69	273,514	1.36	169	2.20
≥ 70	138,132	0.54	75	0.81
Unmarried population				
≥ 51	1,088,428	4.05	437	5.29
51–59	676,782	8.54	193	9.87
60–69	273,514	4.27	169	7.16
≥ 70	138,132	1.10	75	1.65
Marital status of cohabitors				
Separated or divorced	771,409	70.87	265	63.04
Widowed	201,144	18.48	108	22.88
Never married	115,875	10.65	51	11.66
Other (not determinable)	–	–	13	2.42

Notes: HRS = Health and Retirement Survey. All percentages are weighted, and HRS percentages are corrected for complex sampling design.

nearly 10% of those aged 51–59 are cohabiting; this decreases about 7% of those 60–69 and nearly 2% of those 70 and older. This is consistent with the prediction that the number of older cohabitors will increase via the process of cohort replacement. As is also shown by the census data, most HRS cohabitors are divorced or separated (63%), followed by widowed (23%), and never married (12%; these percentages do not equal 100% because marital status is indeterminable for 2% of the sample).

Table 2 shows the weighted means of the variables by union status. As anticipated, older adult cohabitors are less likely than first marrieds and remarrieds to be White and are more likely to be Black. Cohabitors are also younger, on average, than all other groups except the divorced. Although cohabitors have a greater likelihood of being employed full time, the household incomes of older cohabitors, first marrieds, and remarrieds do not differ significantly. Also, older cohabitors are less likely than either group of marrieds to own a house or to have health insurance. About 13% of cohabitors have no health insurance, and another 25% rely solely on Medicare. Although cohabitors, first marrieds, and remarrieds experience similar levels of ADLs (levels that are lower than those reported by divorced, widowed, and never marrieds), cohabitors report significantly higher average levels of alcohol consumption than any other group. In terms of social relationships, cohabitors do not fare especially well. They are least likely of any group to report having friends or relatives in the neighborhood (although they do not differ from the divorced in their reports of having friends or from remarrieds in their reports of relatives nearby). This suggests that cohabitors are more isolated socially. Cohabitors also report lower levels of religiosity than any other union status group. Not surpris-

ingly, although cohabitors are slightly less likely than both groups of married persons to have living children they are much more likely than the never married to have children. Taken together, cohabitors appear most similar to the divorced group, which is consistent with our decision to emphasize here comparisons among those who had been previously married.

The remaining analyses focus on cohabitors, remarrieds, and unpartnereds who are divorced or widowed. Table 3 compares these three groups separately by gender. Women are much more likely to be unpartnered (73%) than are men (41 %). Men are twice as likely as women to be cohabiting (6% vs 3%) or remarried (53% vs 24%). Among both women and men, cohabitors are more likely than remarrieds but less likely than unpartnereds to be previously widowed. Consistent with the pattern shown for the full sample, remarrieds are more likely than cohabitors to be White and older, regardless of gender. The race/ethnic composition of cohabitors and unpartnereds is similar, although the former are younger, on average, than the latter. Among women, remarrieds report higher household incomes, on average, than cohabitors, who in turn report higher incomes than unpartnereds. Among men, the household incomes of cohabitors and remarrieds do not differ, but cohabitors report higher incomes than unpartnereds. Remarried and unpartnered women are less likely than cohabiting women to be employed full time. Among men, employment patterns are similar for remarrieds and cohabitors, but unpartnereds are less likely than cohabitors to work full or part time. Cohabiting women are most likely to be without health insurance (16%), but there are no union status differences among men. Women report more ADLs than men, and unpartnereds report the highest levels of ADLs. Alcohol consumption is higher among men than women; it is also higher among cohabitors than any other group. Cohabitors tend to score lower than either remarrieds or unpartnereds on the measures of social relationships, although reports of children are uniformly high across union status and gender. Among cohabitors, women have higher levels of religiosity than men, on average.

Table 4 shows the multinomial logistic regression models predicting cohabitation versus remarriage among those who have been previously married, estimated separately for women and men. The reference category for these comparisons is the unpartnered (i.e., the widowed and divorced). The patterns of association between demographic characteristics and cohabitation versus remarriage are similar for men and women. Those who were widowed are less likely than those who were divorced to be cohabiting or remarried. Older Blacks are less likely than Whites to be remarried, but the probability of being in a cohabiting union is not associated with race/ethnicity. Age is negatively related to both cohabiting and being remarried.

In contrast, economic resources appear to be related quite differently to women's and men's union type. Education is negatively associated with both cohabitation and remarriage among women, but it is not significantly related to union type among men. Cohabiting and remarried women, but not men, are more likely than the unpartnered to be unemployed. Among women, part-time employment and not working are more common among the remarried,

Table 2 Weighted Means by Union Status

Variable	Cohabiting	First Married	Remarried	Divorced or Separated	Widowed	Never Married	Total
Demographic characteristics							
Female	0.47	0.48	0.44	0.61***	0.82***	0.56**	0.56
White	0.75	0.86***	0.88***	0.71	0.81	0.73	0.83
Black	0.14	0.06***	0.06***	0.17	0.12	0.17	0.09
Hispanic	0.09	0.06	0.04***	0.09	0.05*	0.07	0.06
Other Race	0.02	0.02	0.02	0.03	0.02	0.03	0.02
Age	60.96	64.43***	62.26***	61.40	74.93***	62.26***	65.87
Economic resources							
Education	12.23	12.56	12.61	12.25	11.16***	12.34	12.24
Household income	56,083.04	66,298.12	68,042.83	34,419.38***	21,781.00***	29,976.17***	52,506.86
Own home	0.62	0.83***	0.79***	0.50***	0.61	0.48***	0.72
Employed full-time	0.38	0.29***	0.34	0.39	0.07***	0.29**	0.27
Employed part-time	0.11	0.12	0.12	0.13	0.08	0.12	0.11
Unemployed	0.03	0.01***	0.01**	0.02	0.00**	0.02	0.01
Not working	0.48	0.59***	0.53	0.46	0.84***	0.57*	0.61
Retired	0.36	0.43*	0.41*	0.33	0.63***	0.43*	0.45
Social Security receipt	0.49	0.57	0.56	0.38*	0.86***	0.48	0.60
Pension	0.26	0.40***	0.36**	0.19	0.40***	0.25	0.36
Private health insurance	0.55	0.67***	0.68***	0.55	0.33***	0.49*	0.58
Medicare	0.25	0.28	0.25	0.28	0.61***	0.34**	0.34
Other health insurance	0.07	0.02***	0.03***	0.07	0.02**	0.07	0.03
No health insurance	0.13	0.04***	0.05***	0.10	0.03***	0.10	0.05
Health							
ADL	2.51	2.26	2.45	2.86*	3.86***	2.93*	2.71
Alcohol consumption	2.25	1.96***	2.04*	1.91***	1.61***	1.90***	1.90
Social relationships							
Friends in neighborhood	0.52	0.69***	0.64**	0.59	0.73***	0.65*	0.67
Relatives in neighborhood	0.20	0.31***	0.25	0.26*	0.33***	0.33***	0.29
Religiosity	2.21	2.51***	2.41***	2.42***	2.62***	2.47***	2.50
Children	0.92	0.95*	0.96***	0.90	0.91	0.17***	0.91
N	437	9,617	3,225	1,948	3,899	571	19,727

Notes: Means are weighted using the HRS person-level weight, and standard errors are corrected for the complex sampling design. T Tests for significant differences from cohabitors: * $p < 0.05$; **$p < 0.01$; ***$p < 0.001$.

whereas being retired is negatively associated with remarriage. None of these factors is associated with cohabitation among women, nor are they related to men's union type. Women without health insurance are more likely to be cohabiting, whereas, among men, the absence of health insurance is unrelated to union type. Alcohol consumption is positively related to cohabitation among women, but it is not associated with men's union status. Neither the presence of friends nor of relatives in the neighborhood is associated with cohabitation or remarriage. Among women, religiosity is negatively associated with cohabitation, whereas among men, it is positively related to remarriage. The presence of children is positively associated with cohabitation and remarriage among men and with remarriage among women.

Discussion

The prevalence of cohabitation has grown dramatically in recent decades, and this growth has been evident across all age groups (Bumpass & Lu, 2000; Chevan, 1996). Nonetheless, the cohabitation experiences of older adults have been largely overlooked (Cooney & Dunne, 2001). Combining data from Census 2000 and the 1998 HRS, we constructed a national portrait of older adult cohabitors that reveals both the characteristics of this group and how this group compares with older adults in other union statuses.

The data reported here suggest that, in terms of social and demographic characteristics, older cohabitors and remarried persons differ in many of the same ways that younger cohabitors and married persons do. Blacks are less likely to be married.

Table 3 Weighted Means by Union Status and Gender Among the Previously Married

	Women			Men		
Variable	Cohabiting	Remarried	Unpartnered	Cohabiting	Remarried	Unpartnered
Demographic characteristics						
Previously widowed	0.31	0.14†††	0.69†††	0.23	0.10***†††	0.43***†††
White	0.80	0.89††	0.78	0.76	0.87†††	0.76
Black	0.11	0.07†	0.14	0.13	0.06†††	0.15
Hispanic	0.09	0.03††	0.06	0.07	0.05**	0.07
Other race	0.00	0.02	0.02	0.04	0.02	0.02
Age	60.34	62.39††	70.75†††	62.25*	63.95***†	67.14***†††
Economic resources						
Education	11.94	12.44	11.53	12.59	12.74***	11.68††
Household income	42,020.53	61,655.08†††	22,090.85†††	70,696.54*	73,116.19***	39,277.48***†
Own home	0.61	0.79†††	0.59	0.65	0.79††	0.51***††
Employed full-time	0.34	0.24††	0.16†††	0.40	0.41***	0.28***††
Empoyed part-time	0.16	0.15	0.11	0.06*	0.09***	0.08*
Unemployed	0.03	0.01†	0.01†††	0.03	0.01†	0.02*
Not working	0.48	0.59	0.72†††	0.51	0.49***	0.62***††
Retired	0.32	0.36	0.50†††	0.41	0.45***	0.55††
Social Security receipt	0.54	0.60	0.71†††	0.45	0.52***	0.57***†
Pension	0.24	0.38†††	0.32	0.26	0.34**	0.32
Private health insurance	0.55	0.68††	0.39†††	0.55	0.67†††	0.48***
Medicare	0.24	0.24	0.52†††	0.28	0.26	0.40***†
Other health insurance	0.05	0.03	0.04	0.09	0.03†††	0.04†
No health insurance	0.16	0.05†††	0.05†††	0.08*	0.04	0.08***
Health						
ADL	3.17	2.93	3.78†	1.99**	2.07***	2.62***†
Alcohol consumption	2.11	1.87†	1.59†††	2.38	2.18***†	2.09***††
Social relationships						
Friends in neighborhood	0.54	0.65†	0.69†††	0.50	0.63†	0.65†
Relatives in neighborhood	0.20	0.26†	0.30†††	0.23	0.23*	0.31
Religiosity	2.38	2.56††	2.65†††	2.8	2.30***†††	2.27***††
Children	0.95	0.96	0.91	0.95	0.96	0.90††
N	175	1,506	4,473	198	1,749	1,374

Notes: All respondents in this analysis were previously married (i.e., divorced or widowed). Analyses were weighted and corrected for the complex sampling design.
Significant differences between sexes within union status: $^{*}p < .05$; $^{**}p < .01$; $^{***}p < .001$.
Significant differences from cohabiting within sex: $^{\dagger}p < .05$; $^{\dagger\dagger}p < .01$; $^{\dagger\dagger\dagger}p < .001$.

Cohabitors (particularly women) have lower incomes and are less likely to own their homes than are remarried persons. They are also more likely than remarried to use alcohol. Finally, they score lower than older remarrieds on most of the measures of social relationships used in this study, including religiosity and having friends and relatives who live nearby.

In some respects, cohabitors compare favorably to the unpartnered. Cohabitors' household incomes are higher, and they are more likely to be employed full time and to have private health insurance than are the unpartnered. On the other hand,

cohabitors (especially women) are more likely than the unpartnered to have no health insurance at all. Cohabitors also score lower than the unpartnered on all of the measures of social relationships used in this study, except having children.

The picture that emerges from these comparisons is one of fairly systematic disadvantage among older cohabitors, especially in comparison to their remarried counterparts. As is the case among younger persons (Clarkberg, 1999; Oppenheimer, 2003; Smock, 2000; Smock et al., 2005), cohabitation may be chosen by individuals whose economic circumstances make

Table 4 Multinomial Logistic Regression Predicting Union Status for Men and Women Among the Previously Married

| | Women | | | | | | Men | | | | | |
| | Cohabiting | | | Remarried | | | Cohabiting | | | Remarried | | |
Variable	b	OR	SE	b	OR	SE	b	OR	SE	b	OR	SE
Demographic characteristics												
Previously widowed	−0.931***	0.39	0.18	−2.706***	0.07	0.14	−0.648*	0.52	0.27	−2.297***	0.10	0.14
Black	−0.186	0.83	0.28	−0.896***	0.41	0.16	0.036	1.04	0.24	−1.012***	0.36	0.15
Hispanic	−0.098	0.91	0.40	−1.025***	0.36	0.21	0.244	1.28	0.28	−0.235	0.79	0.23
Age	−0.118***	0.89	0.01	−0.072***	0.93	0.01	−0.045**	0.96	0.02	−0.017*	0.98	0.01
Economic resources												
Education	−0.125**	0.88	0.04	−0.121***	0.89	0.03	−0.004	1.00	0.03	−0.018	0.98	0.02
Household income (logged)	0.609*	1.84	0.23	0.977***	2.66	0.22	0.213**	1.24	0.10	0.394**	1.48	0.14
Own home	−0.014	0.99	0.19	0.782***	2.19	0.10	0.598	1.82	0.21	1.261***	3.53	0.10
Employed part-time	0.031	1.03	0.26	0.442*	1.56	0.17	−0.515	0.60	0.41	−0.201	0.82	0.24
Unemployed	1.005*	2.73	0.49	1.491**	4.44	0.46	0.455	1.58	0.79	−0.202	0.82	0.61
Not working	0.368	1.45	0.33	1.647***	5.19	0.19	0.341	1.41	0.37	−0.307	0.74	0.23
Retired	0.170	1.19	0.29	−0.532***	0.59	0.12	−0.338	0.71	0.35	0.148	1.16	0.27
Social Security receipt	1.413***	4.11	0.31	1.394***	4.03	0.18	0.717*	2.05	0.35	1.188***	3.28	0.18
Pension	−0.235	0.79	0.24	0.111	1.12	0.12	−0.030	0.97	0.24	0.068	1.07	0.12
Medicare	−0.179	0.84	0.31	−0.471***	0.62	0.13	0.192	1.21	0.24	−0.382**	0.68	0.14
Other health insurance	−0.082	0.92	0.43	−0.418	0.66	0.28	1.310***	3.71	0.36	−0.064	0.94	0.35
No health insurance	0.844**	2.33	0.28	−0.036	0.96	0.19	0.093	1.10	0.37	−0.262	0.77	0.23
Health												
ADL	0.050	1.05	0.03	−0.005	1.00	0.02	−0.059	0.94	0.04	0.016	1.02	0.02
Alcohol consumption	0.364**	1.44	0.13	0.007	1.01	0.06	0.156	1.17	0.09	−0.035	0.97	0.04
Social relationships												
Friends in neighborhood	−0.333	0.72	0.20	0.053	1.05	0.10	−0.490	0.61	0.25	0.008	1.01	0.12
Relatives in neighborhood	−0.311	0.73	0.16	0.046	1.05	0.09	−0.179	0.84	0.22	−0.131	0.88	0.10
Religiosity	−0.326**	0.72	0.11	0.118	1.13	0.08	−0.267	0.77	0.14	0.262***	1.30	0.06
Children	0.431	1.54	0.45	0.809***	2.25	0.21	0.742*	2.10	0.30	0.871***	2.39	0.25
$F(44, 9)$	31.06***						23.98***					

Notes: All respondents in this analysis were previously married (i.e., divorced or widowed). The reference category was unpartnered. Analyses were corrected for the complex sampling design.
*$p < .05$; **$p < .01$; ***$p < .001$.

marriage more risky. This raises the question of whether cohabitation has similar consequences to remarriage for older persons. Studies show, for example, that older married persons (especially men) are more likely than unmarried persons to engage in healthy behaviors (Schone & Weinick, 1998); researchers do not know yet whether the same is true of cohabitors.

The disadvantage associated with cohabitation appears especially pronounced among women, who may derive fewer benefits than men do from cohabitation. Among men, cohabitors are more likely than unpartnereds to own a home; among women, cohabitors and unpartnereds do not differ in this respect. Among women, the proportion of cohabitors with no health insurance is 3 times larger than that of remarrieds and unpartnereds; among men, there are no significant union status differences in this respect. Although cohabiting and remarried men enjoy statistically similar high household incomes, cohabiting women report an average household income of roughly

two thirds that of remarried women. It is therefore not surprising that more cohabiting women than either remarried or unpartnered women are employed full time (among men, cohabitors and remarrieds are equally likely to work full time). Taken together, our findings indicate that union status may be more consequential for women than men. Simply put, there are fewer union status differences among men than among women. As researchers continue to explore the gendered consequences of remarriage, divorce, and widowhood, our results reveal the importance of incorporating cohabitation into this research, too.

There are still many unknowns about later life cohabitation. Cohabitation, of course, entails less commitment than remarriage. Does this lesser commitment allow cohabiting persons to "bailout" when their partners become infirm or disabled, and do they take advantage of this possibility? Do older cohabitors share their resources in the same ways that married couples do, or do they hoard their own because the union may be fragile? This is important because cohabitors tend to have fewer resources per capita than remarried persons. To the extent that cohabitation is an alternative to remaining unpartnered, it may be a key source of support for older persons. Similar to marrieds, cohabitors presumably enjoy access to a regular sex partner. To the extent that cohabitation is a substitute for remarriage among the divorced and widowed, it may make older adults' lives less secure and their support networks more vulnerable to disruption.

In order to fully ascertain the implications of cohabitation for policy and practice, researchers need answers to at least some of these questions. For some older persons, a cohabiting partner may be a critical resource, providing help in times of need, material support that alleviates the strains of poverty, and emotional support to assuage loneliness. Or the partner may disappear just when the need for support is greatest. Until researchers know more about what motivates older persons to cohabit, as well as the factors that predict entry into and exit from cohabitation, it is difficult to accurately assess the implications of cohabitation.

As the older adult population continues to grow, and especially as the baby boomers age into this group, it becomes increasingly important that researchers assess the ramifications of cohabitation among older adults. Baby boomers were the first generation to cohabit in significant numbers as young adults, and consequently society can anticipate an increase in older adult cohabitation as the boomers age into older adulthood. Unfortunately, baby boomers are not represented in the 1998 HRS, which is a sample of persons born in 1947 and earlier. Early boomers (those born in 1948–1953) will be folded into the 2004 panel of the HRS.

The present study indicates that cohabitation among older adults is more common than researchers realized and is likely to increase in the future. We are not alone in this prediction; others researchers have noted that a declining share of older adults will be married in the coming decades, and thus a larger share will be at risk for cohabitation (e.g., Allen et al., 2000; Cooney & Dunne, 2001; De Jong Gierveld, 2004). The determinants of the formation and dissolution of older adult cohabiting relationships await future research. In the meantime, the present analyses demonstrate that cohabitors are a distinct group, comparable neither to remarrieds nor to other unmarrieds. As described in this article, the ramifications of this emerging relationship form for the well-being of older adults are not entirely clear. Moreover, because we were not able to ascertain whether older adult cohabitors weighed the decision to cohabit against remaining unpartnered or getting remarried, we compared cohabitors to both of these groups. Whether cohabitation typically operates as an alternative to singlehood or as a substitute for marriage is not readily apparent, because cohabitors—especially women—are unlike those in other union statuses across several key dimensions, including several indicators of economic resources and social relationships. For this reason, future gerontological research would benefit from expanding the formulation of marital status to include cohabitation so that researchers can begin to uncover the implications of cohabitation for the health and well-being of older adults.

Acknowledgments

The research for this paper was supported by Grant R03-AG024512 from the National Institute on Aging and by Bowling Green State University's Center for Family and Demographic Research, which has core funding from Grant R21-HD042831 from the National Institute for Child Health and Human Development. The Health and Retirement Study is conducted by the University of Michigan and is sponsored by the Grant U01AG09740 from the National Institute on Aging. We thank Kelly Balistreri for her help with the Census 2000 data and I-Fen Lin for her comments on an earlier version of the manuscript.

Address correspondence to Dr. Susan L. Brown, Department of Sociology and Center for Family and Demographic Research, Bowling Green State University, Bowling Green, OH 43403. Email: brownsl@ bgnet.bgsu.edu

References

Allen, K. R., Blieszner, R., & Roberto, K. A. (2000). Families in the middle and later years: A review and critique of research in the 1990s. *Journal of Marriage and the Family, 62,* 911–926.

Angel, J. L., Angel, R. J., McClellan, J. L., & Markides, K. S. (1996). Nativity, declining health, and preferences in living arrangements among elderly Mexican Americans: Implications for long-term care. *The Gerontologist, 36,* 464–473.

Brown, S. L., Bulanda, J. R., & Lee, G. R. (2005). The significance of nonmarital cohabitation: Marital status and mental health benefits among middle-aged and older adults. *Journal of Gerontology: Social Sciences, 60B,* S21–S29.

Bulcroft, K. A., Bulcroft, R. A., Hatch, L, & Borgatta, E. F. (1989). Antecedents and consequences of remarriage in later life. *Research on Aging, 11,* 82–106.

Bulcroft, R. A., & Bulcroft, K. A. (1991). The nature and functions of dating in later life. *Research on Aging, 13,* 244–260.

Bumpass, L. L., & Lu, H. (2000). Trends in cohabitation and implications for children's family contexts in the United States. *Population Studies, 54,* 29–41.

Burch, T. K. (1990). Remarriage of older Canadians. *Research on Aging, 12,* 546–559.

Casper, L. M., & Cohen, P. N. (2000). How does POSSLQ measure up? Historical estimates of cohabitation. *Demography, 37,* 237–245.

Chevan, A. (1996). As cheaply as one: Cohabitation in the older population. *Journal of Marriage and the Family, 58,* 656–667.

Clarkberg, M. (1999). The price of partnering: The role of economic well being in young adults' first union experiences. *Social Forces, 77,* 945–968.

Clarkberg, M., Stolzenberg, R. M., & Waite, L J. (1995). Attitudes, values, and entrance into cohabitational versus marital unions. *Social Forces, 74,* 609–632.

Cooney, T. M., & Dunne, K. (2001). Intimate relationships in later life: Current realities, future prospects. *Journal of Family Issues, 22,* 838–858.

De Jong Gierveld, J. (2004). Remarriage, unmarried cohabitation, living apart together: Partner relationships following bereavement or divorce. *Journal of Marriage and the Family, 66,* 236–243.

Hatch, R. G. (1995). *Aging and cohabitation.* New York: Garland. *Health and Retirement Study:* 1998 [Public use dataset]. Ann Arbor: University of Michigan.

King, V., & Scott, M. E. (2005). A comparison of cohabiting relationships among older and younger adults. *Journal of Marriage and the Family, 67,* 271–285.

Oppenheimer, V. K. (2003). Cohabiting and marriage during young men's career-development process. *Demography, 40,* 127–149.

Pinquart, M., & Sorenson, S. (2005). Ethnic differences in stressors, resources, and psychological outcomes of family caregiving: A meta-analysis. *The Gerontologist, 45,* 90–106.

Raley, R. K. (1996). A shortage of marriageable men? A note on the role of cohabitation in black–white differences in marriage rates. *American Sociological Review, 61,* 973–983.

Schone, B. S., & Weinick, R. A. (1998). Health-related behaviors and the benefits of marriage for elderly persons. *The Gerontologist, 38,* 618–627.

Smock, P. J. (2000). Cohabitation in the United States: An appraisal of research themes, findings, and implications. *Annual Review of Sociology, 26,* 1–20.

Smock, P. J., Manning, W. D., & Porter, M. (2005). "Everything's there except money": How money shapes decisions to marry among cohabitors. *Journal of Marriage and the Family, 67,* 680–696.

Talbott, M. M. (1998). Older widows' attitudes towards men and remarriage. *Journal of Aging Studies, 12,* 429–449.

Thornton, A., Axinn, W. G., & Hill, D. (1992). Reciprocal effects of religiosity, cohabitation, and marriage. *American Journal of Sociology, 98,* 628–651.

Thornton, A., & Young-DeMarco, L. (2001). Four decades of trends in attitudes toward family issues in the United States: The 1960s through the 1990s. *Journal of Marriage and the Family, 63,* 1009–1037.

U.S. Census Bureau. (2001). Profiles of general demographic characteristics. In *Census of population and housing, United States.* Washington, DC: U.S. Census Bureau. Retrieved December 10, 2005, from www.census.gov/prod/cen2000/rmdex.html

U.S. Census Bureau. (2002). *Statistical abstract of the United States.* http://www.census.gov/prod/www/statistical-abstract.html

U.S. Census Bureau. (2003). *Statistical Abstract of the United States, Mini-Historical Statistics.* http://www.census.gov/statab/www/minihis.html

Wherry, L., & Finegold, K. (2004). Marriage promotion and the living arrangements of black, Hispanic, and white children. In *New federalism: National survey of America's families* (publication No. B-61). Washington, DC: The Urban Institute.

Wilmoth, J. M. (1998). Living arrangement transitions among America's older adults. *The Gerontologist, 38,* 434–444.

Wilmoth, J. M. (2001). Living arrangements among older immigrants in the United States. *The Gerontologist, 41,* 228–238.

Wu, Z. (1995). Remarriage after widowhood: A marital history study of older Canadians. *Canadian Journal of Aging, 14,* 719–736.

Xie, Y., Raymo, J. M., Goyette, K., & Thornton, A. (2003). Economic potential and entry into marriage and cohabitation. *Demography, 40,* 351–367.

A Practical Guide To Better Health

We Can Control How We Age

What does it take to age successfully—to maintain both a sound body and mind? A landmark Harvard study has followed individuals from their teens into their 80s. It arrives at some optimistic conclusions:

LOU ANN WALKER

How do some people age so successfully? Many of us assume it takes genes or dumb luck. So here's the surprise. Arguably the longest and most comprehensive study of human development ever undertaken is just revealing its final results: *We are very much in control of our own aging.* The secret to a long and happy life, it seems, does not lie as much in our stars as in ourselves.

The Study of Adult Development at Harvard Medical School comprises three projects begun in the 1920s, '30s, and '40s. These careful scientific studies analyze three very different demographic groups: one of Harvard men (the Grant Study), another of inner-city Boston men and the third of gifted California women. In all, 824 men and women have been followed from their teens into their 80s. Over the decades, these people were given psychological tests and asked to evaluate their lives and feelings. They responded to numerous questionnaires, interviews by psychiatrists and physical examinations by doctors.

The study is a medical rarity because it examines the lives of the well, not the sick. "Old age is like a minefield," the study's director, Dr. George E. Vaillant, told PARADE. "If you see footprints leading to the other side, step in them." These results show a clear path that Baby Boomers and Gen X-ers can follow to lead a long, happy life.

The study divides individuals between 60 and 80 years old into two main groups: (1) the "Happy-Well," those who are physically healthy and find life satisfying; and (2) the "Sad-Sick," those with various ailments who do not seem to enjoy life. And it analyzes those who died during the course of the study (the "Prematurely Dead").

Living with a Full Heart

The Harvard study found these four attributes vital to successful aging:

- ORIENTATION TOWARD THE FUTURE. The ability to anticipate, to plan and to hope.
- GRATITUDE, FORGIVENESS AND OPTIMISM. We need to see the glass as half-full, not half-empty.
- EMPATHY. The ability to imagine the world as it seems to the other person.
- THE ABILITY TO REACH OUT. "We should want to do things *with* people, not do things *to* people or ruminate that they do things to us," says Dr. George E. Vaillant. In other words, we need to "leave the screen door unlatched."

It's *not* in our genes...

A major finding was that good genes did not account for better aging. Nor did income. Good care obviously is important, said Dr. Vaillant, "but the trick is not going to the hospital in the first place."

The study disputes the assumption that with aging comes decay. When 30- and 55-year-old brains are compared, the older one is better developed. Advancing age impairs some motor skills, but maturation can make people sharper at emotional tasks.

Seven Keys To Aging Well
What are the secrets to a long, happy life? Dr. George E. Vaillant points out seven major factors that, at 50, predict what life's outcome will be at 80:

1 NOT SMOKING OR QUITTING EARLY: Those who quit the habit before 50 were, at 70, as healthy as those who had never smoked. And heavy smoking was 10 times more prevalent among the Prematurely Dead than among the Happy-Well. "Smoking," said Vaillant, "is probably the most significant factor in terms of health."

Coping With Life's Stresses
Those who learn early how to roll with the punches are much happier in their later years, despite real problems.

2 THE ABILITY TO TAKE LIFE'S UPS AND DOWNS IN STRIDE: If you can make lemonade out of lemons, then you have an adaptive coping style, also known as "mature defenses." Mature defenses don't actually ensure good health at an older age. But a person will suffer less from life's real problems if he or she has the ability to roll with the punches. "Life ain't easy," Vaillant said. "Terrible things happen to everyone. You have to keep your sense of humor, give something of yourself to others, make friends who are younger than you, learn new things and have fun."

An Active Lifestyle
The long-term results of regular exercise are both physical and psychological well-being.

3 ABSENCE OF ALCOHOL ABUSE: "Abusing alcohol destroys both your physical and mental health," Vaillant noted. (He added that a partner's alcoholism can destroy a marriage, which also may have an impact on how one ages.)

4 HEALTHY WEIGHT: Obesity is a risk factor for poor health in later life.

A Strong Marriage
A good marriage contributes to a long and happy life. The study also found that, overall, marriages improved with time—if people were willing to work out the bumps.

5 A SOLID MARRIAGE: This is important for both physical and psychological health. Happy-Well people were six times more likely to be in good marriages than were the Sad-Sick.

6 PHYSICAL ACTIVITY: The study specified that the Happy-Well usually did "some exercise." The benefits of fitness also extended to mental health.

Continuing Education
The more years of school people have, the more they tend to age successfully.

7 YEARS OF EDUCATION: Vaillant speculated that people to whom "self-care and perseverance" are important are also more likely to continue their educations. These individuals, he surmised, are able to take the long view. "People seek education because they believe it is possible to control the course of their lives," he said. In the study, people with less education also were more likely to be obese. Their physical health at age 65 was close to that of the more-educated group at 75.

People who had four or more of these seven factors at age 50 were one-third less likely to be dead by 80. People who had three or fewer of these factors at 50—even though they were in good physical shape—were three times as likely to die during the following 30 years.

...but in ourselves.

Many of the study's findings focus on psychological health. As we age, we should try to develop more mature coping styles, Vaillant concluded from the results. "Our defenses are always more mature when we are not hungry, angry, lonely, tired or drunk," he noted.

"Taking people inside oneself" emotionally is important, he said, adding, "Popular people can be extraordinarily lonely and depressed. The paradox is that they starve, yet there's plenty of food." He pointed to the example of Marilyn Monroe, who made Arthur Miller and others feel cared for yet was unable to feel that love within herself.

Although developmental psychologists often say that personality is formed by age 5, the study found otherwise. By 70, it's how we nurture ourselves throughout our lifetimes that takes precedence over nature. Interestingly, Vaillant discovered that many people who aged well unconsciously reinterpreted early events in their lives in a more positive light as they grew older. Those who clung to negative events were less happy adults. Forever blaming parents for a rotten childhood seems to impede maturity.

"What goes *right* in childhood predicts the future far better than what goes wrong," he noted. Especially important was a feeling of acceptance.

As one ages, remaining connected to life is crucial—as is learning the rules of a changing world. On the other hand, Vaillant said, "One task of living out the last half of life is excavating and recovering those whom we loved in the first half. The recovery of lost loves becomes an important way in which the past affects the present."

The study's results will be published by Little, Brown in January in a book titled *Aging Well: Surprising Guideposts to a Happier Life from the Landmark Harvard Study of Adult De-*velopment. In addition to facts and figures, the book is filled with life stories of the men and women studied.

Vaillant, who has been called "a big, handsome, humorous psychiatrist," looks a decade younger than his 67 years. He and his wife of 30 years, Caroline, live in Vermont. In addition to his research, he maintains a small clinical practice at Boston's Brigham and Women's Hospital. He calls himself an "oppositional character" who loves "proving other people wrong."

I asked Vaillant what he hopes the results of this study will accomplish. "A heightened appreciation of the positive," he shot back. Then he added: "Worry less about cholesterol and more about gratitude and forgiveness."

UNIT 3

Societal Attitudes Toward Old Age

Unit Selections

Key Points to Consider

- What are the prevalent images Americans have of older people?

- Why do most Americans fear getting old?

- What are the basic arguments made by Erdman Palmore against the widespread negative views of older Americans?

- Were single women found to be lonely, shy, unhappy, and insecure?

- As the work force ages, what changes in employer attitudes toward older workers will have to take place in order for business to keep and maintain the critical skills of these workers?

Student Website

www.mhcls.com/online

Internet References

Further information regarding these websites may be found in this book's preface or online.

Adult Development and Aging: Division 20 of the American Psychological Association
http://www.iog.wayne.edu/APADIV20/APADIV20.HTM

American Society on Aging
http://www.asaging.org/index.cfm

Canadian Psychological Association
http://www.cpa.ca/

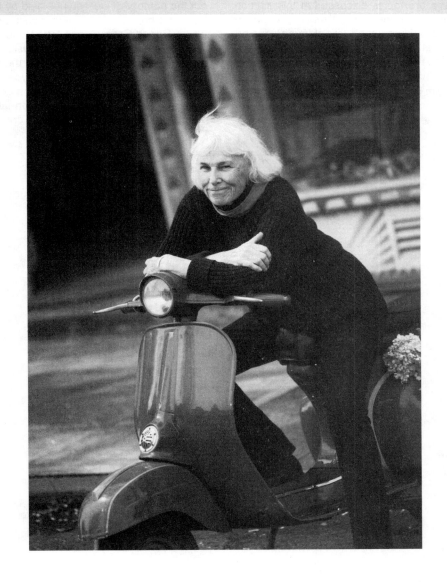

There is a wide range of beliefs regarding the social position and status of the aged in American society today. Some people believe that the best way to understand the problems of the elderly is to regard them as a minority group, faced with difficulties similar to those of other minority groups. Discrimination against older people, like racial discrimination, is believed to be based on a bias against visible physical traits. Since the aging process is viewed negatively, it is natural that the elderly try to appear and act younger. Some spend a tremendous amount of money trying to make themselves look and feel younger.

The theory that old people are a minority group is weak because too many circumstances prove otherwise. The U.S. Congress, for example, favors its senior members and delegates considerable prestige and power to them. The leadership roles in most religious organizations are held by older persons. Many older Americans are in good health, have comfortable incomes, and are treated with respect by friends and associates.

Perhaps the most realistic way to view the aged is as a status group, like other status groups in society. Every society has some method of "age grading," by which it groups together individuals of roughly similar age. ("Preteens" and "senior citizens" are some of the age-grade labels in American society.)

Because it is a labeling process, age grading causes members of the age group, as well as others, to perceive themselves in terms of the connotations of the label. Unfortunately, the tag "old age" often has negative connotations in American society.

The readings included in this section illustrate the wide range of stereotypical attitudes toward older Americans. Many of society's typical assumptions about the limitations of old age have been refuted. A major force behind this reassessment of the elderly is that there are so many people living longer and healthier lives and in consequence playing more of a role in all aspects of our society. Older people can remain productive members of society for many more years than has been traditionally assumed.

Such standard stereotypes of the elderly as frail, senile, childish, and sexually inactive are topics discussed in this section. Mary Pipher, in "Society Fears the Aging Process," contends that young people often avoid interacting with older persons because it reminds them that someday they will get old and die. She further argues that the media most often portrays a negative and stereotypical view of the elderly.

David Crary, in "Ageism in America," outlines the basic arguments made by Dr. Palmore, a retired professor from Duke, against the widespread negative stereotypes of older Americans. In "The Secret Lives of Single Women," the author points out the number of stereotypes held by the public of older single women. She then discusses the accuracy or inaccuracy of these views. Robert Grossman in "The Under-Reported Impact of Age Discrimination and Its Threat to Business Vitality," believes that the legal system is slanted toward the employers who perpetuate many of the negative stereotypes and views of the older workers. He sees age discrimination in the workplace as a more serious problem in the future, when labor shortages will make older workers and their skills more critical and more in demand.

Society Fears the Aging Process

Americans fear the processes of aging and dying, Mary Pipher contends in the following viewpoint. She claims that younger and healthier adults often avoid spending time around the aging because they want to avoid the issues of mortality and loss of independence. In addition, she contends that negative views of the aging process are portrayed in the media and expressed through the use of pejorative words to describe the elderly. Pipher is a psychologist and author of several books, including *Another Country: Navigating the Emotional Terrain of Our Elders,* the book from which this viewpoint was excerpted.

MARY PIPHER

We segregate the old for many reasons—prejudice, ignorance, a lack of good alternatives, and a youth-worshiping culture without guidelines on how to care for the old. The old are different from us, and that makes us nervous. Xenophobia means fear of people from another country. In America we are xenophobic toward our old people.

How Greeting Cards Reflect Culture

An anthropologist could learn about us by examining our greeting cards. As with all aspects of popular culture, greeting cards both mirror and shape our realities. Cards reflect what we feel about people in different roles, and they also teach us what to feel. I visited my favorite local drugstore and took a look.

There are really two sets of cards that relate to aging. One is the grandparent/grandchild set that is all about connection. Even a very dim-witted anthropologist would sense the love and respect that exist between these two generations in our culture. Young children's cards to their grandparents say, "I wish I could hop on your lap," or, "You're so much fun." Grandparents' cards to children are filled with pride and love.

There is another section of cards on birthdays. These compare human aging to wine aging, or point out compensations. "With age comes wisdom, of course that doesn't make up for what you lose." We joke the most about that which makes us anxious. "Have you picked out your bench at the mall yet?" There are jokes about hearing loss, incontinence, and losing sexual abilities and interest. There are cards on saggy behinds, gray hair, and wrinkles, and cards about preferring chocolate or sleep to sex. "You know you're getting old when someone asks if you're getting enough and you think about sleep."

Fears of Aging and Dying

Poking fun at aging isn't all bad. It's better to laugh than to cry, especially at what cannot be prevented. However, these jokes reflect our fears about aging in a youth-oriented culture. We younger, healthier people sometimes avoid the old to avoid our own fears of aging. If we aren't around dying people, we don't have to think about dying.

We baby boomers have been a futureless generation, raised in the eternal present of TV and advertising. We have allowed ourselves to be persuaded by ads that teach that if we take good care of ourselves, we will stay healthy. Sick people, hospitals, and funerals destroy our illusions of invulnerability. They force us to think of the future.

Carolyn Heilbrun said, "It is only past the meridian of fifty that one can believe that the universal sentence of death applies to oneself." Before that time, if we are healthy, we are likely to be in deep denial about death, to feel as if we have plenty of time, that we have an endless vista ahead. But in hospitals and at funerals, we remember that we all will die in the last act. And we don't necessarily appreciate being reminded.

When I first visited rest homes, I had to force myself to stay. What made me most upset was the thought of myself in a place like that. I didn't want to go there, literally or figuratively. Recently I sat in an eye doctor's office surrounded by old people with white canes. Being in this room gave me intimations of mortality. I thought of Bob Dylan's line: "It's not dark yet, but it's getting there."

We know the old-old will die soon. The more we care and the more involved we are with the old, the more pain we feel at their suffering. Death is easier to bear in the abstract, far away and clinical. It's much harder to watch someone we love fade before our eyes. It's hard to visit an uncle in a rest home and realize he no longer knows who we are or even who he is. It's hard to see a grandmother in pain or drugged up on morphine. Sometimes it's so hard that we stay away from the people who need us the most.

Our culture reinforces our individual fears. To call something old is to insult, as in *old hat* or *old ideas.* To call something young is to compliment, as in *young thinking* or *young acting.* It's considered rude even to ask an old person's age. When we meet an adult we haven't seen in a long time, we compliment her by saying, "You haven't aged at all." The taboos against acknowledging age tell us that aging is shameful.

Many of the people I interviewed were uncomfortable talking about age and were unhappy to be labeled old. They said, "I don't feel old." What they meant was, "I don't act and feel like the person who the stereotypes suggest I am." Also, they were trying to avoid being put in a socially undesirable class. In this country, it is unpleasant to be called old, just as it is unpleasant to be called fat or poor. The old naturally try to avoid being identified with an unappreciated group....

The Elderly Are Treated Poorly

Nothing in our culture guides us in a positive way toward the old. Our media, music, and advertising industries all glorify the young. Stereotypes suggest that older people keep younger people from fun, work, and excitement. They take time (valuable time) and patience (in very short supply in the 1990s). We are very body-oriented, and old bodies fail. We are appearance-oriented, and youthful attractiveness fades. We are not taught that old spirits often shimmer with beauty.

Language is a problem. Old people are referred to in pejorative terms, such as *biddy, codger,* or *geezer,* or with cutesy words, such as *oldster, chronologically challenged,* or *senior citizen.* People describe themselves as "eighty years young." Even *retirement* is an ugly word that implies passivity, uselessness, and withdrawal from the social and working world. Many of the old are offended by ageist stereotypes and jokes. Some internalize these beliefs and feel badly about themselves. They stay with their own kind in order to avoid the harsh appraisals of the young.

Some people do not have good manners with the old. I've seen the elderly bossed around, treated like children or simpletons, and simply ignored. Once in a cafe, I heard a woman order her mother to take a pill and saw the mother wince in embarrassment. My mother-in-law says she sees young people but they don't see her. Her age makes her invisible.

In our culture the old are held to an odd standard. They are admired for not being a bother, for being chronically cheerful. They are expected to be interested in others, bland in their opinions, optimistic, and emotionally generous. But the young certainly don't hold themselves to these standards.

Accidents that old drivers have are blamed on age. After a ninety-year-old friend had his first car accident, he was terrified that he would lose his license. "If I were young, this accident would be perceived as just one of those things," he pointed out. "But because I am old, it will be attributed to my age." Now, of course, some old people are bad drivers. But so are some young people. To say "He did that because he's old" is often as narrow as to say, "He did that because he's black" or "Japanese." Young people burn countertops with hot pans, forget appointments, and write overdrafts on their checking accounts. But when the old do these same things, they experience double jeopardy. Their mistakes are not viewed as accidents but rather as loss of functioning. Such mistakes have implications for their freedom.

Media Stereotypes

As in so many other areas, the media hurts rather than helps with our social misunderstandings. George Gerbner reported on the curious absence of media images of people older than sixty-five. Every once in a while a romantic movie plot might involve an older man, but almost never an older woman. In general, the old have been cast as silly, stubborn, and eccentric. He also found that on children's programs, older women bear a disproportionate burden of negative characteristics. In our culture, the old get lumped together into a few stereotyped images: the sweet old lady, the lecherous old man, or the irascible but soft-hearted grandfather. Almost no ads and billboards feature the old. Every now and then an ad will show a grandparent figure, but then the grandparent is invariably youthful and healthy.

In *Fountain of Age,* Betty Friedan noted that the old are portrayed as sexless, demented, incontinent, toothless, and childish. Old women are portrayed as sentimental, naive, and silly gossips, and as troublemakers. A common movie plot is the portrayal of the old trying to be young—showing them on motorbikes, talking hip or dirty, or liking rock and roll. Of course there are exceptions, such as *Nobody's Fool, On Golden Pond, Mr. and Mrs. Bridge, Driving Miss Daisy, Mrs. Brown,* and *Twilight.* But we need more movies in which old people are portrayed in all their diversity and complexity.

The media is only part of much larger cultural problems. We aren't organized to accommodate this developmental stage. For example, being old-old costs a lot of money. Assisted-living housing, medical care, and all the other services the old need are expensive. And yet, most old people can't earn money. It's true that some of our elders are wealthy, but many live on small incomes. Visiting the old, I heard tragic stories involving money. I met Arlene, who, while dying of cancer, had to fear losing her house because of high property taxes. I met Shirley, who lived on noodles and white rice so that she could buy food for her cat and small gifts for her grandchildren. I met people who had to choose between pills and food or heat.

The American Obsession with Independence

Another thing that makes old age a difficult stage to navigate is our American belief that adults need no one. We think of independence as the ideal state for adults. We associate independence with heroes and cultural icons such as the Marlboro man and the Virginia Slims woman, and we associate dependence with toxic families, enmeshment, and weakness. To our postmodern, educated ears, a psychologically healthy but dependent adult sounds oxymoronic.

We all learn when we are very young to make our own personal declarations of independence. In our culture, *adult* means "self-sufficient." Autonomy is our highest virtue. We want relationships that have no strings attached instead of understanding, as one lady told me, "Honey, life ain't nothing but strings."

These American ideas about independence hurt families with teens. Just when children most need guidance from parents, they turn away from them and toward peers and media.

They are socialized to believe that to be an adult, they must break away from parents. Our ideas about independence also hurt families with aging relatives. As people move from the young-old stage into the old-old stage, they need more help. Yet in our culture we provide almost no graceful ways for adults to ask for help. We make it almost impossible to be dependent yet dignified, respected, and in control.

As people age, they may need help with everything from their finances to their driving. They may need help getting out of bed, feeding themselves, and bathing. Many would rather pay strangers, do without help, or even die than be dependent on those they love. They don't want to be a burden, the greatest of American crimes. The old-old often feel ashamed of what is a natural stage of the life cycle. In fact, the greatest challenge for many elders is learning to accept vulnerability and to ask for help.

If we view life as a time line, we realize that all of us are sometimes more and sometimes less dependent on others. At certain stages we are caretakers, and at other stages we are cared for. Neither stage is superior to the other. Neither implies pathology or weakness. Both are just the results of life having seasons and circumstances. In fact, good mental health is not a matter of being dependent or independent, but of being able to accept the stage one is in with grace and dignity. It's an awareness of being, over the course of one's lifetime, continually interdependent.

Rethinking Dependency

In our culture the old fear their deaths will go badly, slowly, and painfully, and will cost lots of money. Nobody wants to die alone, yet nobody wants to put their families through too much stress. Families are uneasy as they negotiate this rocky terrain. The trick for the younger members is to help without feeling trapped and overwhelmed. The trick for older members is to accept help while preserving dignity and control. Caregivers can say, "You have nurtured us, why wouldn't we want to nurture you?" The old must learn to say, "I am grateful for your help and I am still a person worthy of respect."

As our times and circumstances change, we need new language. We need the elderly to become elders. We need a word for the neediness of the old-old, a word with less negative connotations than *dependency,* a word that connotes wisdom, connection, and dignity. *Dependency* could become mutuality or *interdependency.* We can say to the old: "You need us now, but we needed you and we will need our children. We need each other."

However, the issues are much larger than simply which words to use or social skills to employ. We need to completely rethink our ideas about caring for the elderly. Like the Lakota, we need to see it as an honor and an opportunity to learn. It is our chance to repay our parents for the love they gave us, and it is our last chance to become grown-ups. We help them to help ourselves.

We need to make the old understand that they can be helped without being infantilized, that the help comes from respect and gratitude rather than from pity or a sense of obligation. In our so-ciety of disposables and planned obsolescence, the old are phased out. Usually they fade away graciously. They want to be kind and strong, and, in America, they learn that to do so means they should ask little of others and not bother young people.

Perhaps we need to help them redefine kindness and courage. For the old, to be kind ought to mean welcoming younger relatives' help, and to be brave ought to mean accepting the dependency that old-old age will bring. We can reassure the old that by showing their children how to cope, they will teach them and their children how well this last stage can be managed. This information is not peripheral but rather something everyone will need to know.

Further Readings

Henry J. Aaron and Robert D. Reischauer. *Countdown to Reform: The Great Social Security Debate.* New York: Century Foundation Press, 2001.

Claude Amarnick. *Don't Put Me in a Nursing Home.* Deerfield Beach, FL: Garrett, 1996.

Dean Baker and Mark Weisbrot. *Social Security: The Phony Crisis.* Chicago: University of Chicago Press, 1999.

Margret M. Baltes. *The Many Faces of Dependency in Old Age.* Cambridge, England: Cambridge University Press, 1996.

Sam Beard. *Restoring Hope in America: The Social Security Solution.* San Francisco: Institute for Contemporary Studies, 1996.

Robert H. Binstock, Leighton E. Cluff, and Otto von Mering, eds. *The Future of Long-Term Care: Social and Policy Issues.* Baltimore: Johns Hopkins University Press, 1996.

Robert H. Binstock and Linda K. George, eds. *Handbook of Aging and the Social Sciences.* San Diego: Academic Press, 1996.

Jimmy Carter. *The Virtues of Aging.* New York: Ballantine, 1998.

Marshall N. Carter and William G. Shipman. *Promises to Keep: Saving Social Security's Dream.* Washington, DC: Regnery, 1996.

Martin Cetron and Owen Davies. *Cheating Death: The Promise and the Future Impact of Trying to Live Forever.* New York: St. Martin's Press, 1998.

William C. Cockerham. *This Aging Society.* Upper Saddle River, NJ: Prentice-Hall, 1997.

Peter A. Diamond, David C. Lindeman, and Howard Young, eds. *Social Security: What Role for the Future?* Washington, DC National Academy of Social Insurance, 1996.

Ursula Adler Falk and Gerhard Falk. *Ageism, the Aged and Aging in America: On Being Old in an Alienated Society.* Springfield, IL: Charles C. Thomas, 1997.

Peter J. Ferrara and Michael Tanner. *A New Deal for Social Security.* Washington, DC Cato Institute, 1998.

Arthur D. Fisk and Wendy A. Rogers, eds. *Handbook of Human Factors and the Older Adult.* San Diego: Academic Press, 1997.

Muriel R. Gillick. *Lifelines: Living Longer: Growing Frail, Taking Heart.* New York: W. W. Norton, 2000.

Margaret Morganroth Gullette. *Declining to Decline: Cultural Combat and the Politics of the Midlife.* Charlottesville: University Press of Virginia, 1997.

Charles B. Inlander and Michael A. Donio. *Medicare Made Easy.* Allentown, PA: People's Medical Society, 1999.

Donald H. Kausler and Barry C. Kausler. *The Graying of America: An Encyclopedia of Aging, Health, Mind, and Behavior.* Urbana: University of Illinois Press, 2001.

Eric R. Kingson and James H. Schulz, eds. *Social Security in the Twenty-First Century* New York: Oxford University Press, 1997.

Thelma J. Lofquist. *Frail Elders and the Wounded Caregiver.* Portland, OR: Binford and Mort, 2001.

Joseph L. Matthews. *Social Security, Medicare, and Pensions.* Berkeley, CA: Nolo, 1999.

E. J. Myers. *Let's Get Rid of Social Security: How Americans Can Take Charge of Their Own Future.* Amherst, NY: Prometheus Books, 1996.

Evelyn M. O'Reilly. *Decoding the Cultural Stereotypes About Aging: New Perspectives on Aging Talk and Aging Issues.* New York: Garland, 1997.

S. Jay Olshansky and Bruce A. Carnes. *The Quest for Immortality: Science at the Frontiers of Aging.* New York: W. W. Norton, 2001.

Fred C. Pampel. *Aging, Social Inequality, and Public Policy.* Thousand Oaks, CA: Pine Forge Press, 1998.

Peter G. Peterson. *Gray Dawn: How the Coming Age Wave Will Transform America—And the World.* New York: Times Books, 1999.

Peter G. Peterson. *Will America Grow Up Before It Grows Old?: How the Coming Social Security Crisis Threatens You, Your Family, and Your Country.* New York: Random House, 1996.

John W. Rowe and Robert L. Kahn. *Successful Aging.* New York: Pantheon Books, 1998.

Sylvester J. Schieber and John B. Shoven. *The Real Deal: The History and Future of Social Security.* New Haven, CT: Yale University Press, 1999.

Ken Skala. *American Guidance for Seniors—And Their Caregivers.* Falls Church, VA: K. Skala, 1996.

Max J. Skidmore. *Social Security and Its Enemies: The Case for America's Most Efficient Insurance Program.* Boulder, CO: Westview Press, 1999.

Richard D. Thau and Jay S. Heflin, eds. *Generations Apart: Xers vs. Boomers vs. the Elderly.* Amherst, NY: Prometheus Books, 1997.

Dale Van Atta. *Trust Betrayed: Inside the AARP.* Washington, DC: Regnery, 1998.

James W. Walters, ed. *Choosing Who's to Live: Ethics and Aging.* Urbana: University of Illinois Press, 1996.

David A. Wise, ed. *Facing the Age Wave.* Stanford, CA: Hoover Institutional Press, Stanford University, 1997.

Periodicals

W. Andrew Achenbaum. "Perceptions of Aging in America," *National Forum*, Spring 1998. Available from the Honor Society of Phi Kappa Phi, Box 16000, Louisiana State University, Baton Rouge, LA 70893.

America. "Keep an Eye on the Third Age," May 16, 1998.

Robert Butler. "The Longevity Revolution," *UNESCO Courier,* January 1999.

Issues and Controversies on File. "Age Discrimination," May 21, 1999. Available from Facts on File News Services, 11 Penn Plaza, New York, NY 10001-2006.

Margot Jefferys. "A New Way of Seeing Old Age Is Needed," *World Health,* September/October 1996.

Ann Monroe. "Getting Rid of the Gray: Will Age Discrimination Be the Downfall of Downsizing?" *Mother Jones,* July/August 1996.

Bernadette Puijalon and Jacqueline Trincaz. "Sage or Spoilsport?" *UNESCO Courier,* January 1999.

Jody Robinson. "The Baby Boomers' Final Revolt," *Wall Street Journal,* July 31, 1998.

Dan Seligman. "The Case for Age Discrimination," *Forbes,* December 13, 1999.

Ruth Simon. "Too Damn Old," *Money,* July 1996.

John C. Weicher. "Life in a Gray America," *American Outlook,* Fall 1998. Available from 5395 Emerson Way, Indianapolis, IN 46226.

Ron Winslow. "The Age of Man," *Wall Street Journal,* October 18, 1999.

Ageism in America

As boomers become seniors, bias against the elderly becomes a hot topic

DAVID CRARY

Greeting-card and novelty companies call them "Over the Hill" products: the 50th Birthday Coffin Gift Boxes featuring prune juice and anti-aging soap; the "Old Coot" and "Old Biddy" bobblehead dolls; the birthday cards mocking the mobility, intellect and sex drive of the no-longer-young.

Many Americans chuckle at such humor. Others see it as offensive, as one more sign of pervasive ageism in America.

It's a bias some also see in substandard conditions at nursing homes, in pension-plan cutbacks by employers, in the relative invisibility of the elderly on television shows and in advertisements.

"Daily we are witness to, or even unwitting participants in, cruel imagery, jokes, language, and attitudes directed at older people," contends Dr. Robert Butler, president of the International Longevity Center-USA and the person who coined the term "ageism" 35 years ago.

That ageism exists in a society captivated by youth culture and taut-skinned good looks is scarcely debatable.

But as the oldest of the 77 million baby boomers approach their 60s, the elderly and their concerns will inevitably move higher on the national agenda.

Already, there is lively debate as to whether ageism will ease or grow worse in the coming decades of boomer senior citizenship. Erdman Palmore, a professor emeritus at Duke University who has written or edited more than a dozen books on aging, counts himself—cautiously— among the optimists.

"One can say unequivocally that older people are getting smarter, richer and healthier as time goes on," Palmore said. "I've dedicated most of my life to combating ageism, and it's tempting for me to see it everywhere.... But I have faith that as science progresses, and reasonable people get educated about it, we will come to recognize ageism as the evil it is."

Palmore, 74, lives what he preaches—challenging the stereotypes of aging by skydiving, whitewater rafting, bicycling his age in miles each birthday. He recently got a tattoo on his shoulder, though the image he chose was the relatively discreet symbol of the American Humanist Association.

"What makes me mad is how aging, in our language and culture, is equated with deterioration and impairment," Palmore said. "I don't know how we're going to root that out, except by making people more aware of it."

To the extent that ageism persists, there will soon be many more potential targets. The number of Americans 65 and older is projected to double over the next three decades from 35.9 million to nearly 70 million, comprising 20 percent of the population in 2030 compared to less than 13 percent now.

The 85-and-over population is the fastest growing segment— projected to grow from 4 million in 2000 to 19 million in 2050 as part of an unprecedented surge in longevity. Americans now turning 65 will live, on average, an additional 18 years.

Some researchers believe that ageism, in the form of negative stereotypes, directly affects longevity. In a study published by the American Psychological Association, Yale School of Public Health professor Becca Levy and her colleagues concluded that old people with positive perceptions of aging lived an average of 7.5 years longer than those with negative images of growing older.

Levy said many Americans start developing stereotypes about the elderly during childhood, reinforce them throughout adulthood, and enter old age with attitudes toward their own age group as unfavorable as younger people's attitudes.

"It's possible to overcome the stereotypes, but they often operate without people's awareness," Levy said. "Look at all the talk about plastic surgery, Botox—the message is, 'Don't get old.'"

For thousands of American workers, it's the same message they claim to hear on the job. The U.S. Equal Employment Opportunity Commission has received more than 19,000 age discrimination complaints in each of the past two years, and has helped win tens of millions of dollars in settlements. However, attorneys say age discrimination often is hard to prove. Only about one-seventh of the EEOC age cases were settled to the complainant's benefit.

New Yorker Bill DeLong, 84, was fired three years ago from his longtime job as a waiter at a Shea Stadium restaurant, but he continues to seek out charitable volunteer assignments and still works as a waiter occasionally at special events.

"I didn't give up," he said. "A lot of my contemporaries give up too soon."

Seventy-eight-year-old Catherine Roberts stays active with New York City's Joint Public Affairs Committee for Older Adults, a coalition that encourages seniors to advocate on their own behalf on legislative and community issues.

"I don't have time to get old," said Roberts, who came to New York from Maine in 1955. "I'm too busy."

Yet despite her upbeat outlook, she resents how some of her peers are treated. "We're a culture that worships youth," she said. "Seniors are getting pushed aside. I see people in my building whose families ignore them—they fall through the cracks."

For many older people, ageism surfaces most painfully in the context of health care. A report by the Alliance for Aging Research, presented to a Senate committee last year, said the elderly are less likely to receive preventive care and often lack access to doctors trained in their needs.

Only about 10 percent of U.S. medical schools require work in geriatric medicine. The American Geriatrics Society says there are only about 7,600 physicians nationwide certified as geriatric specialists—not enough to meet demand and far below the 36,000 the society says will be needed by 2030.

While the society says the best way to attract more doctors to the field is to make Medicare practice more lucrative, some experts believe that many medical students also have negative attitudes toward the elderly that should be challenged.

In one such effort, the National Institute on Aging, working with Johns Hopkins Medical School and a Baltimore museum, teamed elderly people and first-year medical students in an art program in which they drew, made collages, sang songs and shared stories. A survey showed the students gained a more positive view of seniors and of geriatrics as a possible specialty.

Ageism also manifests itself in advertising. Though adults of all ages drink beer and buy cars, for example, TV and print ads for those products almost invariably feature youthful actors and models.

According to AARP, the lobbying group for people 50 and over, Americans in that age bracket account for half of all consumer spending but are targeted by just 10 percent of marketing. The dynamic is particularly potent in television, where network executives gear programming toward 18-to-34-year-olds because advertisers will pay more to reach those viewers. Jim Fishman, group publisher for AARP Publications oversees the organization's three magazines. He predicts advertisers will increasingly tilt their messages toward older consumers as the baby boomers enter their 60s.

"By and large, the wealth that resides in the older segment of the population is disposable wealth—the kids are done with college, the mortgage is paid off," Fishman said. "This older market is huge and feeling largely ignored."

Looking ahead, Fishman foresees people of all ages, elderly included, gaining the ability to look more attractive than in the past thanks to developments ranging from Botox to fitness programs. He also expects a more deep-rooted change in society's view of aging as the 65-and-older ranks are filled with increasing numbers of computer-savvy boomers, eager for civic engagement and lifelong education programs.

Still, David Wolfe, whose book "Ageless Marketing" advises advertisers how to reach over-50 consumers, says ageism is likely to persist. "There will always be people in society who can't come to terms with other people's aging because they can't come to terms with their own aging," he said.

The Secret Lives of Single Women

Are unattached women sad, lonely, and financially troubled—as the stereotype would have it? In a myth-busting survey, thousands told us that despite some very real hardships, they've never been happier

Sarah Mahoney

It is often said that females are complex and mysterious creatures, hard to understand and completely unpredictable. But older single women seem to have a mythology all their own. They are lonely, they long for love, they are terribly afraid of dying destitute. When Bella DePaulo, Ph.D., a psychology professor at the University of California, Santa Barbara, and author of the forthcoming book *Singled Out* (St. Martin's Press, 2006), asked 950 college students to describe married people, they used words like "happy, loving, secure, stable, and kind." The descriptions of singles, on the other hand, included "lonely, shy, unhappy, insecure, inflexible, and stubborn."

Are the stereotypes true? Is the picture that bleak? Or are these women in fact loving their independence and having the time of their lives? What really goes on behind the closed doors of the millions of single women in America? To find out, AARP recently polled more than 2,500 women ages 45 and older for its landmark "AARP Foundation Women's Leadership Circle Study." Though this group is large and diverse, the results, presented on the following pages, may surprise you.

Mind you, these are not rare birds: of the 57 million American women 45 and up, nearly half—25 million—are unmarried (outnumbering entire populations of countries such as North Korea, Taiwan, and Australia). There are several reasons for this: American women marry later, their divorce rate is high, and, not to put too fine a point on it, those who are married are likely to outlive their mates. As a result, American women are now likely to spend more years of their lives single than with a significant other, according to DePaulo. Instead of having some single stretches in between relationships, she says, "the reality is relationships are now what happens between longer periods of singleness."

Nor are these singles birds of a feather. Is today's typical older unwed female a lot like Carrie Bradshaw, *Sex and the City's* free-spirited patron saint of the deliberately single? Or is she more like Dorothy Zbornak, the wisecracking 50-ish Golden Girl who left her cheating husband to live with a pair of ditzy roommates and her acid-tongued mother? Could she even be Thelma or Louise—two baby-boomer heroines who couldn't

decide if they'd be better off dead or single and, in the end, chose both? The answer: a little of this and a little of that, and in some cases, all of the above.

Whatever their type, it's clear that words like *lonely*, *shy*, and *insecure* no longer apply. Fully half the women in our study say they are happier than they've ever been. Are they sad now and then? Sure—aren't we all? Do they occasionally lose sleep worrying about the future? Yes, and with good reason: being a single older woman comes with its own economic challenges. But that doesn't stop the majority from believing that midlife offers an opportunity for growth, for learning, and the chance to do the things they've always wanted to do. In fact, says DePaulo, "many single women are living lives of secret contentment."

Now, let's take a closer look at the facts and fiction about single older women in the United States today.

Myth #1: All single women are desperate to find a mate. Reality: Open to a nice relationship? You betcha. But obsessed with finding a partner? Hardly.

Given the option, many single women wouldn't mind a committed relationship with a cuddly, caring partner—preferably someone with minimal emotional baggage and the kind of income to support a nice summer house, facts supported by an AARP survey, "Lifestyles, Dating & Romance: A Study of Midlife Singles." It finds that 31 percent of single women 40 through 69 are in an exclusive relationship, and another 32 percent are dating nonexclusively. But it also finds that a surprising number couldn't care less. About one in 10 have no desire to date at all, and another 14 percent say that while they'd date the right guy if he came along, they aren't going to knock themselves out trying to find him. (The remaining 13 percent are, indeed, looking.)

In fact, most of those who aren't dating seem disinclined to change that situation anytime soon. Among 40-plus women who hadn't been on a date in the past three years, 68 percent say they just aren't interested in dating or being in a romantic relationship, though 61 percent of them would reconsider if they met someone interesting. Those who do date say it requires a philosophical balance between putting on a game face on Saturday night and not getting stressed if nothing develops. "I'm dating, and I'd like to find a good relationship," says Flo Taylor, 54, a TV producer in Pittsburgh. "But if it doesn't happen for me, I'm fine with that, too."

Myth #2: Single women are lonely.
Reality: Everyone is lonely sometimes—even married people. But most single women (as well as women with spouses) actually enjoy their solitude.
Living alone can be lonely. AARP's "Sexuality at Midlife and Beyond" survey found that 28 percent of single women said that within the past two weeks they had felt lonely occasionally or most of the time, compared with only 13 percent of married women in the same category. Slightly more single women (93 percent) than their married sisters (87 percent), however, said they felt their independence was important to their quality of life. "I love the freedom, and the fact that I know so many other single women I can network with," says Flo.

The key, says Brenda Bufalino, 68, a dancer and choreographer who lives in New York City, is to accept that some days will be lonely—no matter who you are. "The other day my granddaughter asked me, 'Nana, don't you ever get lonely?'" Bufalino, who's been divorced since 1973, answered her, "Sure, but I got lonely sometimes when I was married, too."

Myth #3: Older women are clueless about finances and don't know how to invest.
Reality: Women are more timid investors than men are, but they're the opposite of clueless and actually make fewer investing mistakes than men do.
It's true that women—both married and single—are more risk-averse and less knowledgeable about investing than men: in a recent Oppenheimer Funds survey, 63 percent of women, versus 41 percent of men, admitted they didn't know how a mutual fund worked.

For single women part of the explanation may be that they have too little money to buy funds. About 39 percent of unmarried women 45 and older are classified by the Census Bureau as "low-income," versus just 20 percent of all women in that age group. But even when they have some money to save, women who have the sole responsibility for household investment decisions invest less in mutual funds than do male decision makers or males and females who make decisions jointly. The Investment Company Institute reports that in households where women are making the investment choices, the mutual fund assets are smaller and less diverse—that is, women investors tend to invest less money and own fewer funds than do the other two groups.

If there is some truth to the cash-under-the-mattress stereotype, it's out of fear rather than an unwillingness to learn, says Ginita Wall, founder of the Women's Institute for Financial Education in San Diego and coauthor of the book *It's More Than Money, It's Your Life* (Wiley, 2004). "Especially for widows, who often get a sum of life insurance, and divorced women, who often get a portion of their ex's retirement account, it can be very hard for them to make decisions. They procrastinate and keep thinking, 'This is the last money I'm ever going to have, so I have to be careful with it.'"

More promising is the fact that women are more likely than men to rely on advice from finance professionals, a finding that is replicated in surveys from brokerage houses Oppenheimer and Merrill Lynch. And because they ask for advice, women in-

vestors actually have an edge over men in at least one respect: a recent Merrill Lynch study found that while women knew and cared less about investing than men did, they also made fewer investing mistakes—such as holding a losing stock too long or failing to research the tax implications of an investment—than men did, and didn't repeat them as often.

"Women are more likely to seek information than men are," says Wall. "But just because single women know something intellectually, it doesn't mean it's easy for them emotionally."

Myth #4: Unlike their female counterparts who were born before the women's movement, baby-boomer career women have it made financially.
Reality: Many single women—particularly those under age 60—carry dangerously high levels of debt.
Once again, credit famously single TV character Carrie Bradshaw for drawing attention to a phenomenon that Esther M. Berger, a Beverly Hills certified financial planner and money manager, calls "the *Sex and the City syndrome*." Berger specializes in high-income women, a number of whom work long hours and earn big bucks "but have more or less invested their entire net worth in clothing and shoes. They often live, quite literally, from paycheck to paycheck."

It's not ignorance, exactly—these are women who manage big corporate budgets. "Part of it is a sense of entitlement," says Berger. "They work hard and feel they deserve to spend lavishly on trips and clothes. They tend to trade immediate gratification for long-term planning." Case in point: some 60 percent of the 45-plus single women in the AARP Foundation women's study haven't figured out how much money they'll need in retirement, and 68 percent don't even have a long-term spending plan.

Debt makes everything worse. While women over 60 tend to shy away from debt, baby-boomer women embrace it. Experian, one of the three premier credit-reporting agencies, notes that the average female in the age range of 45 through 59 carries $11,414 in revolving debt, compared with the $6,521 that 60-plus women carry. And, according to the AARP Foundation's women's study, divorced women and women ages 45 through 49 were the least likely to pay off their credit cards each month.

As a result, many single baby-boomer women live with plenty of financial fear: some 27 percent of the single women in the AARP Foundation women's study admit that if they were hit with an unexpected bill of a few thousand bucks—like a leaky roof or a sudden medical emergency—they would have no idea how to pay for it. Patty Leeson, 47, for example, who works for a real-estate association in Kansas City, Kansas, wound up with uncovered medical expenses of $1,000 last year and is still struggling to catch up. "It's scary that I can't pay," says Patty, who has never been married and doesn't date. "I do feel that I don't have the security married people do, and there are plenty of times I wish I had someone to help me with the bills." And when she thinks ahead to the future? "Sometimes I panic," she admits.

Myth #5: Retirement is a time for single women to slow down and get a few more cats.
Reality: Often it's an exciting chance for reinvention.
It's true that in terms of happy-right-now measurements, single women, overall, don't fare as well as married women or those

with a live-in partner. Though 50 percent of single women say they are happier now than they have ever been, as mentioned earlier, an even greater 75 percent with partners say the same thing, according to the AARP Foundation women's study.

Despite the challenges, though, mature unmarried women are starting to build a culture all their own. And as the proud-to-be-me baby boomers begin to swell their ranks, attitudes are changing. "Single women are starting to realize how much time they have to create a meaningful life," says author Suzanne Braun Levine, who spoke to hundreds of women for her book *Inventing the Rest of Our Lives: Women in Second Adulthood* (Viking, 2005). "If you figure that the first adulthood lasts from 25 to 50, you have statistically at least that much time ahead of you until you're 75, and many women live much longer."

Indeed, some 63 percent of single women who live alone say their older years are the time to pursue their dreams and do things they've always wanted to do. And 80 percent of single women agree that as they've gotten older, they're more free to be themselves. As women reinvent themselves, the results can be surprising. When Carol Wheeler's husband died—just nine days before she would have been eligible to collect his Social Security—she was stunned. They had met and married while she was in her 60s. They had enjoyed the best of city life: a rent-controlled apartment in Manhattan, season tickets to the opera, plenty of time with their grown children. Now, on a Social Security check of just $1,000, Carol had to face facts: "I said to myself, 'I can't go on pretending I'm living the same life without him.'"

So she took a trip to Mexico, checking out the charming mountain town of San Miguel de Allende as a possible retirement destination. Using some money her husband had left her, she bought "an absolute wreck" of a house, which cost far less than anything she could have found in the States, and then renovated it. Now she gets by quite nicely on her Social Security income. And she loves almost everything about Mexico—the way walking on the charming cobblestone streets keeps her fit, her new friends (mostly American women), and how she has been able to fill her little home with brightly colored masterpieces from local artisans. "I lived my whole life with white walls," says Carol, now 70. "Here, everything is bright—I painted my house in mango and rose colors, and the people are so friendly. I'm enchanted."

Myth #6: When it comes to their appearance, older single women say "the heck with it."
Reality: To the contrary, women without partners are keenly aware that appearances matter in our society. But most don't go to extremes to look younger than they really are.

Turns out those stereotypes about single women desperately trying to hang on to their looks as they age—remember Blanche DuBois, shrinking from bright lights in *A Streetcar Named Desire*?—are a bunch of hooey. Nancy Etcoff, Ph.D., a psychology instructor at Harvard Medical School, studied 3,200 women in 10 countries and found that women's perception of how good-looking they are doesn't erode (or improve) as the years roll by. Just as many women (16 percent) think of themselves as attractive at 65 as at 18, says Etcoff, author of *Survival of the Prettiest* (Anchor, 2000). The same goes for women who regard themselves as average (72 per-

cent) or less physically attractive than others (13 percent). "But single women do pay more attention to appearance," she says. "In the dating world physical appearance is always important. You are judged in part by how you look."

With men and women of all ages flocking to plastic surgeons, it's thus no surprise that older single women are getting their share of nips and tucks as well. The American Society of Plastic Surgeons doesn't track the marital status of patients, but surgeons say there are definitely a fair number of single older women who feel surgery can give them an advantage with men. "When women in their 60s come to me for neck- and face-lifts, most are single," says Jeannette Martello, M.D., a plastic surgeon with a busy practice in South Pasadena, California.

Take Annette Bilobran, a 62-year-old retired nurse in Schenectady, New York, who recently had a neck- and face-lift. Long divorced, she believes surgery helps her get dates. "You always see guys gathered around the younger women," she says. "Now I feel like I have a bit more of an advantage." Darrick Antell, M.D., the New York City plastic surgeon who worked on Annette, says he's even seen cases where women demanded that money for a face-lift be written into a divorce settlement.

But women are sprucing themselves up for other reasons, too—it's not all about men. Now that they are working longer, "most women are just engaging in defensive aging," says Antell. In other words, they are taking active measures to slow the signs that they are getting older. For patients 51 to 64—most of whom are women—eyelid surgery, liposuction, and nose reshaping are the most common procedures; the 65-plus group tends to opt for eyelid surgery, face-lifts, and hair transplants, according to the American Society of Plastic Surgeons. June Benedict, a 73-year-old widow from New Wilmington, Pennsylvania, recently had a face-lift with her identical twin, Joan. "At this age," says June, "some people would say, why should we bother? It's not that I have an interest in dating—I don't. I just wanted a little improvement. Now I look like me, only better."

Myth #7: A single woman's worst fear is that she'll wind up old, sick, and alone.
Reality: Winding up alone, with no partner to care for them late in life, is increasingly likely for all women, married or single. But it's not something they lose sleep over.

The majority of single women (81 percent) aren't overly concerned about the prospect of growing old alone, according to the AARP Foundation women's study. Among those who do worry, divorced women (25 percent) fret more than widows (19 percent) and married women (17 percent). And in fact some single women recognize that their single status will actually protect them from the heartbreaking (and often health-breaking) ordeal of caring for a sick husband in his declining years.

For older women, married or single, life can prove challenging whether they fret about it or not. "Married women may enter their 60s better off than women who are single, divorced, or widowed," says Cindy Hounsell, executive director of the Women's Institute for a Secure Retirement. "But through divorce or death, they lose their husbands and many financial benefits of being married. By age 85 the majority are single. That's the astonishing thing—most of us are going to be single."

The truth is that with no spouse to help care for them, women are more likely than men to wind up in nursing homes. And they are also more likely to get chronic illnesses than men are, says Heidi Hartmann, Ph.D., a labor economist and president of the Institute for Women's Policy Research. If the abstract fear of winding up alone doesn't worry single women, the concrete threat of becoming dependent on caregivers does. According to the AARP Foundation women's study, some 41 percent of women who live alone worry that they might lose their independence in a health crisis, versus 35 percent of women who live with a spouse or other adults. A related fear, shared equally by married and single women alike, is imposing on their children at some point in the future. About 31 percent of women who live alone, and 30 percent of women who live with others, say they are at least moderately worried about eventually becoming a burden to their family.

Myth #8: The older they get, the more single women regret the lack of family ties.
Reality: Unmarried women have strong family relationships, and many have stronger social support systems than married women do.

"It always surprises me when people say, 'Don't you wish you had a family?'" says Michele Horon, 57, a corporate-communications coordinator who lives in Bethlehem, Pennsylvania, and has never been married. "I do have a family. My mother lives with me, and I've got siblings and tons of nieces and nephews, and we're very close," she says. Even beyond blood family, contented single women knit together their own support systems of friends, colleagues, neighbors, and other people, says E. Kay Trimberger, Ph.D., a sociologist and author of *The New Single Woman* (Beacon Press, 2005), who tracked 27 single women for almost a decade. "Community really means a lot to these women and gives them geographical stability," she says. "In some cases, women in my study even turned down significant career opportunities because they didn't want to move away from these connections."

Among women living alone, 88 percent of the women in the AARP Foundation women's study say they have friends they can depend on in times of crisis. Experts like Trimberger expect women, especially those in the baby-boomer age group (42 through 60), to keep up those connections as they age. The study also found, for example, 41 percent of single women 45 through 59 said that as they got older they would be open to living with women friends.

Myth #9: Single women are sex-starved.
Reality: They may be hungry at times, certainly, but most have a greater appetite for other forms of sustenance in their lives.

When it comes to sex, single women have all kinds of ways of dealing with—and without—it. A relatively low number, just 22 percent, of the 45-plus single women in AARP's "Sexuality at Midlife and Beyond" study were sexually active in the past six months, and only 18 percent had a regular sex partner. But either way, they weren't hung up about it. "After age 50 a number of single women want fun sex," says author Levine. "This is a no-holds-barred period of their lives—they're more sexually adven-

turous and easygoing, and while sex isn't the biggest deal in the world, they're more willing to take pleasure when it comes." Of the single women in AARP's sexuality study, 15 percent had watched adult films with a partner, 14 percent had used sex toys, 10 percent had had phone sex, and 7 percent had exchanged frisky notes or e-mails. And in the past six months 26 percent had masturbated.

But sexual urges aren't the main driving force for older women dating, at least in the same way they are for men. Some 11 percent of the men in the AARP lifestyles, dating, and romance survey, for instance, said the main reason they date is to fulfill their sexual needs, versus a mere 2 percent of the women. And 24 percent of single women in the same survey agreed that they could be happy never having sex again. "Since menopause, I don't feel the need," says Michele Horon. Her last relationship ended five years ago. "That's not to say I wouldn't be turned on. I certainly could be, but sex is just last on my list."

Myth #10: Single women aren't as healthy as married women.
Reality: Generally true, but now single women are taking charge of their health just as they're taking control of other parts of their lives.

For decades health researchers have consistently found that married women are healthier than single women. But the most negative health outcomes for women have been associated with those who are divorced or widowed. Very little attention has been paid to the long-term health outcomes of women who are contentedly single. One surprising finding to come out of the AARP Foundation women's survey, however, is that single women tend to think of themselves as healthy—46 percent said their health is excellent or very good. In addition, 90 percent of the single women in the study said they're very or somewhat confident that they're doing all they can to keep themselves healthy. "These findings seem promising," says Jean Kalata, AARP research analyst and principal researcher for the AARP Foundation women's study, "but we need more research into single women and the effects of happiness on health."

So, is being single the new happy ending for American women? Of course not. But it doesn't mean life is over. As more unmarried women embrace the challenges and opportunities that come with living alone, they are writing new chapters in self-discovery, says Florence Falk, Ph.D., a psychotherapist in New York City and author of *On My Own: The Art of Being a Woman Alone* (Harmony Books), due out in January 2007. "Many women are surprised at how learning to be alone, in the best sense of the word, opens them up to a bigger world. Even with the speed bumps, being single can lead them to better relationships, more creativity, new friendships, and a deeper sense of self and community."

Writer **SARAH MAHONEY** lives in Durham, Maine. Her last story for AARP The Magazine was *"10 Secrets of a Good, Long Life"* (July-August 2005).

The Under-Reported Impact of Age Discrimination and Its Threat to Business Vitality

The Age Discrimination in Employment Act (ADEA, 29 USCA, 621) is credited with helping eliminate many blatant forms of age discrimination in employment. For example, before the ADEA was enacted 37 years ago, it was common for employment ads to list age limitations, indicating people over 40 need not apply. Across the board, mandatory retirement policies went unchallenged. Despite advancements in these areas since the founding of the Age Discrimination in Employment Act, it remains to be seen whether the ADEA has completed the job it set out to do. Has it proven to be an effective tool for eliminating the unreasonable prejudices that make it difficult for older workers to achieve their full potential? Has it provided adequate compensation for victims of discrimination? The following article takes a snapshot of the current work environment to gain a perspective. Based on extensive interviews with academics, employment lawyers, advocates for older workers, and older workers themselves, it reveals the need for reforms. It finds that, in a legal environment slanted toward employers, older workers continue to face bias and stereotyping, that most victims of discrimination are not made whole, and that society's lack of concern for this type of discrimination may prove more costly in the future as employers look more to older workers to fill projected workforce gaps.

ROBERT J. GROSSMAN
School of Management, Marist College, Poughkeepsie, NY 12601, United States

1. The ADEA: An Introduction

Thirty-seven years ago, Congress passed the Age Discrimination in Employment Act (ADEA) which makes it illegal for an employer or union to discharge, refuse to hire, or otherwise discriminate on the basis of age. Looking back, it is easy to forget the overt discrimination faced by older workers at the time. It was common for employment ads prior to 1967 to list age limitations, indicating people over 40 need not apply. Mandatory retirement policies, applicable to almost everyone but Supreme Court Justices, went unchallenged. Although some states had antidiscrimination laws on the books, they were not enforced, giving employers a free hand to discriminate. But now, almost four decades later, it bears asking whether the ADEA has done more than address age discrimination in its most blatant manifestations. Is it really effective in preventing age bias? Has it been successful in "alleviating serious economic and psychological suffering of persons between the ages of 40 and 65 caused by unreasonable prejudice?" (Polstorff v. Fletcher (1978, ND Ala) 452 F Supp 17). What role has it played in transforming the U.S. culture to be more accepting and appreciative of older workers?

2. Stereotypes Survive

Despite protestations to the contrary, there seems to be little indication that attitudes have changed significantly since the enactment of the ADEA. The notion that older people have had their day and should make room for the next generation continues to be deeply ingrained. "We think maybe it's okay because it's an economic issue, not a civil rights issue," says Laurie McCann, Senior Attorney for AARP in Washington, D.C. "Until we view it as just as wrong and serious, we may not be making the inroads we need to address the intractable, subtle discrimination that is so pervasive. I don't think employers want to discriminate; they don't hate older workers. It's the stereotypes. They may not even know they harbor these biases, but they do" (McCann, 2003).

Such attitudes are evident in the case of Ann Klingert, a 64-year-old resident of the Bronx, who recalled with astonishment the public response to an article in a local New York City newspaper regarding an EEOC lawsuit she had filed. Klingert filed with the EEOC after she was fired by Woolworths and then prohibited from applying for newly created part-time jobs which were filled mostly by student applicants. "When the lawsuit was reported in a local New York City newspaper, *Our Town*, people were outraged," she said. "They wrote letters to the editor saying things like 'why don't you just retire and just take your social security and go away'" (Klingert, 2003).

Although most employers are sensitive to the issues of sexism and racism, "the idea that you cannot teach an old dog new tricks does not seem to carry the same taboo status in society and the workplace," says Todd Maurer, Associate Professor of Industrial-Organization Psychology at the Georgia Institute of Technology. Maurer says that generalizing is dangerous in the range of older workers; perhaps even more so than in other categories. "One size does not fit all," he says. "There can be older individuals who are both interested and able when it comes to learning. Research has found large differences within older groups in things like training performance and in abilities like memory and reaction time" (Maurer, 2003). However, too often, as in the case of Maryland resident Mort Beres, employers are influenced more by stereotypes than skills or experience. When Beres, then in his late 50s, lost his job, the prior owner of small businesses and successful salesman in the auto parts manufacturing industry knew he had skills that should have been in demand, yet he was turned away repeatedly. Any offers he did receive were salaried at much less than he had earned previously, and the positions were often demeaning in nature. Beres held on as long as he could, but admitted that, out of desperation, he took some sketchy jobs. "You take every jerky job you can get just to have some income; some of them make you nauseous" (Beres, 2003).

Eventually, Beres found his niche, working as a trainer and sales rep for Irvine, California-based BDS Marketing. Assigned to the Canon account at a Best Buy in Maryland, his job was to help store personnel sell Canon printers, for which he was paid a salary plus commission. After 5 years on the job, working with a series of regional supervisors, at age 67, Beres achieved a noteworthy record by helping his store become one of the top five in the territory. However, when a new supervisor took over, Beres's star began to fall. "He'd call me and make stupid comments about my age, like 'you're too old, I think it's time for a change." Finally, Beres got the axe. When he asked why he had been fired, the manager told him, "I'm not telling you and I don't have to." Beres recalls hanging up and thinking about what had happened. "I got angry; really angry. It was a little, unimportant job, but they had no right to treat me that way." *(BDS Marketing's Vice President for Human Resources, Jeffrey Sopko, refused to comment specifically but denied Beres's version of what happened and claimed that there were other reasons for Beres's dismissal).*

Beres's plight is not uncommon, yet society appears to be less outraged at age bias than other types of discrimination. "It seems more politically correct to discriminate against older people," says Mindy Farber, Managing Partner at Farber Taylor, LL.C. in Rockville, Maryland. Farber recalls hiring a new associate for the firm who was in her mid-fifties. "It was shocking. I was surprised how open people were about talking about the wisdom of my decision in light of her age. If I had hired an African American, they would have been silent. Here they told me straight out that I had made a mistake" (Farber, 2003).

Table 1 Workers over age 45 reporting presence of age discrimination (*n* =1500)

Do not Know	2%
No	31%
Yes	67%

Source: AARP Work and Careers Study Summary (2002).

3. Perspective: How Older Workers See It

From their perspectives, older workers see little evidence that they are competing on a level playing field. Sixty-seven percent of employed workers aged 45 to 74 surveyed by AARP in 2003's *Staying Ahead of the Curve* said that age discrimination is a fact of life in the workplace (AARP, 2003) (Table 1). This percentage is even higher among African Americans and Hispanics, both at 72%. Age is viewed as so critical to employees that respondents listed it, along with education, as more important in how workers are treated than are gender, race, sexual orientation or religion. Sixty percent said they believe that older workers are the first to go when employers make cuts.

A 2002 Conference Board survey of 1,600 workers aged 50 and older found that 31 percent of workers intending to retire within five years said they would stay on if given more responsibilities. Twenty-five percent said they were leaving because they were being held back or marginalized because of their age (The Conference Board, 2002). Linda Barrington, Labor Economist at The Conference Board, says the high percentage of dissatisfied workers is cause for concern. "It's twice as big as I might have expected," she says. Perceptions, of course, are not necessarily reality, but Barrington says that does not matter. "Perceptions affect the way you work; if you're feeling undervalued, that discouragement will affect your work. Is it perception or reality? Either way, it has to be dealt with" (Barrington, 2003).

It also bears noting that far fewer of the respondents said they have suffered personally from ageism. About 9% say they believe they have been passed up for a promotion because of their age, 6% said they were fired or laid off because of age, 5% said they were passed up for a raise because of age, and 15% attributed their not being hired for a job to their age. However, the survey only queried current workers and did not include individuals in the same age category who were no longer in the workforce.

4. Advantage: Employers

Compared to its sister statutes aimed at race, religion, gender, and disability, the ADEA offers less protection. Court interpretations have proven to be less rigorous and more employer-friendly, ceding to employers the right to make bonafide business decisions even when age is linked. In practice, instead of preventing discrimination, the law serves as a roadmap for employers, enabling all but the obtuse to avoid liability and shield all but the most egregious ageist actions from public scrutiny.

Under the ADEA, if there is a valid reason for an action, it is considered acceptable if age happens to be an accompanying factor. "If you can show you would have done it anyway, you're off the hook," says Harlan Miller, an employment attorney with Miller, Billips, and Ates (Miller et al., 2003) in Atlanta, Georgia. As a result, it is almost impossible to catch a crafty employer discriminating. "I can always get around it if I'm smart. Only idiots get nailed," agrees David Neumark, a nationally recognized expert on the ADEA and Senior Fellow at the Public Policy Institute of California in San Francisco (Neumark, 2003).

Employers are not infallible, however, and they still mess up on occasion. Often when they do, it is because of retaliation: reacting badly to an employee whose initial complaint does not rise above the threshold set by the ADEA. "We tell them to go back and complain about their treatment," says James Rubin, an employment attorney with Farber Taylor. "Then the employer does something really bad. It's not the original claim; it's the reprisal. You can bring an action based on the reprisal even if the original claim is weak" (Rubin, 2003).

Employers also get caught when the rationale for their business decision falls apart. "Typically, the employer comes in with some kind of bogus selection process that says they're trying to keep the most competent," Miller says. "Gulfstream Aerospace's decision to cut from 200 to 230 of its nearly 2000 management-level employees during the period from August through December, 2000, is a case in point. Gulfstream had a rating device based on flexibility and adaptability; code words for old or young…and not subject to any kind of objective analysis. Our analysis showed a complete correlation between age and those factors" (Miller et al., 2003).

On the other hand, if it is legitimate, an employer's business argument can carry the day. "Is it discrimination to fire someone if it is based on economic foundations?" asks Bob Smith, Professor of Labor Economics, ILR at Cornell University in Ithaca, New York. "It's not a slam dunk that they've been mistreated just because they say they are. There may be good reasons why they're singled out. They often are paid too much and have shorter time to work, making them a poorer investment. Why should I expect my employer to invest more in me than someone who will be there longer? Just because they complain, doesn't mean there's discrimination" (Smith, 2003).

5. Avoiding Scrutiny

Employers' incentives to avoid litigation are compelling from financial and public relations perspectives. Generally, when employers get wind that employees are disgruntled and plan to complain or sue, they move to settle by enticing them into retirement with incentives and buyouts, awarded contingent upon their agreeing to confidentiality clauses that prevent discussion of the situation.

The Older Worker Protection Act clarified for employers what they need to say and do when they reach termination agreements with workers. The act requires an employer to give workers 21 days to consider a buyout proposal, to advise them of their right to seek legal counsel, and even to rescind the agreement 10 days after the fact if they have a change of heart.

Until recently, a properly negotiated settlement would foreclose a former employee from further litigation. Now, there has been at least one case where the EEOC has been able to sue on behalf of workers who previously signed releases.

In a typical settlement, the employer denies discrimination, attributing the settlement to "business decisions." In a recent survey by Jury Verdict Research, plaintiffs' lawyers estimated that 84% of their clients' claims were settled, while defense lawyers reported 79% (Jury Verdict Research, 2002).

Often, employees are relieved to accept the face-saving exit. In reality, their options are meager. They are scared if they are still working or owed pensions, and lack money if they have been terminated. According to Howard Eglit, Professor of Law at Chicago-Kent College, it costs, on average, about $50,000 for a lawyer if cases go beyond early negotiations with an employer. Most attorneys will not handle such cases on a contingent basis because they know the chances of winning are slim. Employers, on average, can count on spending $100,000 in legal fees from the time a complaint is filed with the EEOC until trial (Eglit, 2003).

Although the amounts paid to ease workers into retirement or silence complaints are private, high-profile EEOC settlements reveal just how well workers actually do when they press the ADEA to the limit. In March, 2003, the EEOC announced a class action settlement with Gulfstream Aerospace, owned by General Dynamics, on behalf of 66 workers for $2.1 million dollars, an average of approximately $33,000 for each manager the EEOC claimed had been wrongfully terminated. Ninety-three percent, many of whom may never work again full-time, accepted the deal and faded away, careers in shambles.

As meager as the settlement proved to be, there would not have been a case without former Gulfstream Aerospace manager Eddie Cosper of Rincon, Georgia. His role suggests that, behind every major class action, there is an activist who serves as a catalyst in pushing for remediation.

When Gulfstream Aerospace cut more than 200 of its nearly 2000 management employees, most of whom worked in Savannah, it had not bargained on Cosper's pride and persistence. Aged 54 and with the company for 28 years, Eddie Cosper was proud, professional, and still moving up. "I was still ambitious. Every time I put out a fire, I kept getting a promotion," he recalls. However, Cosper reached a dead-end when General Dynamics took over the company in 1999. His seasoning suddenly turned sour. "The VP would tell me, 'You're like father time; you've been here forever. Wouldn't you like to retire and do something different?'" Soon Cosper found himself reassigned to nights, with responsibility for 40 people instead of the 300 he usually had. Then, 30 days later, he was terminated. "My performance reviews were all above average," he says. "I had the highest ranking of all the four managers in my category." How did he feel when his career went up in smoke? "It's like a burning sensation in your gut. You say, why me? I put my whole life into something and it's been taken away for no reason. In the beginning, I felt sorry for myself, then I got angry. I did the numbers and realized I wasn't the only older person being targeted. So I started talking to others and built a network and database." Communication was key. "People who don't have that network have no clue," he says. "Every Joe Blow could get hit cold and not know what's happening. Probably half the people in our suit were along for the ride. If I hadn't reached them, they wouldn't have realized they were discriminated against and would have gotten nothing."

The EEOC's settlement with Footlocker is another example of a remedy that fell short of the mark. When the company settled with 764 former Woolworth employees, the complainants, mostly low-paid hourly workers, walked off with an average of $4,000 per person. Overall, the $3.4 million was a small price to pay for a 40,000-worker retailing giant like Footlocker (EEOC, 2002). A tougher question is why they let the matter fester as long as they did. Many companies buy themselves out of trouble, right or wrong (Eglit, 2003). According to Jury Verdict Research, the median settlement for age cases from 1994 to 2000 was $65,000, $5,000 higher than the median reported for all types of discrimination, age included (Jury Verdict Research, 2002).

6. Complaints Grow

If age discrimination had been decreasing throughout the years, even allowing for more people being aware of their right to complain and more older workers proving their mettle to those who question their ability, it would be reasonable to expect the number of complaints to be trending down. Instead, there are more cases. The EEOC logged 19,921 age discrimination complaints in 2002, an increase of 14.5% from the previous year and accounting for 23.6% of all discrimination claims filed with the agency (U.S. Equal Employment Opportunity Commission, ADEA Charges, 2003).

Some EEOC complainants, either uncertain as to the true basis of the discrimination against them or believing there is more than one basis, file multiple charges. EEOC data reveals that instances of ADEA claimants who alleged an additional type of discrimination are declining. The data suggests there is no move on the part of complainants making their case on some other basis of discrimination (gender, race, religion, or national origin) to add age simply in order to bolster the case, even though it was not thought to be the primary or even substantial basis of the discrimination. For the 3-year period of 1997 to 1999, an average of 17.9% of ADEA claimants made an additional charge. From 2000 to 2003, the average percentage dropped to 15.8%. In addition, states Farber, private lawyers are seeing similar increases in age complaints in proportion to race, gender, and disability (Farber, 2003).

7. Profile

Overall, the majority of claimants tend to be white males, 55 and older at the middle management level. However, the number of women filing claims has doubled in the last few years, a trend that Eglit estimates will continue as women earn more, hold more desirable jobs, and can afford to hire counsel. "The ADEA offers two essential remedies: reinstatement and back pay. If you weren't getting much and your job wasn't worth much, why sue? Now, even with the glass ceiling, women

Table 2   Age bias charge filings with EEOC nationwide by age group of charging parties fiscal years 1999–2002[a]

Fiscal year/age	Age 40–49	Age 50–59	Age 60–69
1999	3367	5949	3526
2000	3941	6620	4609
2001	3779	7584	4603
2002	4219	8455	5686

Source: EEOC, Office of Communications and Legislative Affairs (2003).
[a] Note: the three age ranges combined do not comprise the total ADEA charge filings with the EEOC per year, as a small number of charges which are not listed are filed by individuals 70 and older.

have good jobs and can afford to hire an attorney and sue" (Eglit, 2003) (Table 2).

In 2002, 53% of the cases related to job loss; wrongful discharge, 8,741 and involuntary layoff, 1,463. "They're easier to prove," Eglit says. "If you've been working at a place for 20 years, look around and see five other people fired, you have a case." (Eglit, 2003) It happened in the Woolworth's/Footlocker case, says Michelle Le-Moal-Grey, EEOC attorney. "When they were fired, workers spoke by phone and began to see a pattern forming in their store and beyond" (LeMoal-Grey, 2003).

Of the EEOC claimants between ages 40 and 69, 46% were in their fifties, 31% in their 60s and 23% in their 40s. About 25% of claims were based on failure to hire, an increase of 200% since 1999. As these cases are harder to prove and because damages are limited, it is difficult to find a private attorney for hire without having to pay up-front. "If you're not hired, how do you know what the reason was? It's not so easy to figure it out," Eglit observes (Eglit, 2003).

About 12% of the claimants cited harassment; antagonism, or intimidation, creating a hostile work environment; an increase of 31.5% since 1999. Constructive discharge would be an example, says Dorothy Stubblebine, an expert witness for both plaintiffs and defendants, and President of DJS Associates in Mantua, New Jersey. "Tyically, the older person is pushed out by giving him a really hard time. He's given the worst assignments 'til he can't take it any more" (Stubblebine, 2003) (Table 3).

8. Chances for Success

Whatever the claim and whomever the claimant, few gamblers would bet on the probability of prevailing in an ADEA suit. EEOC data reveals that for most claimants, the filing with the EEOC is a dead-end. Last year, of the cases before it, the agency found "reasonable cause" only 4.3% of the time, "no reasonable cause" 52% of the time, and closed cases for "administrative" reasons 33.5% of the time. Only 6.5% of cases were eventually settled. In contrast, for claimants charging all types of discrimination, age included, the EEOC found reasonable cause 7.2% of the time, found no reasonable cause 59.3% of the time, and closed cases for administrative reasons 26% of the time (U.S. Equal Employment Opportunity Commission, 2003) (Tables 4 and Table 5).

Table 3 Age discrimination charge filings with EEOC nationwide fiscal years 1998–2002

Year[a]	FY 1998	FY 1999	FY 2000	FY 2001	FY 2002
Discharge	7054	6733	6851	7376	8741
Harassment	1871	1758	1966	2146	2311
Hiring	1953	1647	1990	3116	4889
Layoff	1036	1149	1128	1107	1810
Promotion	1547	1590	1666	1623	1463
Terms of Employment	2510	2357	2610	3440	3181
TOTAL	15,191	14,141	16,008	17,405	19,921

Source: EEOC, Office of Communications and Legislative Affairs (2003).
[a] Fiscal years run from October 1 through September 30.

Table 4 EEOC resolution of ADEA claims fiscal years 1998–2002

	FY 1998	FY 1999	FY 2000	FY 2001	FY 2002
Total ADEA Claims	15,191.	14,141	16,008	17,405	19,921
Settlements (%)	4.7	5.3	7.9	6.6	6.5
Withdrawals with benefits (%)	3.6	3.7	3.8	3.6	3.6
Administrative closures (%)	26.1	23.3	22.0	26.1	33.5
No reasonable cause (%)	61.7	59.4	58.0	55.3	52.1
Reasonable cause (%)	3.9	8.3	8.2	8.2	4.3

Source: EEOC, Office of Research, Information, and Planning (2003).

Table 5 EEOC resolution of all discrimination claims fiscal years 1998–2002

	FY 1998	FY 1999	FY 2000	FY 2001	FY 2002
Total Claims	79,591	77,444	79,896	80,840	84,442
Settlements (%)	4.6	6.2	8.5	8.1	8.8
Withdrawals with benefits (%)	3.2	3.7	4.0	4.1	4
Administrative closures (%)	26.7	24.1	20.5	20.7	20.6
No reasonable cause (%)	60.9	59.5	58.3	57.2	59.3
Reasonable cause (%)	4.6	6.6	8.8	9.9	7.2

Source: EEOC, Office of Research, Information, and Planning (2003).

For plaintiffs who win at trial, damages are legally limited to reinstatement, loss of pay, or, where there is a finding of willful discrimination, double the lost salary. In contrast, race and gender plaintiffs have the opportunity to be awarded more lucrative punitive damages. "Why shouldn't someone who's old be compensated for pain and suffering just like someone who's fired for their religion, race, or gender?" Miller asks. "There's nothing worse than, after 30 years' service, to be fired at 58" (Miller et al., 2003).

The solution for many attorneys is to bypass the ADEA and, where possible, sue under local or state statutes. "Everybody tries to stay out of Federal Court," Farber says. "Plaintiffs get their audience but they lose before they can get to a jury. It's so bad that a fellow attorney once told me that if I went to Federal Court when there were other options available, I would be guilty of malpractice." Farber says a plaintiff's chances to reach a jury brighten considerably in state or local courts. Virtually everyone on a jury can identify with the plight of an older worker. "Everybody on the jury is getting older and has a mother and father" (Farber, 2003).

If they get to a state or federal jury, Jury Verdict Research in its study, *Employment Practice Liability: Jury Award Trends and Statistics,* reports a 78% success rate overall for age cases in 2000. In Federal District Courts, from 1994 to 2000, the median verdict was $269,350, tops for all types of discrimination. However, the chances of plaintiffs getting there with the EEOC in their corner are limited. The Office of

General counsel states that during the 5-year period from 1997 to 2001, the EEOC filed 205 lawsuits based on the ADEA, leaving plaintiffs who push ahead with claims the EEOC determines are without merit with the risk and expense of proceeding toward litigation on their own (Office of General Counsel, 2002). Jury Verdict Research indicates that the median verdict for more numerous privately initiated state cases was about the same (Jury Verdict Research, 2002).

9. Justification

Critics point out that there may be valid reasons for determining that older workers are less desirable employees. There is no question that technological changes have significantly altered the way we work, especially in white-collar jobs, explains Camille Olson, Chair of the Labor and Employment Practice Group, Seyfeith Shaw, in Chicago, Illinois. "Persons in their 20s and 30s who are comfortable with technology are more responsive and more adaptable to change. Can people in their 40s and 50s without this background feel that they belong in the workplace? You feel that time has passed you by. Does that affect your motivation, your ability to do things? It does" (Olson, 2003).

"A lot of people who think they've been screwed over have it wrong," agrees AARP's McCann. "Though I'm an advocate, I'd be the first to admit that when someone gets fired or doesn't get promoted, they yell foul. An age discrimination claim is the last resort for older white males. "If you're a 55 year old male who's lost your $70,000 job, what do you do? The odds of finding any job, let alone a comparable job, are slim, so you fight" (McCann, 2003).

"If a person has lost a step or two and doesn't project or have the kind of energy to move forward, the fact that he isn't promoted may show that's where he belongs," explains Ed King, Executive Director of the National Senior Citizen Law Center, a former EEOC mediator in Hawaii. "The question is whether the employer is stereotyping or it is legitimate" (King, 2003).

It is undeniable that age has its advantages; plusses that advocates for older workers tend to downplay. "They do better; get paid more. Their employment rates are high and they get cared for in retirement," Neumark observes. However, he says, it is not all roses and caviar for workers in their 50s or 60s. Once they are unemployed, it is hard for them to find work. They are out of work longer, have difficulty finding jobs with comparable responsibilities and wages, and tend to become disheartened and "retire" (Neumark, 2003).

Adding to the debate is the difference of opinion as to whether age 40, which seemed appropriate in the 1960s, should still be the turning point for providing a person with ADEA coverage. Some experts ask, Why not? There needs to be some beginning point, and 40 is reasonable. Others disagree, arguing that 45 or 50 are more realistic ages when discriminatory treatment is most likely to occur. Whatever the threshold, it has been clear until recently that all people from 40 on up had to be treated similarly, but no longer.

In an opinion issued February 24, 2004, on General Dynamics Land Systems versus Cline, the U.S. Supreme Court held that the ADEA does not prevent an employer from favoring older employees over younger employees. The court upheld an agreement between General Dynamics and the United Auto Workers union that provided for continued retirement health benefits for employees then over 50 years of age but eliminated that benefit for all other employees. The plaintiffs were between the ages of 40 and 50, and were denied the benefits available only to workers over the age of 50.

10. No Special Treatment

Should an employer invest extra to help support an older worker? Offer more and different training? Provide less stressful assignments? The issue, Olson says, is whether under the ADEA an employer needs to take affirmative efforts to assist individuals who do not naturally have the same skills, while at the same time paying them more. Clearly, Olson says, the law never contemplated affirmative action. The law is there only to make sure older people are not treated differently (Olson, 2003).

"The ADEA is about equal treatment, not about preferential treatment," agrees Lynn Clemens, Attorney, Office of Legal Counsel at EEOC. "There are no affirmative obligations on the employer's part. That notion goes against the act." Regardless, advocates are making the case that there are other benefits to be gained by retaining older workers anyway, although they are paid more and have fewer skills. Olson says she does not buy it unless there is a compelling business case. "The issue is whether you need to invest in targeted training, making older workers more productive because you need them to stick around" (Olson, 2003).

11. Call for Action

Meanwhile, William Rothwell, Professor of Workforce Education and Development at Penn State University observes that Bureau of Labor Statistics projections show that while 13 percent of American workers today are 55 and older, that figure will increase to 20% by the year 2015. At the same time, the nation is expected to experience a drop in the percentage of younger workers aged 25 to 44.

With this information in mind, Rothwell says the current economic slump is the calm before the storm. When the economy turns around and there is more demand for products and services, the worker shortage will be the number one issue. "Employers in the U.S. will be forced to go back to their retiree base and deploy it more effectively than ever before. If we can't get labor from anywhere else, we'll look to the most obvious population who knows everything about our business" (Rothwell, 2003).

Unless we get serious about addressing the stereotypes and focus on reducing the alienation that older workers feel, these workers, as well as retirees, may be unreceptive and unprepared to step up when the market finally swings in their favor. Reforming the ADEA is the first step. To better combat age discrimination, we must move quickly to put more teeth into the law. If we do not, when we go to the well, it may just be dry.

References

AARP. (2003). *Staying ahead of the curve.*

Barrington, L. (2003 April 10). Telephone interview. New York, NY.

Beres M. (2003 April 22). Telephone interview. Rockville, MD.

EEOC Press Release. (2002, November 15). *EEOC settles major age bias suit; foot locker to pay $3.5 million to former Woolworth employees.*

Eglit, H. (2003 April 10). Telephone interview. Chicago, IL.

Farber, M. (2003 April 21). Telephone interview. Rockville, MD.

Jury Verdict Research. (2002). *Employment practice liability verdicts and settlements: Jury award trends and statistics.*

King, E. (2003 April 15). Telephone interview. Washington, D.C.

Klingert, A. (2003 May 1). Telephone interview. Bronx, NY.

LeMoal-Grey, M. (2003 April 28). Telephone interview. New York, NY.

Maurer, T. (2003 April 17). Telephone interview. Atlanta, GA.

McCann, L. (2003 April 17). Telephone interview. Washington, D.C.

Miller, Harlan, Principal, Miller, Billips & Ates. (2003). Atlanta, GA. (18 April).

Neumark, D. (2003 April 8). Telephone interview. San Francisco, CA.

Office of General Counsel. (2002, August 13). The U.S. Equal Employment Opportunity Commission. *Study of the litigation program fiscal years 1997–2001,* Table 2.

Olson, C. (2003 April 10). Telephone interview. Chicago, IL.

Rothwell, W. (2003 April 17). Telephone interview. University Park, PA.

Rubin, J. (2003 April 21). Telephone interview. Rockville, MD.

Smith, B. (2003 April 17). Telephone interview. Ithaca, NY.

Stubblebine, D. (2003 April 4). Telephone interview. Mantua, NJ.

The Age Discrimination in Employment Act of 1967. (1967). Pub. L. 90–202, as amended. Volume 29 of the United States Code beginning at section 621.

The Conference Board. (2002). *Voices of experience: Mature workers in the future workplace.*

United States Supreme Court. (2004, February 24). *General Dynamics Land Systems,* v. cline, No. 02–1080.

U.S. Equal Employment Opportunity Commission. (2003). *Age discrimination in employment act charges,* FY 1992-FY 2002.

UNIT 4

Problems and Potentials of Aging

Unit Selections

Key Points to Consider

- Why do doctors find it so hard to treat older patients?

- How is a recent Supreme Court ruling going to affect an employer's discrimination against older workers?

- Of the single, continuously married, and people who experienced several marriages, which group was most likely to have cardiovascular problems?

- What was the relationship between frequent abuse and the health of older women?

Student Website

www.mhcls.com/online

Internet References

Further information regarding these websites may be found in this book's preface or online.

Alzheimer's Association
   http://www.alz.org

A.P.T.A. Section on Geriatrics
   http://geriatricspt.org

Caregiver's Handbook
   http://www.acsu.buffalo.edu/~drstall/hndbk0.html

Caregiver Survival Resources
   http://www.caregiver.com

AARP Health Information
   http://www.aarp.org/bulletin

International Food Information Council
   http://www.ific.org/

University of California at Irvine: Institute for Brain Aging and Dementia
   http://www.alz.uci.edu/

Viewed as part of the life cycle, aging might be considered a period of decline, poor health, increasing dependence, social isolation, and—ultimately—death. It often means retirement, decreased income, chronic health problems, and death of a spouse. In contrast, the first 50 years of life are seen as a period of growth and development.

For a young child, life centers around the home, and then the neighborhood. Later, the community and state become a part of the young person's environment. Finally, as an adult, the person is prepared to consider national and international issues—wars, alliances, changing economic cycles, and world problems.

During the later years, however, life space narrows. Retirement may distance the individual from national and international concerns, although he or she may remain actively involved in community affairs. Later, even community involvement may decrease, and the person may begin to stay close to home and the neighborhood. For some, the final years of life may once again focus on the confines of home, be it an apartment or a nursing home.

Many older Americans try to remain masters of their own destinies for as long as possible. They fear dependence and try to avoid it. Many are successful at maintaining independence and the right to make their own decisions. Others are less successful and must depend on their families for care and to make critical decisions. However, some older people are able to overcome the difficulties of aging and to lead comfortable and enjoyable lives.

In "Primary Care for Elderly People: Why Do Doctors Find It So Hard?" the authors point out that geriatric patients often have multiple and compounding adverse medical events that are much more difficult to diagnose and treat than the single illness that most patients seeking medical attention are experiencing.

In "Breakthrough," David Newman contends that older workers filing a discrimination suit against an employer no longer have to prove that they were singled out for unfair treatment but rather that they were the victim of a policy that caused harm to older workers. In "Marital History and the Burden of Cardiovascular Disease in Midlife," the author points out the negative effect that multiple marriage losses can have on the health of older persons.

Alzheimer's disease destroys brain cells controlling memory, communication, reasoning, and behavior, as well as physical control of the body. In "The Disappearing Mind," Geoffrey Cow-

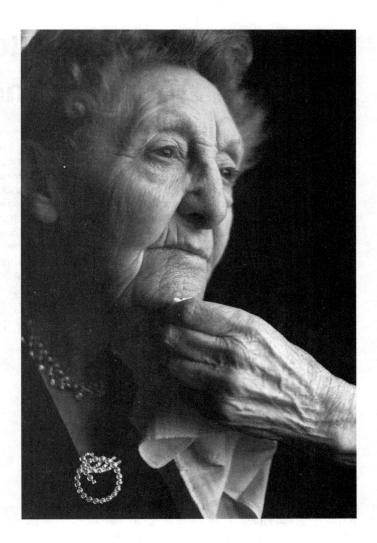

ley describes the current scientific findings of the causes of Alzheimer's disease and the current state of research on the possible cures for the disease. In "The Extent and Frequency of Abuse in the Lives of Older Women and Their Relationship With Health Outcomes," the authors point out the extent of the abuse of older women and the negative impact of abuse on their health.

Primary Care for Elderly People: Why Do Doctors Find It So Hard?

Purpose: Many primary care physicians find caring for elderly patients difficult. The goal of this study was to develop a detailed understanding of why physicians find primary care with elderly patients difficult. ***Design and Method:*** We conducted in-depth interviews with 20 primary care physicians. Using an iterative approach based on grounded theory techniques, a multidisciplinary team analyzed the content of the interviews and developed a conceptual model of the difficulty. ***Results:*** Three major domains of difficulty emerged: (i) medical complexity and chronicity, (ii) personal and interpersonal challenges, and (iii) administrative burden. The greatest challenge occurred when difficulty in more than one area was present. Contextual conditions, such as the practice environment and the physicians's training and personal values, shaped the experience of providing care and how difficult it seemed. ***Implications:*** Much of the difficulty participants experienced could be facilitated by changes in the health care delivery system and in medical education. The voices of these physicians and the model resulting from our analysis can inform such change.

WENDY L. ADAMS, MD, MPH,[1] HELEN E. McILVAIN, PhD,[1] NAOMI L. LACY, PhD,[1] HOMA MAGSI, MD,[1] BENJAMIN F. CRABTREE, PhD,[2] SHARON K. YENNY, RNP, MS,[3] AND MICHAEL A. SITORIOUS, MD,[1]

America is in the midst of a major demographic shift that will have repercussions for health care for some time to come (Manton & Vaupel, 1995). Currently, people aged 65 and older account for 30–40% of primary care physician visits (Schappert, 1999; Stafford et al., 1999; U.S. Bureau of the Census, 1996). As the rapid aging of the population continues toward its projected midcentury plateau, general internists and family physicians will be called upon to provide primary care to an increasing volume of elderly patients. At present, many of these physicians are unwilling or unable to do so. Surveys of primary care physicians show that between 30% and 50% limit the number of elderly patients they admit to their practices (AARP, 1995; Cykert, Kissling, Layson, & Hansen, 1995; Damiano, Momany, Willard, & Jogerst, 1997; Geiger & Krol, 1991; Lee & Gillis, 1993; Lee & Gillis, 1994). To meet the primary care needs of the aging population, researchers and policy makers must understand and respond to this phenomenon.

There have been surprisingly few attempts to determine the reasons physicians limit the number of elderly patients in their practices, and results have been inconsistent. Studies have focused on concerns with Medicare fees and documentation requirements, which clearly are sources of frustration for physicians (Cykert et al., 1995; Geiger & Krol, 1991). However, frustration with Medicare seems to explain only a small part of physicians' willingness to provide care to elderly patients. In one survey of primary care physicians, 65% reported

that low Medicare fees were a very important problem in their practices, but this did not predict whether or not they limited the number of Medicare patients they accepted (Damiano et al., 1997). Some demographic variables are associated with practice limitation, including primary care specialty (Lee & Gillis, 1993; Lee & Gillis, 1994), urban location (Cykert et al., 1995), and type of practice (solo, single specialty, or multispecialty; Cykert et al., 1995). Studies have generally not measured psychosocial or practice level variables that might contribute to physicians' perceived need to limit geriatric practice and no previous qualitative studies have addressed these issues.

Though data are sparse, there are suggestions in the literature that primary care physicians find elderly patients more difficult to treat (Damiano et al., 1997). This may have to do with medical training. In a national survey, only 60% of general and/or family practice physicians and 50% of general internists felt that their formal medical training did a good or excellent job of preparing them to manage care needs for frail elders (Cantor, Baker, & Hughes, 1993). Another survey of primary care physicians in Virginia found that fewer than half thought their current geriatric knowledge was adequate (Perez, Mulligan, & Myers, 1991). Characteristics of the health care system may also contribute to physicians' willingness to provide care to elders. In a survey of Canadian family physicians, respondents endorsed poor reimbursement, time pressure, and inadequate community resources all as sources of frustration in caring for older patients (Pereles & Russell, 1996). Although these studies

Table 1 Characteristics of Participants

Characteristic	Internists (n = 10)	Family Physicians (n = 10)
Age, mean (range)	44.9 (32–69)	49.5 (35–70)
Years since board certification, mean (range)	14.1 (2–37)	14.7 (4–26)
Female, %	60	90
Urban location, %	90	70
Practice 65 or older, mean percent (range)	57 (25–100)	32.8 (15–65)
Size of group	solo practice: 1	solo practice: 2
	2-5 physician group: 5	2–5 physician group: 2
	> 5 physician group: 4	> 5 physician group: 6
Do nursing home practice, %	60	70
Nursing home medical directors, %	40	10

suggest potential contributors to physicians' limitations on practice with elderly patients, a detailed understanding of the problems physicians encounter in geriatric primary care and a clear direction for change are sorely needed.

Given the paucity of data in this area, a research approach that allows in-depth examination of physicians' perspectives is needed. To gain a deeper, more detailed understanding of the key issues, we conducted a qualitative study that explored how physicians view providing primary care to elderly people. This article focuses on the theme that most consistently pervaded the interviews: the increased difficulty of primary care with elderly patients. We present a conceptual model, developed from these data, which suggests vital areas to be addressed to ensure that primary care of elderly people meets current and future needs.

Methods

Design and Participants

We conducted a qualitative in-depth interview study with a diverse sample of 20 practicing general internists and family physicians. The first two respondents were physicians known by one of the authors to have busy internal medicine practices with a relatively high proportion of elderly patients. Subsequently, we selected physicians practicing in the vicinity of Omaha, Nebraska, from a database maintained in the Chancellor's office at the University of Nebraska Medical Center comprising demographic information about all physicians practicing in the state. We used a maximum variation sampling strategy (Kuzel, 1999), in which we selected physicians from the list by gender, age, and specialty to compile a sample representing both men and women, internists and family practitioners, and a wide age range. We approached physicians by an introductory letter followed up by a telephone call. In all, we contacted 141 physicians to recruit the 20 participants.

Demographic and practice information about participants is shown in Table 1. Of the 20 participants recruited, 19 were White and 1 was Hispanic. Eight were women. Ages ranged from 32 to 70 years. Three respondents limited the number of elderly patients they accept into their practices; all three were busy internists with a high volume of elderly patients. In this article, a code letter has been randomly assigned to identify participants.

Procedure

Two of the authors (W. A. and H. M.), both physicians, conducted in-depth interviews (Crabtree & Miller, 1999) with the participants. The average interview lasted 50 min, with a range from 30 to 120 min. Participants appeared to respond in an equally open and forthcoming way to both interviewers. We examined interview content for systematic differences in responses to the different interviewers and were unable to detect any. We were also unable to detect any systematic differences between the responses of the two participants who were previously acquainted with the interviewer and the others, who were not. The interview questions were broad and open ended. We invited the participants to relate personal narratives regarding experiences with geriatric primary care with the initial "grand tour" question: "Please tell me about some of your experiences taking care of elderly people." We then asked them to relate both satisfying and frustrating experiences. The existing literature suggests certain topics important for physician satisfaction that may relate to their views on care of elderly patients. If these did not come up spontaneously, we asked participants to comment on them. We used such prompts for reimbursement issues (Cykert et al. 1995; Damiano et al., 1997; Lee & Gillis, 1993; Lee & Gillis, 1994), time pressure (Burdi & Baker, 1999; Lewis, Prout, Chalmers, & Leake, 1991; Linn, Yager, Cope, & Leake, 1985; Linzer et al., 2000; Mawardi, 1979), confidence in addressing geriatric syndromes (Cantor, Baker, & Hughes, 1993; Perez, Mulligan & Myers, 1991), community resources for elderly patients (Pereles & Russell, 1996; Siu & Beck, 1990), the doctor–older patient relationship (Adelman, Greene, & Ory, 2000; Bates, Harris, Tierney, & Wolinsky, 1998; Greene, 1993; McMurray et al., 1997; Roter, 1991), and frailty and death (Krakowski, 1982; Morrison, Morrison, & Glickman, 1994). We asked the physicians to describe how the doctor-patient relationship was

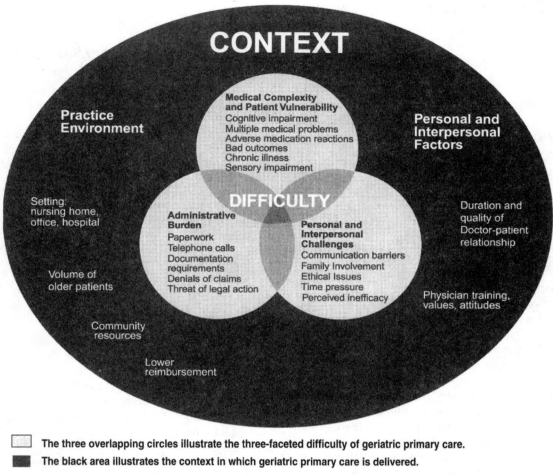

CONTEXT

Practice Environment

Medical Complexity and Patient Vulnerability
Cognitive impairment
Multiple medical problems
Adverse medication reactions
Bad outcomes
Chronic illness
Sensory impairment

Personal and Interpersonal Factors

Setting: nursing home, office, hospital

DIFFICULTY

Administrative Burden
Paperwork
Telephone calls
Documentation requirements
Denials of claims
Threat of legal action

Personal and Interpersonal Challenges
Communication barriers
Family Involvement
Ethical Issues
Time pressure
Perceived inefficacy

Duration and quality of Doctor-patient relationship

Volume of older patients

Physician training, values, attitudes

Community resources

Lower reimbursement

The three overlapping circles illustrate the three-faceted difficulty of geriatric primary care.

The black area illustrates the context in which geriatric primary care is delivered.

Figure 1   The difficulty of primary care for older people and its context.

different with older and younger patients. Other questions did not ask physicians to compare and contrast experiences with older and younger patients, but they frequently made such comparisons when discussing their experiences.

Analysis

We audiotaped and transcribed interviews verbatim. A multidisciplinary team including 2 physicians, a nurse practitioner, a medical anthropologist, a medical sociologist, and a psychologist then analyzed these data. We used a three-stage coding process derived from the sociologic tradition of grounded theory (Strauss & Corbin, 1998). In the initial *open coding* stage, each team member independently read each transcript several times and marked key phrases, terms, or sentences. We then met and discussed the interviews in detail, sharing insights from our various disciplines and assigning topical codes to the text of the interviews. We grouped these codes into categories as it became evident which concepts were emerging as keys to understanding physicians' perspectives on primary care with elderly patients. As the analysis proceeded, we compared the content of each new interview to the existing categories and the coding modified accordingly. In the *axial coding* phase, we developed the categories further and began to define the relationships

among them and their possible implications. In the final *selective coding* process, we developed the conceptual model that is presented here.

We used several techniques common to qualitative research to ensure that standards of rigor were met. To maximize the trustworthiness of our data collection and analysis, we continued recruiting participants until no new major themes were emerging (Patton, 1990). In the process of developing codes and interpreting the data, the diversity of the team kept one point of view from dominating and biasing the results (Creswell, 1998; Lincoln & Guba, 1985). We also routinely searched for disconfirming evidence in the interviews, (Patton, 1990). We conducted follow-up interviews, also known as *member checking* (Lincoln & Guba, 1985), with 5 of our participants. In these interviews, we gave participants written descriptions of the categories of difficulty and contextual conditions we had developed in the analysis process. In the last member checking interview, we presented the evolving conceptual model, similar to Figure 1 in this article. We then asked for discussion and feedback. Although not every point of difficulty was important to every physician, all strongly confirmed the importance of the increased difficulty and the appropriateness of the categories of difficulty presented here.

Results

Overview

Most participants enjoyed their interactions with older patients and emphasized that advanced patient age alone was not problematic. All, however, related experiencing increased difficulty in caring for elderly patients, which fell into three major domains: (i) medical complexity and chronicity, especially patients' vulnerability to adverse events; (ii) personal and interpersonal challenges, including time pressure, communication problems, and ethical dilemmas; and (iii) administrative burden, including more telephone calls and paperwork as well as Medicare's documentation requirements. As illustrated in Figure 1, these categories overlap and interact. For example, a medically complex situation may lead to nursing home placement, which challenges the doctor-patient-family relationship and increases administrative burden. Figure 1 also illustrates that the difficulty was experienced in the context of the practice environment and seen in the light of the personal characteristics of the physician. Although the nature of the difficulty was similar for physicians with small and large volumes of elderly patients, it had more impact on physicians with a high volume.

The Nature of the Difficulty

Medical Complexity and Vulnerability to Adverse Events. —Elderly patients were seen as medically more difficult to care for than younger people. They had more medical conditions, and their illnesses often presented atypically. They were more likely to become seriously ill and were vulnerable to rapid declines in their condition. Multiple medications and the risk of adverse medication reactions also contributed to the difficulty. Participants described diagnostic and therapeutic uncertainty as well as anxiety about causing unintended harm to patients. An internist who had inherited a large volume of elderly patients from a retiring colleague remarked, "There problems were kind of special compared with the general medical population.... The thing that impressed me the most is, their homeostatic mechanisms didn't leave much room for goof-ups" (Dr. C). Another internist described a patient's adverse drug reaction: "I thought, here is something I have done to hurt this patient by giving him this medicine.... What other things can I do to hurt people?... In a lot of ways you've got to be very careful with things" (Dr. I).

Elderly patients often have chronic conditions with symptoms that are difficult to control. "In general, they have more things wrong with them and in general, they're on way more medication and in general, they don't feel good most of the time and they don't sleep at night and they are deteriorating... " (Dr. P). This can lead to a disinclination to see these patients:

> Every time they come in something's aching or hurting or... "My back's a little sore" or "I'm a little stiff, I don't have the energy I used to," "Well, maybe I'm a little depressed." Sometimes they get to be those people that you look at the list and go, "Ah-h-h-h, dog-gone, that name again" (Dr. E).

Many participants described frustration at their perceived inability to help with older patients' chronic conditions. One family physician related,

> No matter what you do, they hurt. No matter what you do, they get agitated. And no drug exists to stop a cognitively impaired patient from falling. You know, yeah, that's frustrating. You bet it is. But hey, somebody needs to take care of these folks (Dr. I.).

An internist reported,

> You know, there are some patients that they're always going to have the same problems year after year after year. They're not going to be fixed. You know, it's their back pain from their osteoporosis and scoliosis and you can't do anything about it, or they may be a little depressed, but they won't take any medicine, and they're chronically constipated and, you know, sometimes those are the most frustrating (Dr. O).

Medical complexity also had a positive side. Several participants enthusiastically told of satisfying experiences in which they had made a difficult diagnosis and helped patients substantially. Regarding a 96-year-old woman with an atypical presentation of ischemic heart disease, a family physician remarked,

> I was able to stabilize her in the hospital, get her feeling good and actually took care of her for another two years or so.... She was so grateful that I had been able to find what was wrong with her, and she became a very dear patient to me... so that was a really good experience (Dr. J).

Adjusting to the increased prevalence of chronic illness and the relative infrequency of cures requires a change of outlook on the physician's part. One young internist seemed to be in the midst of this process when she related,

> But then I was thinking, I need to think of it in a different frame of mind. More of maybe getting them to understand that this is a chronic problem and what can we do to make them feel better as opposed to fix them. (Dr. O).

This may be an adjustment that not all physicians are able to make. Regarding caring for cognitively impaired patients, Dr. I. said,

> I mean in general, there's not a lot that medicine can do about that. Our interventions are somewhat limited, so this just adds to this area of medicine. It takes a special kind of mind set, a special kind of provider to grapple with those on a day-to-day basis.

Personal and Interpersonal Challenges. —Communication barriers, especially those resulting from hearing problems or cognitive impairment, contributed to difficulties with history taking, treatment, and the quality of the relationship. One physician remarked, "[There are] lots of various obstacles to getting the whole story, getting the truth out and sometimes 'cause they don't remember and sometimes they just don't think it's important and sometimes they're just in denial of what's really wrong" (Dr. P). Another commented, "It's sometimes frustrating when you've got an older person who can't hear and won't wear hearing aids and you know, you have to shout so loud that everyone else in the building hears everything you say to them" (Dr. J).

Families often became involved in the care of frail elders. For the physicians we interviewed, this had both positive and negative implications. Involved family members increased the safety of medication use and the home environment. However, their participation increased the length of office visits, the complexity of the doctor-patient relationship, and the difficulty of decision making. Friction with families sometimes arose when it was unclear whose responsibility it was to provide personal care:

> You know, I don't mind dealing with it as long as the family is going to deal with it too. If they act like it's all my problem to deal with Mom or Dad and figure out, you know, a solution at home for care and you know, that's what's irritating because that's not my responsibility (Dr. G).

When older patients were unsafe driving or living alone but wished to continue to do so, the need to balance safety and autonomy was sometimes difficult.

> It's usually a struggle between the family wanting them to move to a more supervised level of care or out of their home and the… parents not wanting to do that, so it's usually a negotiating process, usually a slow process (Dr. Q).

On the whole, physicians found caring for elderly patients who are dying one of the most important and meaningful aspects of practice. Most, however, had experienced serious conflicts with family members in this area. One related,

> The most difficult thing… is just the actual end of life issue when the patient is in the hospital and you have a family there, and the family doesn't get along, and then trying to be a mediator within the family to get some kind of good consensus (Dr. K).

Physicians were challenged to examine their values and balance them with the family's.

> When you internally feel like a family member is making decisions on behalf of the patient that are maybe prolonging the patient's misery… then we are kind of put into the awkward position of having to carry out what they want (Dr. L).

These decisions are frequently emotionally charged. "Our culture is so afraid of death, that usually it isn't that peaceful. It's just wrought with being torn apart by just an incredible amount of argument and bickering between family members. It's terrible" (Dr. P).

Time pressure was a major issue for participants with a large volume of elderly patients. "That's probably the biggest problem I have right now, is managing my time with the older individuals" (Dr. A). Medical complexity, family involvement, ethical decision making, and communication barriers all made caring for frail elders more time consuming. History taking was slower, physical examinations took longer, and mobility impairment slowed down the flow of office activities. Medicare's extensive documentation requirements and lengthy claims processing also make heavy demands on the physicians' time, so do paperwork and phone calls from home health agencies and nursing homes. "[If you see 15 elderly people] it takes time. You feel like you've done a big day's work. You can see 15 young people with sore throats and be done in an hour" (Dr. M). In the current health care environment, where efficiency is highly valued, this presents a major difficulty for physicians. "You have to have sheer volume with Medicare patients but Medicare patients also require most of your time because they need so much, so it's a hard situation out there" (Dr. I).

Administrative Burden. —Nearly all of the physicians felt they spent too much time, effort, and worry on Medicare regulations. Claims were often denied for apparently trivial reasons and resubmitting them requried substantial personnel time. In some situations, "The amount of return is less than the effort made in acquiring the reimbursement" (Dr. Q). Medicare regulations seemed particularly frustrating because they did not seem to relate to the quality of care.

> It has nothing to do with the care the patient got…. You go through a whole long physical exam of stuff that is irrelevant really to the problem at hand,… and spend more time on the paperwork than you do taking care of the patient. And so that's extremely frustrating as well as stupid (Dr. M).

The threat of legal action from Medicare adds additional anxiety to geriatric primary care:

> You wake up in the middle of the night in a cold sweat thinking, "Oh my God! The Office of Inspector General showed up at my office today and wants to go through every file in my charts!" So it's sobering to know what Medicare could do to you and your practice if they chose to. And I'm of the opinion they could probably find improper documentation/coding/billing in every office in this country (Dr. L).

In general, Medicare was seen in an adversarial light, increasing the burden of providing primary care to older patients.

Multifaceted Complexity

In the initial coding process, complexity and difficulty were noted in all 20 interviews. As we returned to the data for the axial coding process, it was evident that participants rarely felt overwhelmed by difficulty in one area alone. In every interview, however, there was a discussion of at least one situation where an elderly patient's medical needs overlapped with psychosocial and/or administrative difficulty. These were the situations in which caring for older patients became seriously problematic. "It's just that you have a number of these things happening all at the same time. Physicians are human. It wears on you" (Dr. N). When considering Figure 1 in a member-checking interview, one participant remarked,

> This helps me understand why these patients are so hard. It's OK if they just have difficulty in one of these areas, but when there's more than one, and especially in that area (pointing to the model) where they have all three, the difficulty is exponential, or logarithmic or something (Dr. B).

Contextual Conditions

The three-faceted difficulty presented above occurred within the context of the practice environment. There was also a context of personal and interpersonal factors. For instance, a complex medical situation that occurred within the context of a long-term doctor-patient relationship was perceived differently from a complex medical situation in the context of a new relationship. Various constellations of these contextual conditions shaped the experience of providing care and how difficult it seemed. In Figure 1, the larger circle represents this context.

Personal and Interpersonal Factors. —All participants found elderly patients more grateful and appreciative than younger patients. Some also enjoyed hearing their stories and experiencing their wisdom. For many, this mitigated the difficulty of their care.

> I enjoy taking care of elderly patients, mostly for the personal interaction with them as opposed to their medical problems. I would look at the medical care of those individuals to be a little more cumbersome than younger people from an operational standpoint. It's harder to do things, more difficult. But the interaction with the individuals is more rewarding I would say (Dr. Q).

When patients are severely cognitively impaired, on the other hand, the limited relationship often made the care seem meaningless. One internist related,

> The very severe cognitively impaired people,... I don't find any particular satisfaction in taking care of them. Whatever was... the essence of their humanity is long since gone and I'm tending to a body, which has no hope of recovery and it's hard for me to get real excited and enthusiastic in that setting (Dr. B).

A family physician said, "You have to tell them the same thing every visit. And they don't remember you. It eliminates some of the camaraderie, if you will, with the patient. That's inevitable" (Dr. L).

Physicians' personal characteristics, values, and training also affected how they viewed geriatric primary care. For instance, older physicians felt closer to their elderly patients:

> I'm not exactly young myself anymore and so I guess I have a fair amount of good feeling towards the elderly. It's easier for me to identify with somebody who is 75 and has lived through some of the things they lived through or the depression, World War II, raising chil-

dren, than a very young person with an earring in their nose and ear and their lip and I'm not sure I have much in common with that person (Dr. H).

Some participants felt a social obligation to care for nursing home patients, whereas others did not.

> It's not that much fun but I just feel like it's something that I have to do for society, part of my job. I could never do that as a full-time job or even have a larger practice in a nursing home (Dr. G).

The Practice Environment. —Certain aspects of the practice environment facilitated or hindered caring for elderly patients. The volume of older patients in the practice had a major impact on how the difficulty was experienced and whether the participant was limiting or was planning to limit the number of new elderly patients. Physicians with a high volume of older patients found it more difficult to incorporate their complex care into the usual flow of work. One internist who had currently cut back her practice related,

> The patients are so complex and they take so much time sometimes and they have side effects from medications and phone calls, that yeah, you get overwhelmed. It's just not physically, humanly possible. It just isn't. You would need to have a smaller patient population to do a good job (Dr. P).

The roles of office staff members and their relationships with the physician and each other also affected how well they were able to cope with a high volume of elderly patients. One geriatrician remarked, "[Nurses] can make you or break you. I mean, if they left, I'd have to leave" (Dr. A).

Community resources were generally perceived as inadequate. None of our participants had ready access to social workers in the office, so arranging home health care, adult daycare, and other community services added to the difficulty of primary care.

> You know, there's no one place, no one clearing house that you can go for those kind of services. You just have to kind of make a patchwork quilt almost of that. It'd be nice to have someplace where you can have one phone call… and say, here's my patient's needs, what can you provide for us? (Dr. C).

Caring for patients in nursing homes was generally regarded as difficult and unpleasant. Prominent difficulties with nursing home care included the logistics of providing care, communication with nursing home staff, and dysfunctional regulations.

> Their regulations are ridiculous, you know, especially the one where they have to call you if somebody scrapes their elbow. Nursing home visits usually aren't the most stimulating… and you have to sift through charts that you're not familiar with and where anything is and I don't know (Dr G).

Although caring for frail elders is difficult and time consuming, Medicare reimbursement is lower than private insurance.

Low fees did not contribute to the difficulty of geriatric primary care, but clearly influenced how physicians responded to it.

> If you told me that I had to run this place on the basis of what I get from Medicare, I would have to tell you I couldn't do it, which is kind of sad, because they claim that they're bankrupt and everything. Where in the hell are they spending their money? They sure ain't giving it to me (Dr. F).

The mismatch between patient needs and the level of reimbursement generates a conflict between the physician's role as healer and his or her role as business person or employee.

> You owe it to your employer to be as productive as you can but you also owe it to your patient to be as helpful as you can and sometimes the two masters can't be served at the same time (Dr. C).

The imbalance between the time required and reimbursement sometimes leads to physicians limiting geriatric practice even if they enjoy it.

> In the real world, communication takes time, whether you're communicating with an elderly person who has a delay between the time that you give them a question and the time they give you an answer, or those that can't understand or deal with complex questions.… It takes longer to take care of patients like that. You superimpose upon this slow reacting patient a worried… family member who has a number of questions.… It adds more time to the office visit and the way Medicare is paying us for office visits. From an economic standpoint it just does not make sense to take care of old people (Dr. C).

Discussion

This study, using face-to-face interviews with practicing physicians, gives an in-depth look at the difficulty involved in providing primary care to elderly patients. The voices of these physicians and the framework we propose for understanding the difficulty they described can inform future efforts to meet the health care needs of our aging population. On the whole, participants enjoyed interactions with their elderly patients, but the high prevalence of multiple medical problems and declining physical and cognitive function among these patients gave rise to interacting medical, interpersonal, and administrative difficulty. Physicians struggled to deal with the difficulty in a practice environment that was not set up to provide the support and resources these patients needed.

We are by no means the first to recognize the mismatch between the chronic care needs of our aging population and the acute orientation of our health care system (Kottke, Brekke, & Solberg, 1993; Wagner, Austin, & Von Korff, 1996). This study vividly demonstrates the real impact of this mismatch on the daily practice of medicine. In so doing, it strongly supports the need for health system change. The recent Institute of Medicine report, *Crossing the Quality Chasm,* calls for efforts to improve health care by approaching it as a "complex adaptive system" (Institute of Medicine, 2001). To effect positive change in such a system, it is essential to recognize which elements can change and which cannot. The three-faceted difficulty at the center of our model must be regarded as a fixed element of the system. Caring for chronically ill elders is and will remain complex and time consuming. There is great potential for positive change in the context in which care is delivered, however.

Our results suggest potential for change in practice organization, health care policy and medical education. In the area of practice organization, a number of interventions to facilitate primary care of chronically ill elders have been proposed and a few have been studied (Boult, Boult, Morishita, Smith, & Kane, 1998; Leveille et al., 1998; Schraeder, Shelton, & Sager, 2001; Netting & Williams, 2000; Wagner et al., 1996). The participation of nurse case managers in primary care practices, for instance, has shown benefits in elderly patient mortality and physician satisfaction (Schraeder et al., 2001). As yet, however, such interventions have met with very little acceptance by health care organizations or third party payers (Boult, Kane, Pacala, & Wagner, 1999; Wagner, Davis, Schaefer, Von Korff, & Austin, 1999). None of our participants had access to such personnel. Perhaps the greatest interpersonal challenge our participants experienced was the expansion of the doctor–patient relationship to include family members and other caregivers. Programs that facilitate communication between families and staff in the nursing home setting have shown great promise (Pillemer, Hegeman, Albright, & Henderson, 1998; Specht, Kelley, Manion, Maas, Reed, & Rantz, 2000). A similar intervention to enhance doctor–patient–family communication could be extremely helpful in the primary care setting.

Regarding health care policy, participants confirmed that Medicare documentation requirements are onerous and fees too low. Simplification of documentation requirement and increased reimbursement for complex nonprocedural care would clearly facilitate caring for elders. Participants also found the infrastructure of support services inadequate and difficult to access. Policy directed at improving community resources to meet the needs of chronically ill elders would also be extremely beneficial.

Changes in medical education could have important impact on physicians, who are themselves modifiable elements of the health care system. On the whole, participants felt confident managing specific illnesses, but lacked confidence in dealing with geriatric issues, such as vulnerability to adverse medical events and cognitive impairment. They experienced the greatest difficulty when the medical problems overlapped with interpersonal challenges and administrative burden. Despite the long recognition of the demographic imperative, few medical schools have mandatory geriatrics rotations and residencies devote minimal time to geriatrics training (Association of Professors of Medicine, 2001). With additional training, physicians could become more skilled and comfortable with the special needs of elderly patients.

This report has both strengths and limitations to consider. The qualitative format allowed participants' views to be explored in depth, adding important information to our understanding of primary care for elderly patients. Because of its intensive nature, however, a qualitative study can include only a small number of participants. Although we found striking consistency in the main themes, it is possible that our participants were systematically different from nonparticipants or physicians in other locales. Larger quantitative studies will determine the generalizability of our findings.

Although primary care for elderly people is rewarding and enjoyable, it is also complex, difficult, and time-consuming. Physicians alone cannot meet the wide range of needs these people have in the current practice environment. Our findings suggest that changes in practice organization, health policy, and medical education will be needed if primary care physicians are to care for a larger volume of elderly patients effectively.

References

AARP. (1995). *Reforming the health care system: State profiles 1995.* Washington, DC: Public Policy Institute.

Adelman, R., Greene, M., & Ory, M. (2000). Communication between older patients and their physicians. *Clinics in Geriatric Medicine, 16,* 1–24.

Association of Professors of Medicine. (2001). Internal medicine: At the nexus of the health care system in responding to the demographic imperative of an aging population. *The American Journal of Medicine, 110,* 507–513.

Bates, A., Harris, L., Tierney, W., & Wolinsky, F. (1998). Dimensions and correlates of physician work satisfaction in a midwestern city. *Medical Care, 36,* 610–617.

Boult, C., Boult, L., Morishita, L., Smith, S., & Kane, R. (1998). Outpatient geriatric evaluation and management. *Journal of the American Geriatrics Society, 46,* 296–302.

Boult, C., Kane, R., Pacala, J., & Wagner, E. (1999). Innovative healthcare for chronically ill older persons: Results of a national survey. *American Journal of Managed Care, 5,* 1162–1172.

Burdi, M., & Baker, K. (1999). Physicians' perceptions of autonomy and satisfaction in California. *Health Affairs, 18,* 134–145.

Cantor, J., Baker, L., & Hughes, R. (1993). Preparedness for practice. Young physicians' views of their professional education. *Journal of American Medical Association, 270,* 1035–1040.

Crabtree, B., & Miller, W. (1999). *Doing qualitative research.* Thousand Oaks, CA: Sage.

Creswell, J. (1998). Standards of Quality and Verification. In *Qualitative Inquiry and Research Design: Choosing Among Five Traditions* (pp. 193–218). Thousand Oaks, CA: Sage.

Cykert, S., Kissling, G., Layson, R., & Hansen, C. (1995). Health insurance does not guarantee access to primary care: A national study of physicians' acceptance of publicly insured patients. *Journal of General Internal Medicine, 10,* 345–348.

Damiano, P., Momany, E., Willard, J., & Jogerst, G. (1997). Factors affecting primary care physician participation in Medicare. *Medical Care, 35,* 1008–1019.

Geiger, W., & Krol, R. (1991). Physician attitudes and behavior in response to changes in Medicare reimbursement policies. *Journal of Family Practice, 33,* 244–248.

Greene, W. (1993). *Econometric analysis.* New York: Macmillan.

Institute of Medicine. (2001). *Crossing the quality chasm: A new health system for the 21st century.* Washington, DC: National Academy Press.

Kottke, T., Brekke, M., & Solberg, L. (1993). Making "time" for preventive services. *Mayo Clinical Proceedings, 68,* 785–791.

Krakowski, A. (1982). Stress and the practice of medicine: II. Stressors, stresses and strains. *Psychotherapy and Psychosomatics, 38,* 11–23.

Kuzel, A. (1999). Sampling in qualitative inquiry. In B. F. Crabtree & W. Miller, *Doing qualitative research* (pp. 33–46). Thousand Oaks, CA: Sage.

Lee, D., & Gillis, K. (1993). Physician responses to Medicare physician payment reform: Preliminary results on access to care. *Inquiry, 30,* 417–428.

Lee, D., & Gillis, K. (1994). Physician responses to Medicare payment reform: An update on access to care. *Inquiry, 31,* 346–353.

Leveille, S., Wagner, E., Davis, D., Grothaus, L., Wallace, J., LoGerfo, M., et al. (1998). Preventing disability and managing chronic illness in frail older adults: A randomized trial of a community-based partnership with primary care. *Journal of the American Geriatrics Society, 46,* 1191–1198.

Lewis, C., Prout, D., Chalmers, E., & Leake, B. (1991). How satisfying is the practice of internal medicine? *Annals of Internal Medicine, 114,* 1–5.

Lincoln, Y., & Guba, E. (1985). *Naturalistic inquiry.* Newbury Park, CA: Sage.

Linn, L., Yager, J., Cope, D., & Leake, B. (1985). Health status, job satisfaction, job stress, and life satisfaction among academic and clinical faculty. *Journal of the American Medical Association, 254,* 2775–2782.

Linzer, M., Konrad, T., Douglas, J., McMurray, J., Pathman, D., Williams, E., et al. (2000). Managed care, time pressure, and physician job satisfaction: Results from the physician worklife study. *Journal of General Internal Medicine, 15,* 441–450.

Manton, K., & Vaupel, J. (1995). Survival after the age of 80 in the United States, Sweden, France, England, and Japan. *The New England Journal of Medicine, 333,* 1232–1235.

Mawardi, B. (1979). Satisfaction, dissatisfaction, and causes of stress in medical practice. *Journal of the American Medical Association, 241,* 1483–1486.

McMurray, J., Williams, E., Schwartz, M., Douglas, J., Van Kirk, J., Konrad, R., et al. (1997). Physician job satisfaction: Developing a model using qualitative data. *Journal of General Internal Medicine, 12,* 711–714.

Morrison, R., Morrison, E., & Glickman, D. (1994). Physician reluctance to discuss advance directives. *Archives of Internal Medicine, 154,* 2311–2318.

Netting, F., & Williams, F. (2000). Expanding the boundaries of primary care for elderly people. *Health and Social Work, 25,* 233–242.

Patton, M. (1990). *Qualitative evaluation and research methods.* Newbury Park, CA: Sage.

Pereles, L., & Russell, M. (1996). Needs for CME in geriatrics, part 2: Physician priorities and perceptions of community representatives. *Canadian Family Physician, 42,* 632–640.

Perez, E., Mulligan, T., & Meyers, M. (1991). Interest in geriatrics education among family practitioners and internists in Virginia. *Academic Medicine, 66,* 558–559.

Pillemer, K., Hegeman, C., Albright, B., & Henderson, C. (1998). Building bridges between families and nursing home staff: The partners in caregiving program. *The Gerontologist, 38,* 499–503.

Roter, D. (1991). Elderly patient-physician communication: A descriptive study of content and affect during the medical encounter. *Advances in Health Education, 3,* 15–23.

Schappert, S. (1999). Ambulatory care visits to physician offices, hospital outpatient departments, and emergency departments: United States, 1997. *Vital Health Statistics, 13* (143), 1–39.

Schraeder, C., Shelton, P., & Sager, M. (2001). The effects of a collaborative model of primary care on the mortality and hospital use of community-dwelling older adults. *Journal of Gerontology: Medical Sciences, 56A,* M106–M112.

Siu, A., & Beck, J. (1990). Physician satisfaction with career choices in geriatrics. *The Gerontologist, 30,* 529–534.

Specht, J., Kelley, L., Manion, P., Maas, M., Reed, D., & Rantz, M. (2000). Who's the boss? Family/staff partnership in care of persons with dementia. *Nursing Administrator Quarterly, 24,* 64–77.

Stafford, R., Saglam, D., Causino, N., Starfield, B., Culpepper, L., Marder, W., et al. (1999). Trends in adult visits to primary care physicians in the United States. *Archives of Family Medicine, 8,* 26–32.

Strauss, A., & Corbin, J. (1998). *Basics of qualitative research: Grounded theory procedures and techniques.* Newbury Park, CA: Sage.

U.S. Bureau of the Census. (1996). Current population reports, special studies, P23-190, 65 + in the United States. *Current Population Reports.* Washington, DC: U.S. Government Printing Office.

Wagner, E., Austin, B., & Von Korff, M. (1996). Organizing care for patients with chronic illness. *Milbank Quarterly, 74,* 511–544.

Wagner, E., Davis, C., Schaefer, J., Von Korff, M., & Austin, B. (1999). A survey of leading chronic disease management programs: Are they consistent with the literature? *Managed Care Quarterly, 7,* 56–66.

We are most grateful to all the physicians who donated their time for the interviews. We also thank **JEFF SUSMAN, MD, KURT STANGE, MD,** and **LYNN MEADOWS, PHD,** for their helpful critiques of earlier drafts of this article; **JOHN CRESWELL, PHD,** for methodologic advice; and **LINDA FERRING** for manuscript preparation. This study was approved by the Institutional Review Board at the University of Nebraska Medical Center.

Address correspondence to Wendy L. Adams, MD, MPH, Department of Family Medicine, University of Nebraska Medical Center, 983075 Nebraska Medical Center, Omaha, NE 68198-3075. E-mail: Wadams@ unmc.edu

Notes

1. Department of Family Medicine, University of Nebraska Medical Center, Omaha.

2. Department of Family Medicine, Robert Wood Johnson Medical School, University of Medicine and Dentistry of New Jersey, New Brunswick.

3. VA Nebraska–Western Iowa Health Care System, Omaha, NE.

Breakthrough

A landmark Supreme Court decision is being hailed as 'the Emancipation Proclamation for older workers'

DAVID NEWMAN

The U.S. Supreme Court struck a major blow for age equality in the workplace when it declared last month that a bulwark of civil rights laws against race and sex discrimination should also protect employees who bring suits in federal court under the Age Discrimination in Employment Act (ADEA). Plaintiffs can now bypass what is often the hardest-to-prove aspect of their cases—showing that their employer's discrimination was deliberate—by arguing instead that they were victims of a policy that caused harm to older workers and went beyond "reasonable" business considerations.

Just as important as the practical benefits of the result, which AARP supported in a friend-of-the-court brief, is the long-term effect that the decision, *Smith v. City of Jackson, Miss.*, will have in elevating age discrimination legally closer to the level of race or gender bias. After years of standing on the sidelines, says Washington lawyer Richard Seymour, a former chair of the Employment Rights Division at the American Trial Lawyers Association, the Supreme Court has finally sent a message that age discrimination is a serious problem that must be attacked when it is unintentional as well as when it is intentional. Seymour goes so far as to call the decision "the Emancipation Proclamation for older workers."

"We were thrilled with the decision," says Laurie McCann, an AARP senior attorney. "We were losing this battle in the federal courts, so the victory was somewhat unexpected."

The justices' reasoning for the *Smith* decision is steeped in references to a race discrimination case from 1971 that represents a high-water mark in employment discrimination law. In *Griggs v. Duke Power Co.* the Supreme Court found that even a seemingly neutral job requirement (the case was about making employment conditional on having a high school diploma) counted as discrimination, since its effect was to keep a disproportionate number of qualified black applicants from getting hired, a so-called disparate impact.

The scope of discrimination based on age will be narrower because the ADEA, while generally modeled on race and sex discrimination laws, allows employers to treat older workers differently as long as they do so based on "reasonable factors other than age."

The effect of this provision is apparent in the result in *Smith* itself, a case about whether the city of Jackson could restructure its salaries for police officers in a way that gave the bulk of a new raise package to more junior officers. The plaintiffs—older officers—contended that this kind of pay-raise system, even if devised in good faith, amounted to illegal age discrimination because it worked mostly to the benefit of officers who tended to be younger.

Reversing two lower courts, the Supreme Court agreed that, in theory, a case could go forward even if the city did not intend to discriminate against older officers. (This step is what opens the door to a new standard in future cases.) However, the court went on to say that the city's justification for its policy—that it wanted to make its entry-level salaries competitive with those offered in neighboring towns—was "reasonable" and justified the discrepancy. Even applying the new standard, in other words, the court found that the *Smith* case should be dismissed.

Because *Smith* and similar age discrimination cases focus on broad policies affecting large numbers of workers, they mostly involve big businesses and other employers (like governments) that make employment decisions using objective formulas. That means the Supreme Court's latest decision gives victims of age discrimination a powerful new weapon, McCann says. If they can tell a story with statistics, they no longer need to have a "smoking gun," such as a memo showing hostility to older workers, to persuade a judge to move their case forward to the evidence-gathering phase.

Merely getting to that point is often tantamount to victory. It is during this pretrial phase that a plaintiff's lawyer can force the other side to produce additional evidence—and gain additional leverage to settle—by subpoenaing documents, taking depositions and preparing witnesses.

With most defendants limited to large employers, Seymour says, the number of lawsuits filed may never be overwhelming. But he is also "as confident that we will catch companies doing wrong as I am that the sun will rise tomorrow," predicting there will soon be at least one major suit against a nationwide employer.

That would jibe with what's going on in Minnesota, Michigan and Ohio, which already have disparate impact standards in place at the state level. In Michigan, for example, AARP attorneys joined a suit that alleged bias against older workers in Ford Motor Company's employee ranking system.

Ford had implemented an A-B-C letter system for ranking its 18,000 employees, which it used to justify terminations and salary increases. "The statistics were just staggering," McCann says. "If you were over 40, the chances of getting a C ranking and not getting a raise were much higher. I don't think Ford wanted to defend a disparate impact case given those numbers."

In the end, Ford paid $10.6 million in a settlement with older workers who had brought the suit.

With the matter of proving intent settled, many experts agree the latest decision fails to give lower courts sufficient guidance about what is "reasonable" and "unreasonable" when it comes to issues like salary and experience, factors that are often correlated with age and can figure prominently in employer calculations. That will be the focus in the next wave of litigation. "AARP plans to be very active by filing friend-of-the-court briefs to make sure 'reasonable' isn't drawn too broadly," McCann says.

Paul Mollica, a partner in a Chicago-based firm that specializes in discrimination cases, believes that in the near term the latest decision will allow lawyers to go after "capricious, arbitrary" policies. It remains to be seen, however, what effect the decision will have on employers that have carefully considered their policies and the alternatives.

"We don't yet know what it means for an employer to have made a 'reasonable' business decision," says Tom Goldstein, an appellate court litigator who represented the veteran Jackson police officers at the Supreme Court.

Part of the tangle is trying to reconcile *Smith* with the court's previous rulings in discrimination cases. In 1993 a unanimous Supreme Court rejected the age discrimination claim of a 62-year-old worker who alleged he had been fired by his employer because he was about to become eligible for a pension. Intentional discrimination, the court stated, "captures the essence of what Congress sought to prohibit in the ADEA." Although March's opinion seems to push back against that kind of reasoning, the court notably did not go so far as to overrule it—and in fact took pains to stress that "age, unlike race or [sex] classifications … not uncommonly has relevance to an individual's capacity to engage in certain types of employment."

In *Smith*, Justice Antonin Scalia cast the deciding vote. While emphasizing that he didn't agree with all of the reasoning of the concurring justices, Scalia said he could reach the same result because the Equal Employment Opportunity Commission, the federal agency that has the job of enforcing the ADEA, had already endorsed the position. "This is an absolutely classic case for deference to agency interpretation," Scalia wrote.

When it comes to age, Scalia has given himself room to break away from the other four justices in future cases that ask the court to say more about what kind of discrimination is "reasonable." Scalia's thinking also indicates that he might be willing to shift his position if the EEOC were to shift its interpretation of the statute.

The EEOC is already under fire for a controversial regulation it issued in the age discrimination context (see <u>Retirees Win on EEOC's Benefits Rule</u>), and McCann cautions that "it would be a horrible PR move for them to try to undermine this Supreme Court decision."

DAVID NEWMAN is a contributing editor to *Legal Affairs* magazine.

Marital History and the Burden of Cardiovascular Disease in Midlife

This study examines the effects of marital history on the burden of cardiovascular disease in midlife. With use of data from the 1992 Health and Retirement Study, a series of nested logistic regression models was used to estimate the association between marital history and the likelihood of cardiovascular disease. Results suggest that, in midlife, the continuously married and the never married are among the healthiest in cardiovascular outcomes. People with multiple marital losses are the most vulnerable group. People with multiple marital losses have a higher likelihood of cardiovascular disease and will need significant formal and informal care as they advance into old age.

ZHENMEI ZHANG, PHD[1]

Being married is associated with longer life expectancy and lower rates of chronic health conditions (Pienta, Hayward, & Jenkins, 2000; Waite & Gallagher, 2000). However, during the past several decades, first-marriage rates declined, while rates of never marrying, divorce, and cohabitation increased significantly (Bianchi & Casper, 2000). The legacy of dramatic increases in singlehood, divorce, and cohabitation, combined with longer life expectancy, means that more and more people are entering old age after experiencing multiple marital transitions (Pienta et al.). What are the implications of marital history on the well-being of cohorts currently on the cusp of old age?

Although many researchers have examined marital status and health, the focus has been on the effects of current marital status on health. Drawing on the 1992 Health and Retirement Study (HRS), this study expands on previous research by examining the health consequences of marital history—that is, the number of marriages, the number and type of marital losses, and cohabitation. Previous research has shown that a marital loss is usually harmful to health (Waite & Gallagher, 2000). What remains unclear is (a) whether the negative effects of marital loss can be modified or erased when a person enters a new relationship, and (b) the health implications of experiencing multiple marital breakups.

Enlightened by the life-course perspective, recent research suggests that the timing and sequence of life events—like marriage and marital dissolution—may lead to different life outcomes in later life through cumulative advantages and disadvantages (Dannefer, 1987; O'Rand, 1996; Wilmoth & Koso, 2002). Specifically, negative events can accumulate over the life course through episodes of illness, adverse socioeco-

nomic conditions, and unhealthy behaviors, resulting in differential lifetime exposure to underlying causal factors of diseases (Kuh & Ben-Shlomo, 1997). This so-called cumulative-effects model suggests that different life trajectories can be associated with different disease risks (Kuh & Ben-Shlomo).

A growing body of research supports the cumulative-effects model. Holden and Kuo (1996) found that people who experienced multiple marital transitions had significantly lower incomes and assets than couples in first marriages. Lower socioeconomic status might be one of the pathways linking multiple marital transitions and health. In terms of mortality, research in the United States as well as in Europe has shown that remarried persons have significantly higher mortality than the continuously married (Hemstrom, 1996; Tucker, Friedman, Wingard, & Schwartz, 1996).

An alternative perspective used in the literature on marital status and health—that is, the selection hypothesis—states that health is associated with marital status through the process of marital selection: Individuals suffering from health problems are less likely to marry and stay married than those who are healthy (Fu & Goldman, 1996; Joung, van de Mheen, Stronks, van Poppel, & Mackenbach, 1997; Lillard & Panis, 1996). In addition, previous research has shown that people with higher education and good economic prospects are more likely to get married (Smock, Manning, & Porter, 2005). This positive socioeconomic selection into marriage suggests that the observed advantage in health enjoyed by married couples cannot be entirely contributed to marriage itself. Nonetheless, there is little evidence that the selection process plays a major role in generating the health advantages of married people (Johnson & Wu, 2002; Waite & Gallagher, 2000).

Infrastructural support was provided by National Institute of Child Health and Human Development Population Center Grants 1 R24HD41025 to The Pennsylvania State University and R21HD04283101 to Bowling Green State University.

Address correspondence to Zhenmei Zhang, Department of Sociology, Bowling Green State University, Bowling Green, OH 43403. E-mail: zzhang@bgnet.bgsu.edu

[1]Center for Family and Demographic Research and the Department of Sociology, Bowling Green State University, OH.

Table 1 Descriptive Statistics of Dependent and Key Independent Variables, 1992 HRS

Variable	%
Dependent variables	
Heart disease	12.7
Heart attack	5.6
Stroke	2.6
Key independent variables	
Marital trajectories	
Continuously married (reference)	54.8
Remarried after one divorce	13.4
Remarried after one widowhood	1.9
Remarried after multiple marital losses	4.3
Separated or divorced once	9.1
Separated or divorced with multiple marital losses	4.7
Widowed once	4.5
Widowed with multiple marital losses	1.4
Cohabiting	2.3
Never married	3.7

Notes: HRS = Health and Retirement Study. The means and percentages are weighted.

Previous work in this area often focused on mortality and mental health as the primary health outcomes. The present study examines cardiovascular disease, the main cause of the burden of disability and the leading cause of death in midlife (National Center for Health Statistics, 2004). Two basic questions guide this research: (a) Are various characteristics of the marital history (e.g., current marital status, number and type of marital losses) associated with the likelihood of cardiovascular disease in midlife? and (b) Can socioeconomic status, health behaviors, and social integration explain the links between marital history and cardiovascular morbidity?

Methods

Data

Data from the 1992 HRS were used to examine the association between marital history and the likelihood of cardiovascular disease. The HRS is a nationally representative sample of adults aged 51–61 and their spouses. Individuals in this cohort provide a unique opportunity to examine the effects of marital. history on health because they were subject to high divorce rates throughout their adulthood from the late 1960s to the 1980s (Wilmoth & Koso, 2002). The analytic sample for the current study was restricted to 9,677 age-eligible respondents with complete information on marital history. The mean age of the sample was 55.6, and women accounted for 52.4% of the respondents. About 86.2% of the respondents were White, 10.3% were Black, and the remaining 3.5% belonged to other racial and ethnic groups. The HRS was based on a complex sampling design, and consequently all models were estimated using the statistical software package SUDAAN Version 9.0 (Research Triangle Institute, 2005), which adjusts standard errors to correct for design effects. All models are based on weighted data.

Measures

Dependent Variables. —This study focuses on three cardiovascular outcomes: heart disease, heart attack, and stroke. Respondents reported whether a doctor ever told them that they had a particular cardiovascular problem. A dichotomous indicator of heart disease was created, where 1 = respondent reported that he or she had had a heart attack, coronary heart disease, angina, congestive heart failure, or other heart problems, and 0 = otherwise. The same method was used to create the indicators of heart attack and stroke. Table 1 shows that approximately 12.7% of the sample reported having heart disease, 5.6% reported having had a heart attack, and 2.6% reported having had a stroke.

Independent Variables. —Respondents were classified into one of 10 mutually exclusive marital history groups: (a) continuously married, (b) remarried after one divorce, (c) remarried after one widowhood, (d) remarried after multiple marital losses (either multiple divorces, multiple widowhoods, or a combination of divorce and widowhood), (e) separated or divorced once, (f) separated or divorced with multiple marital losses, (g) widowed once, (h) widowed with multiple marital losses, (i) never married, and (j) cohabiting. Table 1 describes the distribution of the HRS respondents' marital history. In midlife, only about 54.8% of respondents were still in their first marriages, 13.4% were remarried after a divorce, 1.9% were remarried after being widowed, and 4.3% were remarried after experiencing multiple marital dissolutions. A significant proportion of respondents were unmarried: About 9.1% had separated or divorced once, 4.7% were separated or divorced with multiple marital dissolutions, 4.5% had been widowed once, 1.4% were widowed with multiple marital dissolutions, and 3.7% had never married. About 2.3% of the sample was cohabiting. A closer look at the cohabitants reveals that the majority (86.3%) had gone through at least one marital loss. Regardless of current marital status, 41.3% of respondents had experienced at least one marital loss (either separation or divorce or widowhood); as many as 11.3% of respondents had gone through two or more marital losses by midlife.

Three mechanisms may potentially mediate the association between marital history and cardiovascular-disease morbidity: socioeconomic status, health behavior, and social integration.

Four indicators of socioeconomic status were created: education, household income, wealth, and health insurance coverage. Education measured the number of years of schooling completed. Household income measured the household income during 1991. Wealth represented the market value of respondents' assets minus debts. Household income and wealth were adjusted by adding constants to all households to eliminate zero income and negative wealth, respectively, and then logging the values. Respondents were considered uninsured when they were not covered by any health insurance programs.

Four types of health behaviors were examined: smoking status, alcohol consumption, exercise, and body mass index (BMI). Smoking status included current smokers and past smokers, with people who had never smoked as the reference group. Alcohol consumption included 1–2 drinks per day and 3 or more drinks per day, with 0 drinks per day as the reference group. Exercise was coded 1 if the respondent exercised three times a week or more. BMI was measured as a categorical variable including obesity (BMI ≥ 30), overweight (25.0 ≤ BMI ≤ 29.9), and underweight (BMI < 18.5), with normal weight (18.5 ≤ BMI ≤ 24.9) as the reference group.

Social integration was measured by three variables: childlessness, parental survival status, and church attendance. Childlessness was coded 1 if the respondent had no children. Parental survival status was a categorical variable including one living parent and both parents living, with no living parents as the reference category. Church attendance was a categorical variable including attendance one or more times a week, monthly, or yearly, with non-churchgoers as the reference category.

Age, gender, race, and nativity were controlled in this study because previous research has found that they are associated with cardiovascular disease. The risk of such disease increases with age, and men are more likely than women to develop cardiovascular disease (Black, 1992). Blacks are more likely than Whites to have hypertension and stroke, and foreign-born individuals are less likely than their American-born counterparts to have cardiovascular disease (Hayward, Crimmins, Miles, & Yang, 2000; Jasso, Massey, Rosenzweig, & Smith, 2004). Age was measured as a continuous variable ranging from 51 to 61 years old. Gender (1 = female) and nativity (1 = foreign born) were dummy variables. Race was a categorical variable including Black and Other, with White as the reference category. The weighted descriptive statistics for the independent variables are available from the author upon request.

Analytic Strategy

A series of nested logistic regression models was used to examine differences in the odds of cardiovascular disease across marital history groups and to determine whether the effects of marital history were reduced after introducing the hypothesized mechanisms into the model. The main effects of marital history on the likelihood of cardiovascular disease were examined in Model 1, controlling for age, gender, race, and nativity. In Model 2, the four indicators of socioeconomic status were added to Model 1. And in Model 3, health behaviors and social integration were added to Model 2. Finally, the significance of the interaction between gender and marital history was examined by introducing a set of interaction terms for gender and marital history to Model 3. Although prior work indicated that gender differences existed in the association between marital status and a few health outcomes such as mental health and self-assessed health (e.g., Brown, Bulanda, & Lee, 2005; Williams & Umberson, 2004), only one gender difference reached statistical significance in this study. Therefore, the result is not presented in the table but is described later in the article.

Results

Table 2 reports estimated odds ratios from logistic regression models. Model 1 in Table 2 shows that (controlling for age, gender, race, and nativity) the continuously married and the never married—the two groups who did not experience any marital loss—were among the healthiest groups in terms of every cardiovascular outcome examined. Because the continuously married tend to fare better than others, the cumulative-effects model is partially supported. Furthermore, the relative good cardiovascular health of never-married adults casts some doubt on the selection hypothesis, which would predict the never married as one of the most disadvantaged groups.

Three other findings are also consistent with the cumulative-effects hypothesis. First, although a marital loss, divorce in particular was associated with higher risks of several types of cardiovascular disease; the negative effect increased with the number of the losses. For example, Model 1 shows that regardless of current marital status, individuals who experienced one divorce were significantly more likely than the continuously married to report having had a heart attack but did not have significantly higher rates of heart disease or stroke. In contrast, the remarried with multiple marital losses were significantly more likely than the continuously married to report having had heart disease, a heart attack, or a stroke. The odds of having heart disease, a heart attack, or a stroke among the remarried with multiple marital losses were higher by 58%, 80%, and 128%, respectively, than the odds among the continuously married. The odds of having heart disease, a heart attack, or a stroke among the currently divorced with multiple marital losses were higher by 68%, 109%, and 129%, respectively, than the odds of the continuously married. Similar disadvantages were also found for the currently widowed who had experienced multiple marital losses. Second, loss of first-marriage partners to death did not significantly increase the risk of cardiovascular disease for middle-aged people if no additional marital loss followed. For example, persons who had been widowed once and persons who had remarried after one widowhood were not significantly different from the continuously married. Third, the cohabitants were substantially disadvantaged. They were significantly more likely than the continuously married to report having had a heart attack or stroke. Because the majority of cohabitants had gone through at least one marital loss, this finding supports the cumulative-effects hypothesis.

The addition of socioeconomic status in Model 2 of Table 2 reduced but did not explain away the health advantages enjoyed by the continuously married. For example, with the inclusion of socioeconomic status, the odds of heart disease, heart attack, or stroke for the remarried who had experienced multiple losses dropped about 5%, 9%, and 7%, respectively, but were still statistically significant. Socioeconomic status played a much larger role in explaining the higher likelihood of cardiovascular disease among the divorced who had experienced multiple marital losses. Their odds of heart disease, heart attack, and stroke dropped about 16%, 24%, and 24%, respectively, when socioeconomic status was controlled. The results suggest that socioeconomic status is an important mechanism linking marital history and cardiovascular problems. Model 3 introduced health

Table 2 Odds Ratios From Logistic Regression Models: Marital History and CVD, 1992 HRS

Model	Heart Disease	Heart Attack	Stroke
Model 1			
Remarried after one divorce	1.13	1.36*	1.07
Remarried after one widowhood	1.28	1.26	0.88
Remarried after multiple marital losses	1.58**	1.80**	2.28**
Separated or divorced once	1.16	1.41*	1.42
Separated or divorced with multiple marital losses	1.68**	2.09**	2.29**
Widowed once	0.99	0.89	1.28
Widowed with multiple marital losses	1.89**	2.20†	1.20
Never married	0.99	1.03	0.74
Cohabiting	1.17	1.95*	2.37*
−2 × Log-likelihood	7,205.00	3,961.47	2,253.28
Model 2			
Remarried after one divorce	1.13	1.36*	1.07
Remarried after one widowhood	1.27	1.22	0.86
Remarried after multiple marital losses	1.50**	1.64*	2.11**
Separated or divorced once	1.02	1.17	1.19
Separated or divorced with multiple marital losses	1.41**	1.58*	1.74†
Widowed once	0.85	0.70	1.03
Widowed with multiple marital losses	1.63*	1.73	0.96
Never married	0.84	0.82	0.58
Cohabiting	1.18	1.82*	2.21*
−2 × Log-likelihood	7,120.02	3,869.56	2,214.63
Model 3			
Remarried after one divorce	1.13	1.33†	1.05
Remarried after one widowhood	1.28	1.21	0.87
Remarried after multiple marital losses	1.49**	1.53†	2.05†
Separated or divorced once	1.06	1.25	1.23
Separated or divorced with multiple marital losses	1.44**	1.59*	1.73†
Widowed once	0.82	0.67	0.99
Widowed with multiple marital losses	1.52*	1.53	0.94
Never married	1.06	1.03	0.83
Cohabiting	1.27	1.97*	2.38*
−2 × Log-likelihood	7,016.40	3,786.25	2,155.13
N	9,677	9,677	9,677

Notes: Model specification: Model 1 controlled for age, gender, race, and nativity; Model 2 added socioeconomic status to Model 1; Model 3 added health behaviors and social integration to Model 2. Continuously married was the reference category for all three models.

*$p < .05$; **$p < .01$; †$p < .1$.

behaviors and social integration to Model 2. Overall, the disparities of the odds of cardiovascular disease across marital-history groups persisted. Health behaviors and social integration did not explain much of the remaining health advantage of the continuously married once socioeconomic status was controlled.

In models not shown here, multiplicative interaction terms for gender and each marital history group were added in Model 3 of Table 2 to examine whether the effects of marital history on the likelihood of cardiovascular disease differed significantly between men and women. Results suggested that the effects of marital history on the risk of cardiovascular disease were similar for men and women with one exception: After controlling for demographic characteristics, socioeconomic status, health behaviors, and social integration, first-time widows were significantly more likely than their male counterparts to report having had a heart attack.

Discussion

This study examined the effects of marital history on the likelihood of cardiovascular disease in midlife. Results suggest that current marital status and the number and type of marital losses are associated with the likelihood of cardiovascular problems, with demographic controls. Consistent with the cumulative-effects model, the continuously married and the never married are among the healthiest in cardiovascular outcomes. People with multiple marital losses are the most vulnerable group, with significantly higher odds of cardiovascular disease than the continuously married. In addition, people who have divorced once, regardless of current marital status, have a higher risk of heart attack. However, first-time widows and widowers do not seem to be at a disadvantage compared with the continuously married. This is consistent with the argument that divorce often involves long-term marital strain and stress before and/or after divorce, whereas widowhood usually exerts acute short-term stress. Long-term stress can lead to cardiovascular problems. The results also show that cohabitants are at high risk of heart attack and stroke. As for the mechanisms linking marital history and cardiovascular health, socioeconomic status plays a significant role in explaining the higher risk of cardiovascular disease among people with multiple marital losses. However, differences in health behaviors and social integration do not explain many of the remaining differences.

There are several limitations to this study. First, because the 1992 HRS did not contain information about the relative timing of marital transitions and the onset of cardiovascular disease (HRS only asked about the year of the most recent heart attack and stroke), no causal inferences can be drawn between marital history and disease. Both health selectivity into stable marriages and cumulative negative effects of marital losses can produce the cardiovascular-disease morbidity patterns observed in this study. It is highly possible that both processes are operating. The relative good cardiovascular health of the never married, however, casts some doubt on the selection hypothesis. In order to disentangle causal processes, longitudinal data with detailed life-course information about respondents' childhood socioeconomic status, personality traits, family history of cardiovascular disease, and health status before and after marital losses are needed. Second, recent studies suggest that different dimensions of marital quality are related to well-being. The incorporation of quality of current and/or previous marriages may shed light on issues such as whether the health disadvantage of the divorced is due more to poor marital quality before the divorce than to events and conditions after the divorce. Nonetheless, the present results suggest that substantial health disparities exist across different marital trajectories in the risk of cardiovascular disease.

As the trend of marital instability shows no sign of abating, and more and more people live longer than ever before, the number of people with multiple marital losses will certainly increase in the future. This group of people, regardless of current marital status, has a higher risk of cardiovascular disease than the continuously married. Considering the debilitating nature of cardiovascular disease, they will need significant formal and informal care as they advance into old age. This study demonstrated the importance of going beyond current marital status in the study of marital status and health in old age as the marital history of baby boomers becomes increasingly complex.

References

Bianchi, S. M., Casper, L. M. (2000). American families. *Population Bulletin 5*(4), 1–40.

Black, H. (1992). Cardiovascular risk factors. In B. L. Zaret, L. S. Cohen, & M. Moser (Eds.), *The Yale University School of Medicine heart book* (pp. 23–35). New York: Hearst Books.

Brown, S. L., Bulanda, J. R., & Lee, G. R. (2005). The significance of nonmarital cohabitation: Marital status and mental health benefits among middle-aged and older adults. *Journal of Gerontology: Social Sciences, 60B*, S21–S29.

Dannefer, D. (1987). Aging as intracohort differentiation: Accentuation, the Matthew effect, and the life course. *Sociological Forum, 2*, 211–236.

Fu, H., Goldman, N. (1996). Incorporating health into models of marriage choice: Demographic and sociological perspective. *Journal of Marriage and the Family, 58*, 740–758.

Hayward, M. D., Crimmins, E. M., Miles, T. P., & Yang, Y. (2000). The significance of socioeconomic status in explaining the racial gap in chronic health conditions. *American Sociological Review, 65*, 910–930.

Hemstrom, O. (1996). Is marriage dissolution linked to differences in mortality risks for men and women? *Journal of Marriage and the Family, 58*, 366–378.

Holden, K. C., & Kuo, D. H. (1996). Complex marital histories and economic well-being: The continuing legacy of divorce and widowhood as the HRS cohort approaches retirement. *The Gerontologist, 36*, 383–390.

Jasso, G., Massey, D., Rosenzweig, M., & Smith, J. (2004). Immigration health: Selectivity and acculturation. In N. B. Anderson, R. A. Bulatao, & B. Cohen (Eds.), *Critical perspectives on racial and ethnic differences in health in late life* (pp. 227–266). Washington, DC: National Academies Press.

Johnson, D. R., & Wu, J. (2002). An empirical test of crisis, social selection, and role explanations of the relationship between marital disruption and psychological distress: A pooled time-series analysis of four-wave panel data. *Journal of Marriage and the Family, 64*, 211–224.

Joung, I. M. A., van de Mheen, H. D., Stronks, K., van Poppel, F. W. A., & Mackenbach, J. P. (1997). A longitudinal study of health selection in marital transitions. *Social Science and Medicine, 46*, 425–435.

Kuh, D., & Ben-Shlomo, Y. (1997). Introduction: A life course approach to the aetiology of adult chronic disease. In D. Kuh & Y. Ben-Shlomo (Eds.), *A life course approach to chronic disease epidemiology* (pp. 3–14). New York: Oxford University Press.

Lillard, L. A., & Panis, C. W. A. (1996). Marital status and mortality: The role of health. *Demography, 33*, 313–327.

National Center for Health Statistics. (2004). *Preventing heart disease and stroke*. Retrieved October 1, 2004, from http://www.cdc.gov/nccdphp/bb_heartdisease/ index.htm

O'Rand, A. M. (1996). The precious and precocious: Understanding cumulative disadvantage and cumulative advantage over the life course. *The Gerontologist, 36*, 230–238.

Pienta, A., Hayward, M. D., & Jenkins, K. R. (2000). Health consequences of marriage for the retirement years. *Journal of Family Issues, 21*, 559–586.

Research Triangle Institute. (2005). SUDAAN 9.0 [Statistical software]. Research Triangle Park, NC: Author.

Smock, P. J., Manning, W. D., & Porter, M. (2005). "Everything's there except money": How money shapes decisions to marry among cohabitors. *Journal of Marriage and the Family, 67*, 680–698.

Tucker, J. S., Friedman, H. S., Wingard, D. L., & Schwartz, J. E. (1996). Marital history at midlife as a predictor of longevity: Alternative explanations to the protective effects of marriage. *Health Psychology, 15*, 94–101.

Waite, L. J., & Gallagher, M. (2000). *The case for marriage: Why married people are happier, healthier, and better off financially.* New York: Doubleday.

Williams, K., & Umberson, D. (2004). Marital status, marital transitions, and health: A gendered life course perspective. *Journal of Health and Social Behavior, 45*, 81–98.

Wilmoth, J., & Koso, G. (2002). Does marital history matter? Marital status and wealth outcomes among preretirement adults. *Journal of Marriage and the Family, 64*, 254–268.

The Disappearing Mind

By the year 2050, as many as 14 million Americans could be suffering from Alzheimer's disease. Scientists are now using imaging technology to diagnose the condition at its earliest stages—and racing to develop new treatments that can stop its terrifying progression. Will they succeed?

GEOFFREY COWLEY

Do senior moments scare you? Eight years ago Nancy Levitt had one that would unsettle anyone. She was in her mid-40s at the time, and watching her father drift into the late stages of Alzheimer's disease (several aunts and uncles had suffered similar fates). Levitt's son was about to graduate from high school, so she called a mail-order company to order fluorescent-light sticks for him and his friends to wear around their necks at a party. When her package arrived in the next day's mail, the receipt and postmark knocked her flat. She had ordered the same gift a few days earlier—and lost all recollection of it. "I just freaked," she says. Suddenly, every forgotten name, misplaced pencil and misspelled word became a prophecy of doom. Was she getting Alzheimer's herself?

When Levitt sought testing at UCLA, researchers gave her the usual cognitive tests—name some simple objects, repeat a list of words—and assured her she was fine. But the occasional lapses continued, so she returned to the same clinic several years later and enrolled in a study aimed at distinguishing early Alzheimer's from run-of-the-mill forgetfulness. This time the researchers didn't just talk to her. They placed her under a scanner and recorded detailed images of her brain, both at work and at rest. Alzheimer's disease has traditionally been diagnosed by exclusion. If you lagged significantly on a memory test—and your troubles couldn't be blamed on strokes, tumors or drug toxicity—you were given a tentative diagnosis and sent on your way. To find out for sure, you had to die and have your brain dissected by a pathologist. Levitt didn't have to do any of that. By looking at the images on his video screen, Dr. Gary Small was able to give her some reassuring news. She didn't have Alzheimer's disease—and the odds were less than 5 percent that she would develop it any time soon. Levitt calls the images "the most wonderful thing I've ever seen."

"Without a good method of early detection, the best Alzheimer's treatment would be worthless."
—Dr. Ferenc Jolesz

Technology is changing all of medicine, but it is positively transforming our understanding of Alzheimer's. Armed with state-of-the-art PET scanners and MRI machines, specialists are learning to spot and track the disease in people who have yet to suffer symptoms. It's one thing to chronicle the brain's disintegration, quite another to stop it, but many experts are predicting success on both fronts. Drugmakers now have two dozen treatments in development. And unlike today's medications, which offer only a brief respite from symptoms, many of the new ones are intended to stall progression of the disease. As Alzheimer's runs its decades-long course, it replaces the brain's exquisite circuitry with mounds of sticky plaque and expanses of dead, twisted neurons. No drug will repair that kind of damage. But if the new treatments work as anticipated, they'll enable us to stop or slow the destruction while our minds are still intact. A decade from now, says Dr. Dennis Selkoe of Harvard Medical School and Boston's Brigham and Women's Hospital, physicians may monitor our brain health as closely as our cholesterol levels—and stave off Alzheimer's with a wave of the prescription pad.

"There are a lot of people who could benefit from today's treatments, but they aren't getting help."
—Dr. Gary Small

Until we can control this awful illness, early detection may seem a fool's errand. "With diagnostics ahead of therapeutics, there's a lot of potential for harm," says University of Pennsylvania ethicist Arthur Caplan. He worries that entrepreneurs will peddle testing without counseling, leaving patients devastated by the findings. He wonders, too, whether employers and insurers will abandon people whose scans show signs of trouble. Advocates counter that early detection can help patients make the most of today's treatments while giving them time to adjust their plans and expectations. With so many people at risk, they say, anything is better than nothing. Some

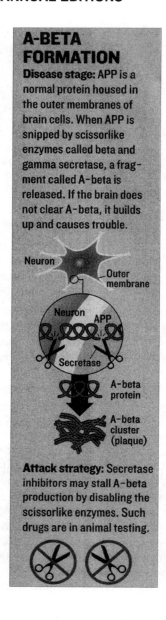

A-BETA FORMATION

Disease stage: APP is a normal protein housed in the outer membranes of brain cells. When APP is snipped by scissorlike enzymes called beta and gamma secretase, a fragment called A-beta is released. If the brain does not clear A-beta, it builds up and causes trouble.

Neuron

Outer membrane

Neuron   APP

Secretase

A-beta protein

A-beta cluster (plaque)

Attack strategy: Secretase inhibitors may stall A-beta production by disabling the scissorlike enzymes. Such drugs are in animal testing.

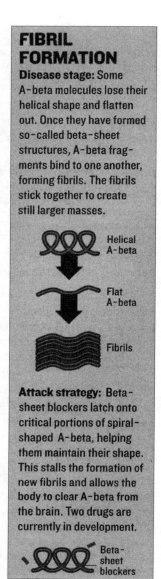

FIBRIL FORMATION

Disease stage: Some A-beta molecules lose their helical shape and flatten out. Once they have formed so-called beta-sheet structures, A-beta fragments bind to one another, forming fibrils. The fibrils stick together to create still larger masses.

Helical A-beta

Flat A-beta

Fibrils

Attack strategy: Beta-sheet blockers latch onto critical portions of spiral-shaped A-beta, helping them maintain their shape. This stalls the formation of new fibrils and allows the body to clear A-beta from the brain. Two drugs are currently in development.

Beta-sheet blockers

4 million Americans have Alzheimer's today, but the number could hit 14 million by 2050 as the elderly population expands.

The diagnostic revolution began during the 1990s, as researchers learned to monitor neurons with an imaging technique called PET, or positron-emission tomography. Unlike an X-ray or CT imaging, PET records brain activity by homing in on the glucose that fuels it. And as Small's team has discovered, it can spot significant pathology in people who are still functioning normally. Instead of glowing with activity, the middle sections of their brains appear dim and torpid. And because Alzheimer's is progressive, abnormal scans tend to become more so with time. In a study published last fall, UCLA researchers scanned 284 people who had suffered only minor memory problems. The images predicted, with 95 percent accuracy, which people would experience dementia within three and a half years.

PET scanning has yet to transform patient care; few clinics have the machines, and Medicare doesn't cover their use. But scientists are now using the technique to see whether drugs already on the market (such as the anti-inflammatory ibuprofen) can slow the brain's decline. And PET is just one of several potential strategies for tracking preclinical Alzheimer's. San Diego researchers have found that seniors who score inconsistently on different mental tests are at increased risk of dementia—even if their scores are generally high. And in a study published this spring, researchers at the Oregon Health Sciences University hit upon three signs of imminent decline in octogenarians. The 108 participants were all healthy at the start of the study, but nearly half were demented six years later. As it turned out, they had entered the study with certain traits in common. They walked more slowly than their peers, requiring nearly two extra seconds for a 30-foot stroll. They lagged slightly on memory tests. And their MRI scans revealed a slight shrinkage of the hippocampus, a small, seahorse-shaped brain structure that is critical to memory processing. The changes were subtle, says Dr. Jeffrey Kaye, the neurologist who directed the study, but they presaged changes that were catastrophic.

Powerful as they are, today's tests show only that the brain is losing steam. The ideal test would reveal the underlying pathology, letting a specialist determine how much healthy tissue has been replaced by the plaques and tangles of Alzheimer's. It's not hard to fashion a molecule that will highlight the wreckage. Unfortunately, it's almost impossible to get such a probe through the ultrafine screen that separates the brain from the bloodstream. If a probe is complex enough to pick out plaques and tangles, chances are it's too large to pass from the bloodstream into the brain. At UCLA and the University of Pittsburgh, researchers have developed probes that are small enough to get through, yet selective enough to provide at least a rough measure of a person's plaque burden. At Brigham and Women's Hospital, meanwhile, radiologist Ferenc Jolesz is trying to open the barrier to bigger, better probes. His technique employs tiny lipid bubbles that gather at the gateway to the brain when injected into the bloodstream. The bubbles burst when zapped with ultrasound, loosening the mesh of that ultrafine screen and allowing the amyloid probe to enter. Lab tests suggest the screen will repair itself within a day, but no one yet knows whether it's safe to leave it open that long.

One way or another, many of us now seem destined to learn we have Alzheimer's disease while we're still of sound mind. The question is whether we'll be able to do anything more constructive than setting our affairs in order and taking a drug like Aricept to ease the early symptoms. Fortunately the possibilities for therapy are changing almost as fast as the diagnostic arts. Experts now think of Alzheimer's not as a sudden calamity but as a decades-long process involving at least a half-dozen steps—each of which provides a target for intervention. Slowing the disease may require four or five drugs rather than one. But as AIDS specialists have shown, the right combination can sometimes turn a killer into a mere menace.

Brain Spotting

For the first time, PET scans can spot plaque in the brains of Alzheimer's patients. The advance will allow for confident early detection of the disease.

PLAQUE BUILDUP Red areas in the brain scan of an Alzheimer's patient show plaque accumulation. The healthy brain shows none.

Alzheimer's brain

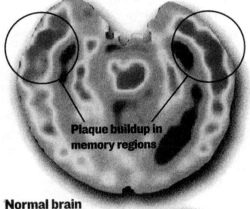

Plaque buildup in memory regions

Normal brain

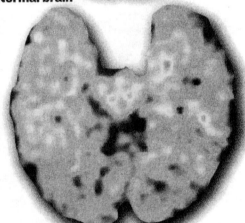

BRAIN ACTIVITY Blue areas in the Alzheimer's patient's memory regions indicate reduced activity caused by the plaque.

Alzheimer's brain   **Normal brain**

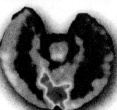   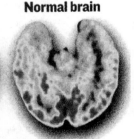

Leading causes of death in the U.S., all ages, 1999

Heart disease	725,192
Malignant tumors	549,838
Vascular disease	167,366
Respiratory disease	124,181
Accidents	97,860
Diabetes	68,399
Pneumonia/flu	63,730
Alzheimer's	**44,536**
Kidney disease	35,525
Blood disease	30,680

Projected cases in the U.S.*

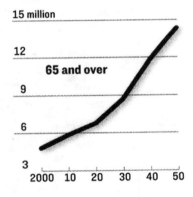

65 and over

Projected cases by age group*

PLAQUE FORMATION

Disease stage: A-beta fibrils bind with proteins like SAP. The SAP reinforces the fibrils, making them less soluble and harder for the body to clear. Fibrils bind with other fibrils and grow into plaques.

SAP

A-beta fibril

A-beta bound to SAP

Attack strategy: Specially designed chemicals bind SAP before it can link to fibrils. This helps prevent fibril accumulation. A few drugs are in early trials.

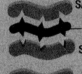

SAP

SAP inhibitor

SAP

SAP bound to inhibitor

SOURCES: GARY W. SMALL, M.D., UCLA; DENIS EVANS, M.D., CDC

Though experts still quarrel about the ultimate cause of Alzheimer's, many agree that the trouble starts with a scrap of junk protein called amyloid beta (A-beta for short). Each of us produces the stuff, and small amounts are harmless. But as A-beta builds up in the brain, it sets off a destructive cascade, replacing healthy tissue with the plaques seen in Alzheimer's sufferers. No one knew where this pesky filament came from until 1987, when researchers discovered it was part of a larger molecule they dubbed the amyloid-precursor protein (APP). Thanks to more recent discoveries, they now know exactly how the parent molecule spawns its malevolent offspring.

APP is a normal protein that hangs from a neuron's outer membrane like a worm with its head in an apple. While performing its duties in and around the cell, it gets chopped up by enzymes called secretases, leaving residues that dissolve in the brain's watery recesses. Occasionally, however, a pair of enzymes called beta and gamma secretase cleave APP in just the wrong places, leaving behind an insoluble A-beta fragment. Some people produce these junk proteins faster than others, but after seven or eight decades of service, even the healthiest brain carries an amyloid burden. When it reaches a certain threshold, the brain can no longer function. That's why Alzheimer's dementia is so rampant among the elderly. Given enough time, anyone would develop it.

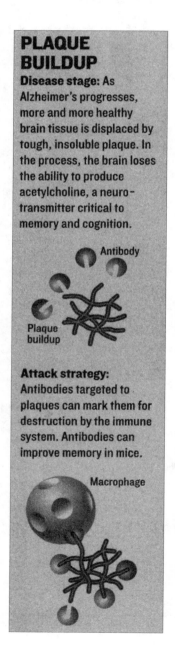

PLAQUE BUILDUP

Disease stage: As Alzheimer's progresses, more and more healthy brain tissue is displaced by tough, insoluble plaque. In the process, the brain loses the ability to produce acetylcholine, a neurotransmitter critical to memory and cognition.

Antibody

Plaque buildup

Attack strategy: Antibodies targeted to plaques can mark them for destruction by the immune system. Antibodies can improve memory in mice.

Macrophage

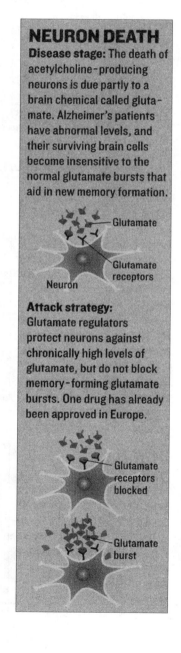

NEURON DEATH

Disease stage: The death of acetylcholine-producing neurons is due partly to a brain chemical called glutamate. Alzheimer's patients have abnormal levels, and their surviving brain cells become insensitive to the normal glutamate bursts that aid in new memory formation.

Glutamate

Glutamate receptors

Neuron

Attack strategy: Glutamate regulators protect neurons against chronically high levels of glutamate, but do not block memory-forming glutamate bursts. One drug has already been approved in Europe.

Glutamate receptors blocked

Glutamate burst

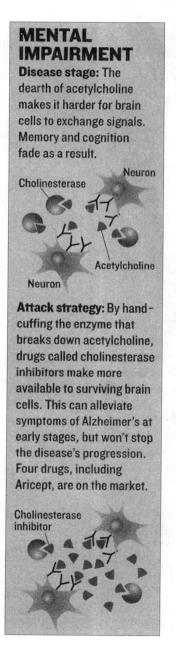

MENTAL IMPAIRMENT

Disease stage: The dearth of acetylcholine makes it harder for brain cells to exchange signals. Memory and cognition fade as a result.

Neuron

Cholinesterase

Acetylcholine

Neuron

Attack strategy: By handcuffing the enzyme that breaks down acetylcholine, drugs called cholinesterase inhibitors make more available to surviving brain cells. This can alleviate symptoms of Alzheimer's at early stages, but won't stop the disease's progression. Four drugs, including Aricept, are on the market.

Cholinesterase inhibitor

The ideal Alzheimer's remedy would simply slow the production of A-beta—by disabling the enzymes that fabricate it. Elan Corp. was the first drugmaker to try this tack. During the mid-'90s its scientists developed several gamma-secretase blockers and tested them in animals—only to find that they sometimes derailed normal cell development, damaging bone marrow and digestive tissues. A few companies are still pursuing gamma blockers, but beta secretase now looks like a safer target for therapy. More than a half-dozen drugmakers are now working on beta inhibitors. "In the industry," says Dr. Ivan Lieberburg of Elan, "we're hoping that the beta-secretase inhibitors will have as much therapeutic potential as the statins." Those, of course, are the cholesterol-lowering medicines for which 35 million Americans are now candidates.

Secretase inhibitors may be our best hope of warding off Alzheimer's, but they're not the only hope. As scientists learn more about the behavior of A-beta, they're seeing opportunities to disarm it before it causes harm. One thing that makes A-beta fragments dangerous is their tendency to bind with one another to form tough, stringy fibrils, which then stick together to create still larger masses. Three companies are now testing compounds designed to keep A-beta from forming fibrils—and at least two other firms are working to keep fibrils from aggregating to create plaque. All of their experimental drugs have helped reduce amyloid buildup in plaque-prone mice, suggesting they might help people as well. But human studies are just now getting underway.

Suppose for a moment that all these strategies fail, and that amyloid buildup is simply part of the human condition. As Selkoe likes to say, there's more than one way to keep a bathtub from overflowing. If you can't turn down the faucet, you can always try opening the drain. Recognizing that most of the people now threatened by Alzheimer's have already spent their lives under open amyloid faucets, researchers are pursuing several strategies for clearing deposits from the brain. One elegant idea is to mobilize the immune system. Three years ago Elan wowed the world by showing that animals given an antiamyloid vaccine mounted fierce attacks on their plaques. Vaccinated mice reduced their amyloid burdens by an astounding 96 percent in just three months. The vaccine proved toxic in people, triggering attacks on normal tissue as well as plaque, but the dream isn't dead. Both Elan and Eli Lilly are now developing ready-made antibodies that, if successful, will target amyloid for removal from the brain without triggering broader attacks by the immune system.

Even later interventions may be possible. As a person's amyloid burden rises, so does the concentration of glutamate in the brain. This neurotransmitter helps lock in memories when it's released in short bursts, but it kills neurons when chronically elevated. At least two teams are now betting they can rescue cells surrounded by amyloid, simply by shielding them from glutamate. One possible life jacket is a drug called Memantine, which is already approved in Europe. It covers a receptor that lets glutamate flow freely into neurons, but without blocking the glutamate bursts needed for learning and memory. New York's Forest Laboratories is now launching an American trial of the drug, and hoping for approval by next year.

If even half these treatments fulfill their promise, old age may prove more pleasant than today's projections suggest. For now, the best we can expect is an early warning and perhaps a year or two of symptomatic relief. That may seem a paltry offering, but it's a far cry from nothing. As Small argues in a forthcoming book called "The Memory Bible," people at early stages of Alzheimer's can do a lot to improve their lives, but few of them get the chance. Three out of four are already past the "moderate" stage by the time their conditions are recognized. Some may find solace in ignorance. But the case for vigilance is getting stronger every day.

With ANNE UNDERWOOD and ANDREW MURR

The Extent and Frequency of Abuse in the Lives of Older Women and Their Relationship with Health Outcomes

Purpose: This study assessed the extent of different types of abuse, repeated and multiple abuse experiences among women aged 60 and older, and their effects on the women's self-reported health. ***Design and Methods:*** A cross-sectional study of a clinical sample of 842 community-dwelling women aged 60 and older completed a telephone survey about type and frequency of abuse, self-reported health status and health conditions, and demographic characteristics. Bivariate and multivariate analyses were performed using SPSS 11.5 and STATA 7.0. ***Results:*** Nearly half of the women had experienced at least one type of abuse—psychological/emotional, control, threat, physical, or sexual—since turning 55 years old. Sizable proportions were victims of repeat abuse. Many women experienced multiple types of abuse and experienced abuse often. Abused older women were significantly more likely to report more health conditions than those who were not abused. Women who experienced psychological/emotional abuse—alone, repeatedly, or with other types of abuse—had significantly increased odds of reporting bone or joint problems, digestive problems, depression or anxiety, chronic pain, and high blood pressure or heart problems. ***Implications:*** It is important that health care and service providers acknowledge psychological/emotional, control, threat, physical, and sexual abuse against older women and understand their health implications. In addition, it is important for providers to be trained in both aging and domestic violence services and resources.

BONNIE S. FISHER, PHD,[1] AND SAUNDRA L. REGAN, PHD[2]

R esearchers' understanding of psychological, physical, or sexual abuses against women and their relationship with physical and mental health conditions is derived almost exclusively from the experiences of teenage girls and pre-menopausal women. Generally, violence-against-women researchers and aging service providers have overlooked older women (Fisher et al., 2003). Even among the most steadfast advocates, only a handful of initiatives and collaborations promoting the intersection of abuse and aging exist (Brandl, 1997; Fisher, Zink, Pabst, Regan, & Rinto, 2004; Vinton, 2003; Wilke & Vinton, 2003).

Recently, however, there has been a renewed interest in examining the extent and nature of abuse against older women. Researchers and advocates from a variety of disciplines have reported that older women experience intimate-partner and do-

mestic violence well into old age (Grossman & Lundy, 2003; Rennison & Rand, 2003; Teaster & Roberto, 2004). It should not be too surprising that, given the paucity of older women abuse studies, our understanding of the health consequences for abused older women is woefully limited. The issues of abuse and its health consequences will not retreat anytime soon. Older women are a fast-growing population as the baby boomers enter into old age and their life expectancy continues to lengthen.

Using data from a clinical sample of 842 community-dwelling women aged 60 and older, this study makes four contributions to researchers' understanding of the extent and nature of abuse against older women and the associated health conditions. First, we measured the extent of abuse experiences in late life—that is, since age 55—to capture the experiences of women who had reached a mature stage of their life cycle. Second, we expanded upon the

This research was supported under award R605H23525 from the Attorney General of Ohio, Betty Montgomery. The points of view in this article are those of the authors and do not necessarily represent the official position of the office of Ohio Attorney General. Thanks to Dr. Therese Zink, Dr. Amy Cassedy, Stephanie Pabst, Barbara Rinto, and Elizabeth Gothelf for their enthusiasm and thoughtfulness as members of the research team. Thank you also to the anonymous reviewers who provided us with the opportunity to improve our research.

Address correspondence to Bonnie S. Fisher, PhD, Division of Criminal Justice, University of Cincinnati, P.O. Box 210389, Cincinnati, OH 45221-0389. E-mail: Bonnie.Fisher@uc.edu

[1]Division of Criminal Justice, University of Cincinnati, OH.
[2]Department of Family Medicine, University of Cincinnati, OH.

types of abuse examined in previous studies to include control and threat abuses. Third, we examined not only the extent of abuse but also the extent of repeat abuse and multiple abuses and their respective frequencies. Last, we investigated the relationships between type of abuse (including repeat abuse) and older women's self-reported general health, number of health conditions, and specific psychological and physical health conditions.

The Extent of Abuse Against Older Women

The estimation of the extent of abuse against older women is a young field of inquiry. Only two national-level studies have been conducted since Pillemer and Finkelhor's (1988) pioneering study revealed that older women had experienced physical violence and verbal aggression since turning 65 years old. First, results from the National Elder Abuse Incidence Study (National Center on Elder Abuse, 1998) reported that 76.3% of surveyed women aged 60 and older had experienced emotional/psychological abuse and 71.4% were victims of physical abuse. Second, the National Crime Victimization Survey estimated that 118,000 intimate-partner victimizations were committed against women 55 years and older during a 9-year period (1993–2001; Rennison & Rand, 2003).

Only a handful of single-state studies have examined the extent of abuse suffered by older women (Grossman & Lundy, 2003; Teaster & Roberto, 2004). To illustrate, using data from the Women's Health Initiative in San Antonio, Texas, Mouton and colleagues (2004) reported that 11% of postmenopausal women had reported abuse within the past year. At the 3-year follow-up, 5% of the women had reported new experiences with abuse.

Collectively these studies reveal that older women are abuse victims into their old age, yet many questions about women's abuse later in life remain largely unanswered. These questions include: (a) What types of abuse do older women experience in their later years? (b) Are these women repeatedly abused, and, if so, which type of abuse do they repeatedly experience? (c) Do these women experience multiple types of abuse, and, if so, what are the patterns? and (d) How often does abuse occur? By better understanding the extent and frequency of abuse against older women, researchers can determine whether linkages exist between the abuse older women experience and their health-related outcomes.

The Associations Between Abuse and Health-Related Outcomes

Researchers have documented that abused women are at risk for several negative health-related consequences.

Self-Reported General Health Status. —Three studies are illustrative of the association between abuse and general health status. First, Koss, Koss, and Woodruff (1991), using a 16-item measure of criminal victimization, reported that victimized women aged 19–69 years old perceived themselves as less healthy than nonvictimized women (i.e., as having more somatic complaints and less physical and mental well-being). Second, investigating a sample of women aged 21–55 years old,

Campbell and colleagues (2002) reported that twice as many women who had experienced intimate-partner violence over a 9-year period rated their health as fair to poor compared with women who had never experienced such abuse. And third, Coker and colleagues (2002) reported that women aged 18–65 years old who had experienced lifetime intimate-partner physical, sexual, or psychological abuse were significantly more likely than nonabuse victims to self-report current poor health.

Number of Self-Reported Health Problems or Conditions. —Researchers have also shown that women who have experienced abuse are more likely to suffer more health problems compared with nonabused women. This includes suffering from more physical and mental health conditions and chronic health problems (see Sutherland, Bybee, & Sullivan, 2002). Campbell and colleagues (2002) reported that abused women had a higher rate of total physical health problems and central nervous system, gynecological, and chronic-stress symptoms compared with women who had never been abused.

Specific Chronic Health Problems or Conditions. — There is mounting evidence that different types of abuse and their co-occurrence are related to specific short- and long-term mental and physical health problems and conditions (Sutherland et al., 2002). The list of negative health effects includes depression, fear, chronic pain, osteoarthritis, gastrointestinal disorders, chronic stress, gynecological symptoms, chest pains, and cardiac problems (Campbell et al., 2002; Coker et al., 2002).

Repeat and Multiple Abuse. —For many women, abuse is not an isolated event; abuse happens repeatedly. Women who suffer repeated abuse experience two or more incidents of the same type of abuse within a specified time period—for some, this is daily (Tjaden & Thoennes, 1998). Women also experience different types of abuse (i.e., multiple forms of abuse). Campbell and colleagues (2002) reported that 33% of the abused women surveyed experienced both physical and sexual abuse.

Research suggests that repeat and multiple abuses take a negative toll on women's health, possibly even more negative than the abuse-nonabuse distinction that is commonly used in the abuse literature. First, there is evidence that women who experience multiple types of abuse report having poor health (Koss et al., 1991). Second, the frequency of different types of abuse may affect some health outcomes but not others. Coker and colleagues (2002) also found that increased psychological intimate-partner-violence scores were strongly associated with self-reported current poor health status. Physical or sexual intimate-partner violence, however, was not related to current poor health status. Further clarifying the relationship between repeat abuse and type of health condition, Coker and associates reported that the frequency of a certain type of abuse was related to specific health conditions. That is, higher psychological intimate-partner-violence scores were significantly related to both the development of a chronic disease and current depressive symptoms. Higher physical or sexual intimate-partner-violence scores were significantly related only to current depressive symptoms.

There is evidence to suggest that experiencing multiple abuses—a combination of two types of abuse—has negative health-related consequences. Hegarty, Gunn, Chondros, and Small (2004) reported that "probably" depressed women were more likely to have experienced physical abuse and emotional abuse or harassment than "not" depressed women.

Overall, the results from these studies suggest that abuse has negative effects on women's health. There is room for further research, including the examination of the abuse–health-consequences relationship for older women. To date, no published research has examined this relationship using a sample of women aged 60 years and older, and only a few published studies have examined abuse that happened after age 55 and its relationship to women's health (see Mouton, 2003; Zink, Fisher, Regan, & Pabst, 2005).

Methods

Sample

In March 2003, we obtained patient lists of women aged 55 and older from five adult primary care clinics affiliated with an academic institution in southwestern Ohio and serving Indiana, Ohio, and Kentucky. We arranged the patient lists into three groups of phone numbers stratified by age: 55–64 years, 65–74 years, and 75 years and older. Trained female interviewers called each woman on the list between March and June 2003. We had obtained a total of 4,261 phone numbers. Each woman, aged 55–90, was called at least three times at different times on different days before being taken out of the sample.

Women gave verbal consent by agreeing to participate in the Women's Health and Relationship Survey (WHRS). Of the 4,261 available numbers, 44% of the women ($n = 1,852$) were not available (answering machine or no answer). In addition, 7% ($n = 297$) of the numbers had been disconnected, and 6% ($n = 261$) were wrong numbers. Approximately 2% ($n = 67$) of the women were deceased, 1% ($n = 45$) were too sick to answer, and 0.4% ($n = 15$) of the women had family members who intercepted the call and would not allow them to participate. Of the 1,724 women reached by phone, 40% ($n = 695$) refused to participate, 1.5% ($n = 26$) were unable to answer the three mental competency questions correctly (their age, birth date, and the current year) to assess their mental status, and 0.5% ($n = 8$) refused to answer the abuse questions. This resulted in 995 usable surveys and an adjusted response rate of 58% (995 out of 1,698).

Only women aged 60 and older ($n = 842$) were included in the current study. All of the women in the sample were community dwelling. None lived in institutional settings, such as a nursing home.

Instrument

The WHRS was adapted from validated instruments and included questions about mental status (Lachs & Pillemer, 1995), health conditions (Tjaden & Thoennes, 1998), abuse (Shepherd & Campbell, 1992; Tjaden & Thoennes) and sociodemographics. The survey administration took 20–45 minutes, depending on whether the woman had experienced abuse.

Measures

Type of Abuse. —The WHRS measured five different types of abuse: (a) psychological/emotional, (b) control, (c) threat of physical abuse, (d) physical, and (e) sexual. The abuse measures combined the uniform definitions regarding intimate-partner violence recommended by the Centers for Disease Control and Prevention with definitions housed within the elder abuse framework recognized by the U.S. National Academy of Sciences (Bonnie & Wallace, 2002; Saltzman, Fanslow, McMahon, & Shelley, 1999/2002).

We measured each of these five types of abuse by using multiple items. A principal components factor analysis performed on the six psychological/emotional and control abuse items confirmed two distinct factors. Three items loaded on one factor, psychological/emotional abuse (.85, .82, and .52); and three other items loaded on a second factor, control abuse (.81, .70, and .66).

Psychological/emotional abuse was a 3-item measure (Cronbach's $\alpha = .64$). Control abuse was a 3-item measure (Cronbach's $\alpha = .59$). Threat abuse was a 2-item measure (Cronbach's $\alpha = .52$). Physical abuse was a 4-item measure (Cronbach's $\alpha = .72$). Sexual abuse was a 3-item measure (Cronbach's $\alpha = .71$). For each abuse item, women were asked if they had experienced the behavior "since you turned 55."

Extent of Abuse. —We created three variables to measure the extent to which women in the sample experienced the five types of abuse. First, we created a dichotomous variable, abuse victim, which measured whether a respondent had experienced any of the five types of abuse since she had turned 55 years old.

Second, we created a measure of repeated abuse. Repeated abuse was a count of the number of women who had experienced two or more abusive behaviors that comprised a specific type of abuse (i.e., the same type of abuse). To illustrate, three behaviors comprise psychological/emotional abuse. Women who reported having experienced two or more of these behaviors were coded as having been repeatedly psychologically/emotionally abused since age 55.

Third, multiple abuse was a measure of the number of women who had experienced any combination of at least two types of abuse. For example, a woman was coded as a victim of multiple abuse if she had experienced either both sexual and physical abuse, or both control and physical abuse.

Frequency of Abuse. —In order to measure the frequency with which abuse occurred, interviewers asked women how often different forms of abuse had happened to them since they had turned 55 years old. Responses were: never, rarely, occasionally, frequently, or very frequently. Of the respondents who had experienced at least one form of abuse within a specific type of abuse, those who reported "rarely" were coded as the Rarely group and those who reported "occasionally, frequently, or very frequently" were coded as the Often group. For example, a woman who had experienced any form of psychological/emotional abuse frequently was coded as often psychologically/emotionally abused. If, within the same type of abuse, she reported one form as having happened rarely and another form as having happened frequently, she was coded using the "highest" frequency category; in this case, coded as being in the Often group.

Health-Related Consequences. —Because one of the primary aims of this study was to examine the relationship between abuse experience and health-related consequences, we used several measures of health outcome. First, we created a dichotomous measure of the status of a woman's health. Interviewers asked respondents to assess their health on a 5-point scale ranging from poor to excellent. For ease of analysis, we collapsed the "poor" and "fair" categories into one category and collapsed "good," "very good," and "excellent" categories into a second category to create the dichotomous measure of self-reported health status. We found that 55% ($n = 429$) of the women rated their health as good to excellent, and 45% ($n = 378$) rated their health as poor or fair.

The second dependent variable, number of self-reported health conditions, was a count of the number of health conditions that a doctor had told each woman that she currently had. The 10 items included: high blood pressure or heart problems; lung problems (e.g., asthma or chronic obstructive pulmonary disease); diabetes or thyroid problems; bone or joint problems (e.g., osteoporosis or arthritis); depression or anxiety; digestive problems (e.g., irritable bowel syndrome or heartburn); stroke or nerve problems (e.g., Multiple Sclerosis or Parkinson's disease); blood problems (e.g., anemia); chronic pain (e.g., migraines or back pain); and any type of cancer. Respondents averaged 3.3 ($SD = 1.8$) health conditions.

Third, we created a dichotomous measure of whether respondents currently had or did not have a specific health condition by asking questions that required respondents to identify which health conditions a doctor had told them they had. These were the 10 health conditions listed in the preceding paragraph. More than half of the respondents reported having high blood pressure or heart problems (75%) or bone or joint problems (65%). Less than half reported having diabetes or thyroid problems (37%), chronic pain (36%), digestive problems (31%), depression or anxiety (30%), lung problems (24%), cancer (13%), stroke or nerve problems (12%), or blood problems (12%).

Control Variables. —Similar to Coker and colleagues (2002) and Campbell and associates (2002), we employed several sociodemographic characteristics as control variables in the multivariate health-related consequences models. Using aged 75 and older (34%, $n = 285$) as the reference group, we created two age dummy variables for 60–64 years old (23%, $n = 191$), and 65–74 years old (44%, $n = 366$; percentages may equal greater than 100% due to rounding). Race/ethnicity was measured as a dichotomy: Black/African American or Other (45%, $n = 373$) and White (reference group, 55%, $n = 453$). Using less than high school education (36%, $n = 297$) as the reference group, we measured respondents' level of education with two dummy variables: high school diploma (31%, $n = 255$), and some college to college graduate (34%, $n = 281$). Using being married/common law (32%, $n = 336$) as the reference group, we measured current marital status with three dummy variables: divorced/separated (18%, $n = 152$), widowed (41%, $n = 342$), and single/never married (9%, $n = 72$). Using less than $20,000 (47%, $n = 389$) as the reference group, we measured annual household income with three dummy variables: $20,000–

$40,000 (15%, $n = 128$), more than $40,000 (10%, $n = 84$), and refused to answer or did not know (28%, $n = 228$). Given the Appalachian heritage in southwest Ohio, we included a dichotomous measure of whether a woman was of Appalachian decent (9%, $n = 79$) or not (91%, $n = 717$).

Data Analysis

Descriptive statistics and bivariate and multivariate data analyses are reported here. Appropriate tests of significance are presented for the bivariate analyses. In order to examine the relationship between type of abuse and health-related consequences, we estimated several multivariate models. Depending on the distribution of the dependent variable, we estimated either a logit model or an analysis of covariance model. We estimated all of the multivariate logit models using STAT A, version 7.0 (StataCorp, 2001). We calculated the descriptive statistics and estimated the analysis of covariance models with SPSS 11.5 for Windows (SPSS Inc., 2002).

Results
The Extent and Frequency of Abuse and Repeat Abuse

Nearly half (47%, $n = 393$) of all women aged 60 and older had experienced at least one type of abuse since the age of 55. Table 1 presents the descriptive results for the extent and frequency of abuse among older women. As is shown in Table 1, a substantial percentage (45%) of older women had experienced psychological/emotional abuse since turning 55 years old. Nearly 12% of older women had been threatened. Less than 5% of women had been victims of control abuse (4%), physical abuse (4%), or sexual abuse (3%).

However, the results on type of abuse experienced mask a more telling result once we look at the extent of repeat abuse. Of women who had experienced a specific type of abuse, between 21% (sexual abuse) and 47% (psychological/emotional abuse) had been victims of repeat abuse. For example, 32% of the physical abuse victims had been victims of repeat physical abuse. This means that these women had experienced two or more forms of physical abuse since turning 55 years old (i.e., any combination of the four different forms of physical abuse, such as being pushed and slapped, being slapped and choked, or being pushed, slapped, or choked).

The frequency of the occurrence of abuse also reveals noteworthy patterns. Of the older women who had experienced a specific type of abuse, in the case of 4 of the 5 types of abuse, more than 45% of the women had experienced abuse often since age 55: control abuse (88%), psychological/emotional abuse (57%), threat abuse (48%), and sexual abuse (46%). Slightly less, but still a substantial proportion (41%), had experienced physical abuse often since age 55.

Asking who perpetrated the abuse also revealed interesting results (not presented here). Interviewers did not ask respondents about the identity of the perpetrator of psychological/emotional abuse due to their concern for the respondent's discomfort with answering the first set of experience questions about psychological/emotional abuse. Interviewers did ask respondents about different categories of perpetrators (i.e., spouse/boyfriend, relative, or non-relative) for the other types of abuse. Almost

Table 1 Abuse Since 55 Years Old: Types of Abuse and Extent and Frequency of Abuse of Women 60 and Older

Type of Abuse Specific Behavior[a]	Extent of Abuse		
	Abuse Victim, % (n)[b]	Repeat Abuse Victim, % (n)	Abuse Occurring Often, % (n)[c]
Psychological/emotional	44.6 (372)	47.3 (176)	57.3 (212)
Called you a name or criticized you	30.2 (245)		
Shouted or swore at you	25.3 (209)		
Been possessive or jealous of someone close to you	17.6 (139)		
Control	4.1 (34)	29.4 (10)	88.2 (30)
Routinely checked up on you in a way that made you afraid	2.5 (21)		
Put you on an allowance	1.7 (14)		
Not letting you go to work or social activities or see or talk with your friends	1.3 (12)		
Threat	11.7 (98)	23.5 (23)	48.0 (47)
Said things to scare you	6.0 (50)		
Threw, hit, kicked, or smashed something	8.5 (71)		
Physical	3.8 (38)	31.6 (12)	40.6 (13)
Pushed, grabbed, or shoved you	2.6 (22)		
Slapped, hit, or punched you	1.7 (14)		
Hit you with an object	1.0 (8)		
Choked or attempted to drown you	0.7 (6)		
Sexual	3.4 (28)	21.4 (6)	46.4 (13)
Pressured you to have sex in a way you did not like or want	2.9 (24)		
Physically forced you to have sex	1.1 (9)		
Attacked the sexual parts of your body	0.5 (4)		

[a]The items listed under each type of abuse are the specific behaviors that comprise the respective type of abuse measure.
[b]Respondents who refused to answer or reported "don't know" to a form of abuse question were not included in the forms of abuse calculations. Only those who refused to answer or reported "don't know" to all the forms of abuse questions within a respective type of abuse were excluded from the type of abuse estimates.
[c]Percent represents those women who responded that at least one form of abuse within the specific type of abuse happened occasionally, frequently, or very frequently.

three-fourths of the women (73%, n = 66) reported that a relative—child, grandchild, or other relative—had threatened them, compared with 21% of women who had been threatened by a spouse/boyfriend and 14% by a non-relative. A majority of the women reported that their spouse/boyfriend had perpetrated control abuse (56%, n = 19) and sexual abuse (73%, n = 19). Physical abuse did not exhibit the same pattern as to who was the perpetrator. Of the physically abused women, 45% (n = 14) reported that a relative had been the perpetrator, compared with 39% (n = 12) who reported that their spouse/boyfriend had. Almost 20% (n = 6) of these women reported that a non-relative had physically abused them.

The Extent and Frequency of Multiple Abuses

Table 2 presents additional insight into the multiple-abuse experiences of older women who had experienced two different types of abuse (i.e., had been victims of multiple abuse). The diagonal in bold shows the unconditional percentages, or the percentage of women who had been victims of the specific type of abuse listed in

each column (same percentages as reported in Table 1). The conditional likelihood for women who had been abused in the specific manner as noted in the columns is presented in the off diagonal. For example, among the women who had been physically abused, 69% had been threatened, 44% reported having experienced control abuse, and 31% reported having been sexually abused. In more than half of the conditional likelihoods (13 out of the 20 pairs), 25% or more women had experienced multiple types of abuse. It appears that multiple abuses were characteristic of the type of abuse from which these victimized women suffered.

Two additional noteworthy multiple-abuse patterns are evident in Table 2. First, psychological/emotional abuse co-occurred with other types of abuse for a large number of older women. Among those older women who had experienced a specific type of abuse, between 86% (threat) and 97% (physical abuse) had experienced psychological/emotional abuse. Second, the conditional likelihoods (in the off diagonal) exceed the unconditional likelihoods in their respective rows. This suggests that many older women were more likely to have experienced multiple

Table 2 The Extent of Multiple Abuse

Type of Abuse	Conditional Type of Abuse				
	Psychological/emotional, % (n)	Control, % (n)	Threat, % (n)	Physical, % (n)	Sexual, % (n)
Psychological/emotional	**44.6 (372)**	91.2 (31)	85.7 (84)	96.9 (31)*	89.3 (25)
Control	8.4 (31)	**4.1 (34)**	18.4 (18)	43.8 (14)*	32.1 (9)*
Threat	22.6 (84)	52.9 (18)	**11.7 (98)**	68.8 (22)*	50.0 (14)
Physical	8.4 (31)	42.4 (14)*	22.7 (22)	**3.8 (38)**	35.7 (10)
Sexual	6.8 (25)	27.3 (9)	14.4 (14)	31.3 (10)*	**3.4 (28)**

Notes: Unconditional likelihoods are shown in the main diagonal in bold. The highest value in each row is indicated by an asterisk. The conditional type of crime is not necessarily temporally prior to the type of row abuse.

types of abuse than one type of abuse. To illustrate, 12% of the women had been threatened, yet from twice (of those who had been psychological/emotionally abused, 23% had also been threatened) to more than five times (of those who had been physically abused, 69% had also been threatened) as many women had experienced multiple abuse in which they had also been threatened.

Extent and Frequency of Abuse Measures Refined

Two noteworthy results convinced us to refine our measures of extent and frequency of abuse. First, the extent of abuse results suggests that many older women had experienced repeat abuse and multiple types of abuse. The results in Table 2 suggest that psychological/emotional abuse occurred in conjunction with other types of abuse (control, threat, physical, or sexual). Nearly 30% (28.7%, n = 110) of abuse victims were multiple-abuse victims who had suffered from psychological/emotional abuse. The remaining abuse victims had experienced only one type of abuse. The majority of older abused women (67%, n = 262) had experienced *only* psychological/emotional abuse, and 5% (n = 21) had experienced *only* control, threat, physical, or sexual abuse since age 55. The analysis of those women who had *only* experienced control, threat, physical, or sexual abuse is not reported here due to the small number of cases.

In order to measure the possible effects that each of these three types of abuse experience may have had on health outcomes, we created two dummy variables that refined the extent-of-abuse measures in light of the multiple-abuse results. These new variables measured whether a woman had experienced (a) only psychological/emotional abuse, and no control, threat, physical, or sexual abuse, or (b) multiple abuses (psychological/emotional abuse plus any another type of abuse). Women who had not experienced any type of abuse since turning 55 years old were the reference group.

To measure repeat abuse, we created a nonrepeat-/repeat-abuse measure for those women who had experienced psychological/emotional abuse. As is shown in Table 1, 176 women (21% of the entire sample) had experienced repeated psychological/emotional abuse. Given the very small number of repeat victims within the other abuse categories, we did not create a nonrepeat-/repeat-abuse measure for these types of abuse.

Second, as the results on frequency of abuse presented in Table 1 suggest, a substantial proportion of older women had experienced abuse often. Taking into account the effects of the frequency with which these women had experienced psychological/emotional abuse or multiple types of abuse (psychological/emotional plus another type of abuse), we created four dummy variables. We further dichotomized each of the two dummy variables for specific type of abuse into two frequency groups: Rarely or Often. We found that 51% of the psychologically/ emotionally abused women and 81% of the multiple-abuse victims experienced abuse often.

Bivariate and Multivariate Results: Type and Frequency of Abuse and Health Outcomes

Demographic Correlates of Type of Abuse. —To examine the bivariate effects of the demographic characteristics used as control variables in the multivariate models, we examined their relationship with the type of abuse (psychological/emotional, repeated, and multiple abuse). The results of the chi-square test of independence showed that, of the demographic variables used as control variables in the multivariate analyses, only race was not significantly associated with any of the measures of abuse: abuse victimization ($\chi^2 = .434$, $df = 1$, $p = 0.51$), repeated psychological/emotional abuse ($\chi^2 = 0.272$, $df = 1$, $p = 0.60$), or multiple abuses ($\chi^2 = .346$, $df = 1$, $p = 0.56$). Level of education was not significantly related to experiencing multiple abuse ($\chi^2 = 0.367$, $df = 3$, $p = 0.94$). Being of Appalachian decent was not related to repeated abuse ($\chi^2 = 0.340$, $df = 1$, $p = 0.59$) or multiple abuse ($\chi^2 = 1.18$, $df = 1$, $p = 0.28$). Marital status was not related to multiple abuse ($\chi^2 = 4.89$, $df = 4$, $p = 0.30$). All of the relationships between the other control variables (e.g., age, income, and marital status) and the type of abuse were significant at $p < .05$ (the exception being the relationship between level of education and multiple abuse). A significantly larger percentage of younger older women (60–64 years old) had been abuse victims, victims of repeated abuse, and victims of multiple abuse compared with women older than age 65.

Type of Abuse and Health Outcomes. —Table 3 presents the effects of experiencing different types of abuse since age 55 on health outcomes. There are several noteworthy results. First, none

Table 3 Types of Abuse Since 55 Years Old and Health-Related Consequences

| | Type of Abuse | | | |
Variable	Abuse Victim, AOR[a] (95% CI)	Single Type of Abuse Victim: Psychological/ emotional, AOR (95% CI)	Repeat Psychological/ emotional Victim, AOR (95% CI)	Multiple Types of Abuse Victim: Psychological/ emotional and Other Types,[b] AOR (95% CI)
Health-related consequence				
Self-reported poor health status	0.96 (0.73–1.25)	1.03 (0.73–1.45)	0.86 (0.58–1.29)	0.83 (0.51–1.32)
No. of self-reported health conditions	3.6***[c] (1.7)	3.7*** (1.6)	3.7*** (1.6)	3.6*** (1.9)
Current health conditions				
Depression or anxiety	2.24*** (1.70–2.96)	1.74*** (1.25–2.44)	1.93*** (1.32–2.82)	1.85** (1.17–2.92)
Digestive problems (e.g., irritable bowel, ulcer, heartburn)	1.60** (1.22–2.09)	1.70*** (1.23–2.37)	1.45* (1.10–2.10)	0.97 (0.61–1.56)
Chronic pain (e.g., back pain, migraines)	1.65*** (1.28–2.15)	1.60*** (1.16–2.22)	1.51* (1.04–2.18)	1.09 (0.69–1.72)
High blood pressure or heart problems	1.22 (0.91–1.64)	1.52* (1.04–2.23)	1.32 (0.85–2.06)	0.72 (0.43–1.20)

Notes: AOR = adjusted odds ratio. Significance of the Wald statistic: *p <.05; **p < .01; ***p < .001.
[a]Adjusted for age, race and ethnicity, education, marital status, income, and Appalachian descent.
[b]Other types include control, threat, physical, and sexual abuse.
[c]The mean has been adjusted for age, race and ethnicity, education, marital status, income, and Appalachian decent. The standard deviation is reported in parentheses. The mean for nonvictims is 3.1 (SD = 1.8).

of the abuse measures were significantly related to older women's self-reported poor health status. Second, older women who had experienced abuse were significantly more likely than nonvictims to self-report more health conditions, on average. Third, regardless of how psychological/emotional abuse was operationalized—as occurring alone, repeatedly, or with other types of abuse—this type of abuse took a negative toll on women's current health. Women who had been psychologically/emotionally abused reported significantly more health conditions, on average, than did women who had not been abused in this manner.

Looking at the effects of abuse on current health conditions reveals that, overall, psychological/emotional abuse, again regardless of how it was operationalized, had negative effects on abused women. First, all types of abuse increased the odds of women reporting depression or anxiety by a factor of almost 2. Second, women who had experienced only psychological/emotional abuse had increased odds of having digestive problems, high blood pressure or heart problems, or chronic pain. Third, repeated psychological/emotional abuse was associated with increased odds of digestive problems and chronic pain. Fourth, women who had experienced any abuse were not significantly more likely to have reported lung, diabetes or thyroid, stroke or nerve, or blood problems, or cancer (p > .05; results not shown here).

Frequency of Abuse. —Table 4 presents the effects of the frequency of different types of abuse since age 55 on health out-

comes. These results show some noteworthy patterns supportive of those reported in Table 3.

First, in this study, frequency of abuse did not significantly predict women's self-reported poor health status. Second, abuse regardless of frequency or type was significantly associated with a number of self-reported health conditions. Women who had experienced either psychological/emotional abuse or multiple abuse reported significantly more health conditions, on average, than nonvictims. Third, having experienced psychological/emotional abuse, regardless of how often, increased women's odds of having digestive problems or chronic pain. Fourth, women who experienced psychological/emotional abuse often had increased odds of having bone or joint problems, depression or anxiety, or high blood pressure or heart problems. Fifth, regardless of the frequency or type of abuse experienced, women's odds of reporting depression or anxiety significantly increased. Notably, for women who had often experienced multiple abuse, the odds of reporting depression or anxiety increased by a factor of 4. Last, the frequency of neither psychological/emotional nor multiple abuse was significantly related to having lung, diabetes or thyroid, stroke or nerve, or blood problems, or cancer (p > .05; results not shown here).

Discussion

These results shed insight on the extent and nature of different types and patterns of abuse against older women. The findings revealed that a substantial proportion, nearly half, of older

Table 4 Frequency of Type of Abuse Since 55 Years Old and Health-Related Consequences

Variable	Single Type of Abuse Victim: Psychological/emotional, AOR[a] (95% CI)				Multiple Types of Abuse Victim: Psychological/emotional and Other Types, AOR[b] (95 CI)			
	Rarely		Often		Rarely		Often	
Health-related consequence								
Self-reported poor health status	0.91	(0.57–1.47)	1.07	(0.69–1.67)	0.51	(0.17–1.52)	0.92	(0.53–1.58)
No. of self-reported health conditions	3.3*[c]	(1.6)	3.8***	(1.5)	3.6*	(2.0)	3.6***	(1.9)
Current health conditions								
Bone or joint problem (e.g., arthritis or osteoporosis)	1.08	(0.70–1.67)	1.58*	(1.01–2.47)	1.62	(0.56–4.70)	1.12	(0.66–1.88)
Depression or anxiety	1.76*	(1.10–2.82)	2.61***	(1.69–4.03)	2.34**	(1.37–3.98)	4.06**	(1.52–10.87)
Digestive problems (e.g., irritable bowel, ulcer, heartburn)	1.77**	(1.13–2.76)	1.62***	(1.19–2.79)	1.41	(0.51–3.92)	1.21	(0.70–2.07)
Chronic pain (e.g., back pain, migraines)	1.70*	(1.09–2.64)	1.81**	(1.19–2.75)	1.46	(0.54–3.97)	1.38	(0.82–2.34)
High blood pressure or heart problem	1.24	(0.76–2.03)	1.77*	(1.03–3.02)	0.59	(0.19–1.90)	0.87	(0.49–1.56)

Notes: AOR = adjusted odds ratio. Significance of the Wald statistic: *$p < .05$; **$p < .01$; ***$p < .001$.
[a]Adjusted for age, race and ethnicity, education, marital status, income, Appalachian descent, and single control, threat, physical or sexual abuse, and multiple abuses.
[b] Adjusted for age, race and ethnicity, education, marital status, income, Appalachian descent, and single psychological/emotional abuse and single control, threat, physical or sexual abuse.
[c]The mean has been adjusted for age, race and ethnicity, education, marital status, income, Appalachian descent, and as per the respective abuses noted in footnotes a and b. The standard deviation is reported in parentheses. The mean for nonvictims is 3.1 ($SD = 1.8$).

women had experienced psychological/emotional, control, threat, physical, or sexual abuse since turning 55 years old. Second, the largest percentage of women had experienced psychological/emotional abuse. Third, a notable percentage of women had experienced multiple types of abuse. Fourth, many older women had experienced abuse repeatedly and often. Lastly, there does seem to be a relationship between abuse and health problems among older women.

As the literature review stated, the effect of abuse on younger women's health is becoming well documented. However, researchers have only begun to unravel the effects of abuse on the health of older women; more study is needed. Within the broader elder abuse literature, researchers have reported that older people who suffer abuse or mistreatment experience a much higher incidence of depression (Pillemer & Finkelhor, 1988; Pillemer & Prescott, 1989); and that experiencing elder abuse or mistreatment is a risk factor for nursing home placement in the older population (Lachs, Williams, O'Brien, & Pillemer, 2002) and higher mortality rates (Lachs, Williams, O'Brien, Pillemer, & Charlson, 1998). The present results are supportive of researchers' overall conclusion: Abuse takes a negative toll on the quality of life of older persons. The current results suggest that both the physical and mental health of older women are negatively affected by abuse.

This study has three main implications for people who serve the health care needs of older women. First, with regard to those practitioners in the health care arena who provide care to older women, it is important that providers acknowledge that abuse is happening and that it is affecting the health of these older women. The present results are a first step toward aiding in the understanding that women who are experiencing abuse may not report lower general health compared with women who are not being abused, yet are more likely to experience detrimental effects to their health if one examines for specific health conditions. Second, because older women who are being abused are more likely than nonvictims to report a higher total number of health conditions and to experience certain health conditions such as depression, anxiety, digestive problems, and chronic pain, these conditions may serve as red flags to health providers to screen for possible abuse within intimate-partner and interpersonal relationships. Third, the type of abuse most frequently experienced by the older women in this study was psychological/emotional abuse. This confirms findings by Harris (1996) that physical and sexual abuse decreases with age, whereas psychological abuse remains. Although great progress has been made in the elder abuse and domestic violence arenas to come to a consensus on uniform definitions of abuse, it is important to continue to define different categories of abuse (e.g., psychological, emotional, and control) because older women may have a more difficult time identifying this behavior as abuse. Zink, Regan, Jacobson, and Pabst (2003), in a qualitative study of abused women, found that in many cases women did not even identify psychological/emotional abuse as abuse. Or women reported that things in their marriage were okay now that it was *only* psychological/emotional abuse and that the physical and sexual abuse had decreased or stopped. However, in the present study, we found that, for those women who were experiencing abuse, the likelihood that they were experiencing different kinds of abuse was high. Consequently, if an older woman does admit to one type of abuse, it is likely that she is experiencing or has experienced other types of abuse as well, and that she experiences abuse more than once and possibly often.

This study also has implications for individuals who provide social services for older women. First, it is important for providers to be trained to look for signs of psychological/emotional abuse in older women, as the present results suggest that (a) this is the type of abuse that is most likely to occur, and (b) this type of abuse is most likely to co-occur with other more severe forms of abuse. It is common for providers who suspect abuse to make referrals to agencies such as adult protective services. However, in the case of domestic abuse, this may be an inappropriate referral. In many states, adult protective services is only allowed to intervene if the victim is physically or mentally impaired, which may not be the case in every instance. Consequently, neither the cause nor the effects of the abuse will be addressed. Many people who provide services to the elderly are taught to think only about caregiver stress as a possible cause of abuse. In such cases, they may make referrals to get aging service providers into the home. In some situations this may exacerbate an already abusive situation. Advocates such as Brandl (1997) and researchers (Fisher et al., 2003; Vinton, 2003) have suggested that professionals in the aging field need to be more informed about the resources available for the victims of domestic violence. Similarly, professionals in the domestic violence field need to become more familiar with the resources available on aging (Fisher et al., 2004; Grossman & Lundy, 2003). As women who are being abused continue to age and live longer, it will become increasingly imperative that more and more crosstraining take place between these two fields. Lastly, this study found that control, threat, physical, and sexual abuse is perpetrated by many people who are routinely involved in their victim's lives. The perpetrator can be a spouse or boyfriend, other relative, or non-relative. Consequently, health care and social service providers need to insist, if possible, for a few minutes alone with the older woman to question her about possible abuse and even the identity of the abuser.

This study is not without limitations. First, this is a cross-sectional study, which limits our ability to make causal inferences about the effects of health and abuse. We are unable to ascertain if abuse is the cause of the increase in health conditions or if having more health conditions puts women at more risk for being abused. Second, many of the potential survey respondents were never reached, and, because of the Health Insurance Portability and Accountability Act regulations, we were unable to find out any information on non-responders. Third, the abuse

and health information is uncorroborated self-report and could not be confirmed through medical record review. The abuse is also self-report; however, because women are unlikely to report abuse, the abuse reported for this study may actually be an underreporting of the abuse taking place. Fourth, interviewers asked women to recall events that may have happened several years ago. It must also be kept in mind that the marital status and abuse relationship is one that must be viewed with caution. Respondents were asked about their current marital status—not their marital status at the time of the abuse. A respondent may have been abused by her spouse a year ago, and the spouse has since died.

Despite its limitations, this study is an important first step in documenting the existence of the different types of abuse happening to older women, its repetitive nature and frequency, and its effect on health. It is imperative that health care and service providers be aware of the health implications of abuse and understand the need for identification and training in both aging and domestic violence. As the population continues to age, awareness of resources available through both aging and domestic violence networks will become necessary.

References

Bonnie, R., & Wallace, R. (Eds.). (2002). *Elder abuse: Abuse, neglect and exploitation in an aging America.* Washington, DC: The National Academies Press.

Brandl, B. (1997). *Developing services for older abused women.* Madison: Wisconsin Coalition Against Domestic Violence.

Campbell, J., Jones, A. S., Dienemann, J., Kub, J., Schollenberger, J., O'Campo, P., et al. (2002). Intimate partner violence and physical health consequences. *Archives of Internal Medicine, 162,* 1157–1163.

Coker, A. L., Davis, K. E., Arias, I., Desai, D., Sanderson, M., Brandt, H. M., et al. (2002). Physical and mental health effects on intimate partner violence for men and women. *American Journal of Preventive Medicine, 23,* 260–268.

Fisher, B. S., Zink, T., Pabst, S., Regan, S., & Rinto, B. (2004). Service and programming for older abused women: The Ohio experience. *Journal of Elder Abuse & Neglect, 15*(2), 67–83.

Fisher, B. S., Zink, T., Rinto, B., Regan, S., Pabst, S., & Gothelf, E. (2003). Overlooked during the golden years: Violence against older women. *Violence Against Women, 12,* 1409–1416.

Grossman, S., & Lundy, M. (2003). Use of domestic violence services across race and ethnicity by women 55 and older: The Illinois experience. *Violence Against Women, 12,* 1442–1452.

Harris, S. (1996). For better or for worse: Spouse abuse grown old. *Journal of Elder Abuse & Neglect, 8*(1), 1–33.

Hegarty, K., Gunn, J., Chondros, R., & Small, R. (2004). Association between depression and abuse by partners of women attending general practice: Descriptive, cross-sectional survey. *British Medical Journal, 328,* 621–624.

Koss, M. P., Koss, P. G., & Woodruff, W. J. (1991). The deleterious effects of criminal victimization on women's health and medical utilization. *Archives of Internal Medicine, 151,* 342–347.

Lachs, M., & Pillemer, K. (1995). Abuse and neglect of elderly persons. *New England Journal of Medicine, 332,* 437–443.

Lachs, M., Williams, C., O'Brien, S., & Pillemer, K. (2002). Adult protective service use and nursing home placement. *The Gerontologist, 42,* 734–739.

Lachs, M., Williams, C., O'Brien, S., Pillemer, K., & Charlson, M. (1998). The mortality of elder mistreatment. *Journal of the American Medical Association, 280,* 428–432.

Mouton, C. (2003). Intimate partner violence and health status among older women. *Violence Against Women, 12,* 1465–1477.

Mouton, C., Rodabourgh, R., Rovim, S., Hunt, J., Talamantes, M., Brzyski, R., et al. (2004). Prevalence and 3-year incidence of abuse among postmenopausal women. *American Journal of Public Health, 94,* 605–612.

National Center on Elder Abuse. (1998). *The National Elder Abuse Incidence Study.* Washington, DC: The Administration for Children and Families and the Administration on Aging, U.S. Department of Health and Human Services.

Pillemer, K., & Finkelhor, D. (1988). The prevalence of elder abuse: A random sample survey. *The Gerontologist, 28,* 51–57.

Pillemer, K., & Prescott, D. (1989). Psychological effects of elder abuse: A research note. *Journal of Elder Abuse & Neglect 1*(1), 65–74.

Rennison, C., & Rand, M. (2003). Non-lethal intimate partner violence: Women age 55 or older. *Violence Against Women, 12,* 1417–1428.

Saltzman, L., Fanslow, J., McMahon, P., & Shelley, G. (2002). *Intimate partner violence surveillance: Uniform definition and recommended data elements, version 1.0.* Atlanta, GA: National Center for Injury Prevention and Control, Centers for Disease Control and Prevention. (Original work published in 1999)

Shepard, M., & Campbell, J. (1992). The abusive behavior inventory: A measure of psychological and physical abuse. *Journal of Interpersonal Violence, 7,* 291–305.

SPSS, Incorporated. (2002). *SPSS 11.5 for Windows.* Chicago: Author.

StataCorp. (2001). *Stata Statistical Software: Release 7.0.* College Station, TX: Author.

Sutherland, C., Bybee, D., & Sullivan, C. (2002). Beyond bruises and broken bones: The joint effects of stress and injuries on battered women's health. *American Journal of Community Psychology, 30,* 609–636.

Teaster, P., & Roberto, K. (2004). Sexual abuse of older women living in nursing homes. *The Gerontologist, 44,* 788–796.

Tjaden, P., & Thoennes, N. (1998). *Prevalence, incidence and consequences of violence against women: Findings from the National Violence Against Women survey* (NCJ172837). Washington, DC: U.S. Department of Justice, National Institute of Justice and Centers for Disease Control and Prevention.

Vinton, L. (2003). A model collaborative project toward making domestic violence centers elder ready. *Violence Against Women, 12,* 1504–1513.

Wilke, D., & Vinton, L. (2003). Domestic violence and aging: Teaching about their intersection. *Journal of Social Work Education, 39,* 225–235.

Zink, T., Fisher, B. S., Regan, S., & Pabst, S. (2005). The prevalence and incidence of intimate partner violence in older women in primary care practice. *Journal of General Internal Medicine, 20,* 884–888.

Zink, T., Regan, S., Jacobson, C. J., & Pabst, S. (2003). Cohort, period and aging effects: A qualitative study of older women's reasons for remaining in abusive relationships. *Violence Against Women, 9,* 1429–1441.

UNIT 5

Retirement: American Dream or Dilemma?

Unit Selections

Key Points to Consider

- What are some of the individual adjustment problems older people often face during their first year of retirement?

- Upon arriving at retirement age, why do some workers choose to continue to work either full-time or part-time?

- What are the advantages to the employers of retaining older employees on a full-time or part-time basis?

- Are persons between 40 and 60 able to save enough for their retirement?

- What incentives could employers develop to keep older persons working longer?

- Are company retirement programs proving to be economically solvent today?

- Given different choices of lifestyles between work and retirement, which older Americans are most satisfied during their later years?

Student Website

www.mhcls.com/online

Internet References

Further information regarding these websites may be found in this book's preface or online.

American Association of Retired People
http://www.aarp.org
Health and Retirement Study (HRS)
http://www.umich.edu/~hrswww/

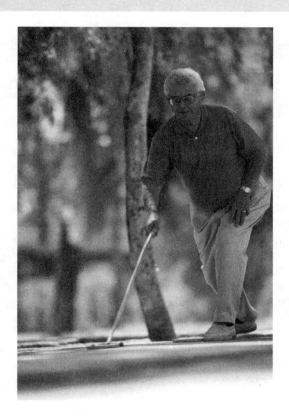

Since 1900, the number of people in America who are age 65 years and over has been increasing steadily, but a decreasing proportion of that age group remains in the workforce. In 1900 nearly two-thirds of those over the age of 65 worked outside the home. By 1947 this figure had declined to about 48 percent (less than half), and in 1975 about 22 percent of men 65 and older were still in the workforce. The long-range trend indicates that fewer and fewer people are employed beyond the age of 65. Some people choose to retire at age 65 or earlier; for others, retirement is mandatory. A recent change in the law, however, allows individuals to work as long as they want with no mandatory retirement age.

Gordon Strieb and Clement Schneider (Retirement in American Society, 1971) observed that for retirement to become an institutionalized social pattern in any society, certain conditions must be present. A large group of people must live long enough to retire; the economy must be productive enough to support people who are not in the workforce; and there must be pensions or insurance programs to support retirees.

Retirement is a rite of passage. People can consider it either as the culmination of the American Dream or as a serious problem. Those who have ample incomes, interesting things to do, and friends to associate with often find the freedom of time and choice that retirement offers very rewarding. For others, however, retirement brings problems and personal losses. Often, these individuals find their incomes decreased; they miss the status, privilege, and power associated with holding a position in the occupational hierarchy. They may feel socially isolated if they do not find new activities to replace their previous work-related ones. Additionally, they might have to cope with the death of a spouse and/or their own failing health.

Older persons approach retirement with considerable concern about financial and personal problems. Will they have enough retirement income to maintain their current lifestyle? Will their income remain adequate as long as they live? Given the current state of health, how much longer can they continue to work?

The next articles deal with changing Social Security regulations and changing labor demands that are encouraging older persons to work beyond the age of 65. In "How to Survive the First Year," Kelly Greene observes that the first year of retirement is the most difficult transition for new retirees. Critical questions that each prospective retiree should address are outlined. Paul Lim in "The Big Squeeze" discussed the ever-increasing financial pressure put on middle-aged Americans as they attempt to save for retirement while paying for their children's education and supporting aging parents. In "Old. Smart. Productive." the author points out the reasons why he believes a significant number of the baby boom generation will work beyond age 65. In "The Broken Promise," the authors point out how federal bankruptcy and related laws have allowed employers to default on their employees' pension funds and programs. In "Work/Retirement Choices and Lifestyle Patterns of Older Americans," the authors examine six different work, retirement, and leisure patterns that older people may choose to determine which is most satisfying to the individual.

"How to Survive the First Year"

KELLY GREENE

Patricia Breakstone, age 63, remembers her first year of retirement from her 38-year career as a state-government analyst in San Diego as a "terrible transition period."

Shortly after leaving her job last spring, she started a long-awaited kitchen renovation, which turned her condo upside-down right when she was starting to spend her days at home for the first time in her adult life. Then her dog was struck by kidney disease, and Ms. Breakstone wound up spending $7,000 in veterinary bills over two months as she tried in vain to nurse her pet back to health.

As the months wore on, "I didn't want to get up in the morning," she says. Finally, a friend goaded her into applying for a part-time job at a bakery near her home, which helped her regain some structure in her days—along with providing a social outlet. "Retirement," she says now, "is a real balancing act."

For all its allure, for all the time that people spend planning and daydreaming about it, the actual act of retiring can turn out to be a wrenching experience. That's what we learned from canvassing dozens of people across the country about their first year outside the office. We wanted to find out—at a time when the 50-plus crowd, in particular, is apprehensive about its future and finances—just how satisfying, or scary, those first 12 months can be.

Among the questions we asked: Did the transition prove to be easy or difficult? If people did any planning beforehand, had it paid off? Did they find themselves spending more or less money than they had anticipated? Had they gone back to work? What did they miss most about their jobs? What was the biggest surprise?

The answers showed that while some people clearly enjoyed leaving work behind, many were disoriented. Just like college freshmen, first-year retirees often change their "majors." Even people who start out with a road map rarely wind up following it the way they expected. And rare is the retiree who spends significantly less money than when he or she was working full time.

But as the first year winds down, many retirees start settling into Plan B—or C, or D, for that matter. That's when post-work life finally starts to get comfortable.

"There doesn't seem to be the big hole that I expected after all those years working," says Steve Holt, age 63, who retired from General Electric Co. in Seattle in late 2001, and moved to Tucson, Ariz., the following May. "I was surprised that it was so easy to find things to do and become involved."

In hopes of providing a shortcut for people contemplating retirement—or retirees still struggling to make it work—here are the first-year lessons we heard most often.

Be Choosy with Your Time

You might expect to have an empty calendar during your early days of retirement. But whether you find that prospect frightening or appealing, your schedule could fill up quickly if you aren't careful—and with things you may not really want to be doing.

Debbie Lynch, for example, was asked to stay on for several months as director of communications and head of an educational foundation at the Aurora, Colo., school system after she officially retired, in November 2001. As the school year drew to a close, she was offered two consulting jobs that would start the following fall, one in fund raising for the local community college, the other helping to set up a foundation for the local chamber of commerce.

"I initially thought, every job that comes along, I have to take," says Ms. Lynch, 54 years old. Despite the fact that she and her husband both have secure pensions, "every once in a while, I think, 'Who will take care of me when I'm old?' I don't have any children." Plus, she wanted to stay connected with the professional friends she had made through the years.

But last summer, between the old job and new consulting work, "I discovered there are a lot of things you can do during daylight hours. It was a real treat to go to the grocery store at 10 a.m.," she says. "It was the first time in years and years that I had that much time. I played a little golf, walked every day, did some long-term cleaning I probably should have done 25 years ago. I just piddled."

When it came time to begin the consulting job, "I started thinking, 'Why did I agree to do this?' " Ms. Lynch recalls. "It was one of the biggest surprises I had. I wasn't ready to get back into being responsible on a regular basis." Although she enjoys her community ties, she regrets the fact that work eats up four days a week. "I really think I would prefer in the long run to do more project-based things that have a beginning and an end. I'm less interested in being tied down to certain days and hours."

Part of the initial temptation to fill up the calendar stems from the fear "that if you say no, nobody's ever going to ask you

On Your Mark, Get Set...

Are you ready to retire? In their book "Don't Retire, Rewire," authors Jeri Sedlar and Rick Miners offer the following questions, developed by Tessa Albert Warschaw, to help people gauge where they stand in their preparations:

Taking Stock

- Have you thought about restructuring or reinventing yourself?
- Have you spent time asking yourself, "What's next?"
- Are you aware of the loss you may feel (i.e., loss of position, power, the game, the deal, a place to go, schedule, agenda, assistants, secretary, etc.)?
- Have you considered whether you will miss the travel and entertainment perks?
- Have you thought about how you will feel doing your own paperwork?
- Have you considered how you will feel?
- Have you thought about whether you will miss all those problems to solve?
- Have you anticipated whether you will miss the triumphs and approvals?
- Have you considered whether you will miss your title?
- Have you thought about whether your spouse will miss your title?

Family Dynamics

- Have you considered the changes in your family dynamic?
- Will your being home more affect your partner?
- Will your family see you as less powerful?
- Will you consider yourself less powerful?
- Will you transfer your "work style" to your home?
- Do you see yourself setting up a command post at home-issuing directives, responsibilities and orders?
- Do you see yourself taking on household duties, running family errands, cooking, etc.)?
- Do you see yourself assisting younger family members or "baby-sitting" the grandchildren or elder parents?
- Will you feel resentment for your partner who hasn't retired and continued to work inside and/or outside the home?

Source: "Don't Retire, Rewire," © 2002, Alpha Books-Penguin Group, USA

to do something again," says Bob Atchley, a Boulder, Colo., gerontologist who has studied retirees since 1963. As a result, retirees can be victimized by time poachers who volunteer them for tasks they might not necessarily want to do but may feel guilty turning down.

"You have to learn the lesson of how to say 'no,' whether it's to the kids saying, 'Oh, you can baby-sit, can't you?' Or someone saying, 'You can co-chair this project. What else do you have to do?'" advises Jeri Sedlar, a New York retirement-transition counselor.

Robert Carpenter, 64, who participates in a "Reinventing Retirement" class at Emory University's Academy for Retired Professionals in Atlanta, says many of his friends are "activity addicted." It's a trap he found himself falling into during his retirement from Georgia Power Co., before he started making a conscious effort to clear time on his calendar.

"I found myself filling up my calendar with 'good' things, which was the enemy of the 'best' things when they came up." For example, when he decided to skip an enrichment course on a recent weekday, he and his wife seized on the sunny weather to check out a nearby lakeside resort for lunch. And after they cleared from their schedules an annual golf tournament that they usually attend, it freed them up to accept an invitation to their granddaughter's fifth birthday party. "That's something we would have rather done anyway," he says.

It's OK to Slow Down

Taking time for yourself can change your outlook on what you want to do with all your newfound free time, as Ms. Lynch in Colorado and many others have found.

"Drift time" is something that many retirees rediscover, says Joel Savishinsky, an anthropologist at Ithaca College in New York, who has studied people during their first year in retirement. One couple he watched would take long bike rides "presumably to go from Point A to Point B in their community, and they rarely made it to Point B. In retirement, if you allow yourself, you have the luxury to be diverted, to digress, to slow down, to change directions. To get off the bike."

And as you're making the adjustment to retirement, that can be especially important. Mary Roberson, who retired as an elementary-school librarian in Dallas last spring, recommends taking some initial time "to just veg." For most people, she says, "those last couple of months before retirement are nonstop. It was incredible how many things had to be done before I turned the library over to the next person."

"I didn't take on any new projects," says Ms. Roberson, 61. "I gave myself time to work in the yard and feel better about the flower beds. I cleaned out a few closets. I sat and had a second cup of coffee and read the whole paper. I needed a couple of unwinding months before I did anything else."

Now, she's starting to take on short-term projects. She recently wrapped up five weeks of work at her son's law firm as he scrambled to prepare for a big trial, "and five weeks is as long as I want to commit to anything," she says.

By all means, try new things and challenge yourself—but don't get stressed out about it. Ed Susank, 58, a retired healthcare benefits consultant with Mercer Human Resource Consulting, says he initially made a list of things he wanted to do after he retired, including "becoming more proficient in a foreign language." But he isn't rushing to cross things off. "I like to have a few pegs around which the rest of it can kind of drape casually."

That's an approach that Dr. Atchley, the gerontologist, considers healthy. "In our world, most people push themselves beyond anything that's good for them physically and mentally," Dr. Atchley says. "So the idea that people actually could cut back quite a bit on the complexity and the level of activity that they're involved in after they retire and still be at the level any full-time person ought to be has a lot to recommend it."

Work Out the Ground Rules

If you have a partner, chances are you'll be spending a lot more time together under one roof when you retire. That could lead to some stomping (albeit unintentional) on each other's toes.

Ken Schumann says that within two months of his retirement last year as director of the North American agriculture business for Ciba Special Chemicals AG, his wife, Patty, came up with three rules for him: "No. 1, I cannot fall asleep in front of the TV from Monday to Friday. No. 2, I cannot follow Patty around and ask what she's doing next. No. 3 is, since I traveled so much and she wasn't used to cooking seven days a week, we needed an outside life, including dinners out. I now have a 3A. I must answer the telephone because the calls are for me for a change."

Mr. Schumann, who is 59 years old and lives in suburban Atlanta, talked about his new rules at a recent meeting of the same Emory class that Mr. Carpenter attends. Their classmates agree that negotiating personal space with your partner is one of the biggest hurdles in the first year.

Among their recommendations: Shell out the bucks for separate phone lines, computers and e-mail addresses. Stake out space in your home that is yours alone. Mr. Carpenter says he has a "cave" with his own TV, computer, and recliner. Also, negotiate the time you spend together—and apart. Derek Moore, 64, a retired aerospace executive with Lockheed Martin Corp. in Marietta, Ga., had planned on selling antiquarian books as a new career, with help from his wife. That pastime ended after five months, because they each realized the project was keeping them from individual interests they considered important. Mr. Moore, for his part, wanted more time to pursue the arts, and he has since taken up painting.

Be Prepared to Switch Gears

Jim Matheson was always bothered by the litter he saw along the road during his 10-mile commute to Worcester, Mass., as an insurance executive. "I swore that when I retired, I was going to get a little pickup trailer, and in the course of a year, I was going to pick up the trash on all 116 miles of roads in our town," he recalls.

Mr. Matheson retired in January 2002, shortly after he turned 55 and could take an early-retirement package. A few months later, he visited the local police department to explain his plan "before someone reported that there was this vagrant along the side of the road." While he was there, the chief told him the department could use some help with its roadside radar-information unit (responsible for the signs that say, "Slow Down, Your Speed Is . . .").

"I said, 'Wait a minute. You're telling me I get to drive the cruiser, right?'" Mr. Matheson recalls. What started out as an effort to pick up bottles and cans evolved into what Mr. Matheson considers the chance of a lifetime: getting behind the wheel of a police car—even if it's only to haul the signs around. The first time he drove the vehicle on a major highway, "traffic backed up for miles behind me," he says. "What a feeling of power."

Sometimes, your retirement plans don't work out the way you envisioned, as with Mr. Moore's book-dealing business. In that case, "if you've tried it and you don't like it, discard it," says Ms. Sedlar, the counselor. She steers many people to volunteermatch.org, a Web site that matches your interests and location to community needs.

But make sure you give a retirement plan, whether it's volunteer or for pay, a fair shake before you move on, Ms. Sedlar adds. She recalls a woman in New York who tried volunteering with a political group. In her first days there, not surprisingly, the woman was assigned several humdrum tasks, including licking envelopes. But rather than giving her new position a chance, the woman quickly "called up and got her old job back," Ms. Sedlar says. "That's the road of least resistance."

Another reason to stay flexible: Sometimes, the retirement gig you were counting on doesn't materialize. Malcolm McNeill took early retirement as a 55-year-old manager with General Electric's GE Capital unit in Cincinnati last year, and then moved to Fort Collins, Colo., planning to teach graduate business courses at Colorado State University, as he had done in the past at other colleges.

"But they are going through the same budget downturn as everyone else," he says, and as a result, he wasn't hired. "That was disappointing. I don't know if colleges know it, but they could hire people like me almost for free."

Mr. McNeill found a way to teach after all. He has volunteered to lead personal-enrichment courses in photography through the Front Range Forum, a retirement-learning institute where "everyone is there because they want to be there."

A Role Model or Two Can Help

Mark Feinknopf, a 66-year-old retired architect, was laid off about a year ago from his job as an urban planner for the Metropolitan Atlanta Rapid Transit Authority. A year earlier, he had started interviewing his mentors, most of them in their 70s and 80s, to find out how they had handled later-life transitions, including retirement and the premature deaths of spouses.

One of those role models, Josiah Blackmore, is a retired president of Capital University in Columbus, Ohio, who now spends his days in the countryside as an alpaca farmer. He and his wife have even opened a retail store on their farm where they're having trouble keeping enough alpaca fiber in stock.

Mr. Feinknopf hasn't decided what he wants to do yet with his own retirement, but talking to more-experienced retirees helped him settle on a goal: "I'm spending the second year trying to . . . find an opportunity to build something of value with other people."

Many retirees seek out role models without even realizing it, says Dr. Savishinsky, the anthropologist. In his studies, he notes, people's thoughts about retirement were "partly based on what they had learned from watching other people go through it," most often their parents and older co-workers. The recent retirees he followed were more likely to fixate on negative role models than positive ones. "Many retirees seem to be concerned with not blowing it," he says. "It was almost more important to know what not to do than it was to have a clear idea of what they wanted to do, which provided a very helpful road map of the people and places or pursuits to avoid."

Indeed, Mr. Matheson thinks many people are afraid to retire early because "they superimpose themselves on their parents and say, 'My father, when he retired, sat in the living room, drank beer and watched TV.' I think we [baby boomers] break that mold. If you can shake yourself loose, you see there's a big bad world out there, and there's a lot of fun stuff to do."

Finding Friends Can Take More Work

Mr. McNeill, the retired GE manager, made an unpleasant discovery when he and his wife moved to Colorado: Making friends their own age was more difficult than he had imagined.

"The thing that's been a little tough for us, and we probably should have foreseen, is most retirees are older than us, and most people's lives revolve around work," he says today. "That's where you make most of your friends."

In the McNeills' case, the solution has come through strong interests they have had for many years. He has immersed himself in photography, making frequent expeditions to Arches National Park near Moab, Utah; she plays the tuba and cello in community music groups.

Mr. Susank and his wife moved to Alexandria, Va., a few years before he retired from Mercer in late 2001, after living in Los Angeles for most of their lives. A big part of their relocation strategy was buying a townhouse in a new complex where everyone would be getting to know one another at the same time. That way, they reasoned, it would be easier to make friends with neighbors than if they moved into an established development where everybody else already had found their barbecuing buddies.

They got lucky, too. "The lady who is right next door to us had a husband in the Navy for many years," says Mr. Susank. "She's done a lot of traveling, and she has introduced us to many people."

Finding friends the same age isn't just a matter of dinner-table company, says Dr. Atchley. "All of the doubts and funny stuff you do yourself that are connected to the transition become a little more obvious when you talk about it. It's funnier when you see it in your friends, too," he says. "You begin to laugh at your own foibles, and that's a good thing. A sense of humor is adaptive."

Don't Expect Spending to Fall

When Mr. Schumann, the former Ciba executive, began thinking about expenses in later life, he used a familiar benchmark. "Everything you read says you spend 20% less in retirement, so I [factored] that in my monthly budget." But he never realized how much of his entertainment expenses—for meals, trips and the like—actually were tied to business and reimbursed by his company.

Today, he says, "I think I'm spending a little bit more in retirement than I was when I was working."

Other retirees mention the loss of similar job-related extras leading to increased retirement spending: company cars, frequent-flier miles—even technical assistance for their home computers.

Then there's the whopper: health insurance. If you're lucky enough to get any coverage at all from your former employer, the premiums and deductibles are likely to rise steeply in coming years. A study of 56 retiree health plans last year by Watson Wyatt Worldwide, a human-resources consulting firm in Washington, found that 17% require retirees to pay the full premiums. And 20% have eliminated such plans altogether for new hires.

When Fred Hattman retired from Milford, Conn., to Nags Head, N.C., two years ago, he took a job delivering the local Coastal Times newspaper three times a week. That way, Mr. Hattman, 64, can pay his share of his health-insurance premiums. It's a sizable expense—$550 a month—even though he's able to piggy-back on his wife's coverage through her full-time job at a local bank. "I knew I had to get some money somewhere to pay for the medical," he says, adding that the cost is "pretty scary, when you consider I'm pretty healthy."

Even for people who have turned in their time cards for good, the reduced costs of business suits, gasoline for the commute, dry cleaning, lunches and other expenses are often offset by the cost of new interests, says Wicke Chambers, a retired communications consultant in Atlanta who teaches the Emory course.

"You suddenly become a gardener," she says. "Or you become a golfer and you take more lessons, and you buy more balls, and you get a new bag."

Not only that, but being around the house more can make people "project-happy," she says. "You decide to redo the kitchen," for instance. "So the spending goes from a lot less in clothes and cleaning and things like that to the 'impulse itch.'"

Retiring Can Be Tough If Your Spouse Still Works

After a one-year trial, some people find that they still haven't eased into retirement, so they dust off their resumes and go back to work. Often, the people who wrestle with their newfound leisure time are those with spouses still on the job.

Marla Church, 60, a lawyer who took a buyout a year ago from Elan Corp. in Atlanta, says her husband "leaves at 6:45 in the morning and comes home at 4:30 in the afternoon. I need to find something productive to do in this period." Especially because her Elan stock has plummeted in value, she says, "I feel guilty if I do watercolors during the day."

At the moment, she's doing consulting work with Elan and is patent attorney of counsel with a local law firm. But she's also exploring the idea of doing "something entirely different," perhaps in the field of archaeology. She's taking a course in geology through the Emory program, at the moment, among other classes. Still, "it's hard to start over again without going back to school for years," she says. "My husband loves his work, and here I am floundering. It's a tough situation."

Myrna Weiss, a retired marketing executive in New York, had started doing many of the activities while she was working that people typically look forward to in retirement. She already was spending at least 10 hours a week volunteering and has gone to the opera and ballet regularly for years. "I don't feel like I've denied myself," she says.

But her spouse, too, still heads for the office each day. "My husband is going to work until he's disabled or horizontal," Ms. Weiss says. "He's happy as a clam."

When she first retired, Ms. Weiss pursued consulting work, but soon found it old hat since she had done a similar stint in the 1980s. Now, to scratch her entrepreneurial itch, she's exploring the chance to invest in and work with a group planning to buy and restructure an existing financial business.

"I'm looking for a niche that is going to keep the adrenaline going," she says. "It's just a matter of my being patient to alight on something that I want to do, versus getting antsy enough to choose anything."

MS. GREENE is a staff reporter in *The Wall Street Journal*'s Atlanta bureau. She can be reached at encore@wsj.com.

The Big Squeeze

The pressure is on baby boomers saving for retirement. Many also face college tuition and caring for a parent

PAUL J. LIM

I n his State of the Union address, President Bush made a pledge to Americans 55 and older. Yes, it's true he plans to overhaul the nation's retirement safety net, he said. But "for you," he promised, "the Social Security system will not change in any way."

How about workers who were born in 1950 or later? What kind of guarantee do they get?

Apparently none in today's retirement world. For workers in their mid-40s and 50s, the specter of Social Security reform adds yet another air of uncertainty to their retirement plans. Already shaken by a three-year bear market at the start of this decade, and a listless market now, workers must also confront an ever-changing global economy and, for many, the squeeze presented by the need to finance college tuitions and care for aging parents. Many of them are facing this uncertain age with only the barest of financial preparation: Forty-one percent of workers ages 45 to 54 have less than $25,000 saved up for retirement.

But even those who have planned by the book are enduring their share of anxiety. For much of their careers, Paul and Margaret Eberts of West Chester, Pa., have done the right thing by saving 10 to 15 percent of their annual income.

The crunch years. But while Paul, 48, and Margaret, 47, make a decent living—he's a family practice physician while she works part time as a physician in occupational medicine—the Eberts aren't so sure they'll be able to keep hitting those targets. That's because "the crunch years" are just a couple years off, says Paul.

Paul and Margaret have four kids: two boys and two girls ages 16, 14, 12, and 10. Between 2007 (when their oldest starts college) and 2017 (when their youngest is expected to finish up her undergraduate work), the Eberts's biggest financial obligation will be paying for college "It's going to be a real question mark whether we'll be able to contribute the max to our retirement plans," during this stretch, says Paul who will be 60 at the end of it.

65% of workers ages 45 to 54 say they're saving for retirement.

"Young boomers are running out of time to save," says Mike Scarborough, president of the Scarborough Group, a retirement planning advisory firm.

Assuming current expectations for Social Security benefits, only around 40 percent of workers born between 1951 and 1960 are on track to have enough money to cover basic expenses in retirement, based on their current savings and investment behavior. That's according to an analysis by the Employee Benefit Research Institute. "And that's just to meet basic living expenses," says EBRI Chief Executive Officer Dallas Salisbury. As anyone reaching middle age knows, life can throw out a curve ball, like an illness or the loss of a job.

Already, the boomer generation has borne the brunt of the seismic shift in the private sector, from traditional pensions—with their promise of income for life—to do-it-yourself retirement plans like 401(k)'s, which put workers at the mercy of the markets.

Even boomers lucky enough to be covered by traditional pensions are waking up to a new reality: It turns out those guaranteed benefits aren't necessarily guaranteed after all. Many pilots and flight attendants at United Airlines, for example, are likely to see their pensions slashed now that the struggling airline has been allowed to offload its pension to the federal Pension Benefit Guaranty Corp. Other employers could follow United's example.

And the boomers need to plan for *long* retirements. Modern medicine and better diets are yielding longer lives. The average American woman today can expect to live until 80, up nearly five years from 1970. Those who make it to 65 can expect to live until nearly 84.

Yet boomers also have to worry about higher expenses in their elongated retirements—and not just because of their propensity to spend. Only 13 percent of private-sector employers offer medical benefits to retired former workers, according to EBRI. And the promise of longer lives through better medicine has come with a price. Healthcare expenses could wind up costing retirees 20 percent of their annual income, according to the employee benefit consulting firm Hewitt Associates. This may explain why three times as many boomers say they fear major illness and healthcare expenses more than dying.

Here's another pressure point: With recent record low mortgage interest rates and surging home values, Americans have been refinancing their mortgages in droves. This includes young boomers like the Eberts.

Last year, the Eberts refinanced their mortgage and took some of their equity out of the home to pay for additions to their house. They redid their kitchen and added a bedroom and a garage for their growing family. To do so, they took an old 30-year mortgage—of which they already paid down 12 years—and replaced it with a new 30-year loan. This means Paul will be around 77 by the time his home is paid off.

Worse still, because of the renovations, the couple's monthly mortgage payments actually increased even though they refinanced at lower rates. "It bothered me a bit to take that on," says Paul, but "we really didn't have a whole lot of options."

Mortgage bonfire. The fact that so many Americans will be carrying mortgages well into retirement means that the old rule of thumb of needing to replace 70 or 80 percent of your preretirement income is out the window. "That may have been true in the old days, when retirees burned their mortgages before retiring," says Rande Spiegelman, vice president of financial planning for the Schwab Center for Investment Research. But today, he says, young boomers should plan on saving enough to replace 100 percent of their preretirement income—minus whatever they are setting aside to build up their nest eggs.

25% of workers ages 45 to 54 plan to retire at age 65, down from 39% just 10 years ago.

If only there were a federal Leave No Young Boomer Behind Act. But, says Daniel Houston, senior vice president for retirement and investor services at the Principal Financial Group, "there are no silver bullets. The Lone Ranger left the last one of those on the prairie."

So what should one do? For starters, young boomers simply have to save more money. Period. This may be difficult for workers who are simultaneously paying their children's college bills. But "if you don't cut your spending voluntarily now, you'll be forced to cut your standard of living in retirement," says Houston.

Consider this: Fifty-five percent of young boomers—those ages 45 to 54—have saved less than $50,000 toward their retirement, not including the value of their primary residences. Two thirds have less than $100,000 saved. And nearly 9 in 10 have less than $250,000.

Yet academic research shows that retirees who want to play it safe can afford to withdraw only 4 percent to 5 percent of their nest eggs each year in retirement—if they want them to last for 30 years or more. Even a person with $250,000 could afford to tap only $10,000 or so annually.

The good news is many young boomers, like David Fooshe, 50, are getting the message. Fooshe, an engineering project manager in Portland, Ore., has always made the maximum contributions allowed in his 401(k)'s and IRAs. But in recent years, he has also begun taking advantage of the so-called catch-up

provisions in tax-deferred retirement plans. Next year, workers 50 and older are allowed to put an additional $5,000 into their 401(k)'s and $1,000 into their IRAs.

It helps to start the saving habit early. The Schwab Center for Investment Research concluded that all workers should start saving 10 percent to 15 percent of their income in their 20s. That way, they can maintain that rate all their working life. If you wait until your 30s to start, then you need to set aside 15 percent to 25 percent of your annual income for the rest of your career. Workers who haven't started by their early 40s will need to sock away 25 percent to 35 percent of their incomes annually to make up for lost time.

For many, this represents a huge undertaking. But keep in mind that if you're maxing out your 401(k) and contributing to an IRA, you may already be close to hitting 15 percent.

You may think you can play catch up with the stock market. Think again.

David Darst, chief investment strategist of Morgan Stanley's individual investor group, says today's young boomers are "facing relatively mundane and mediocre returns in the stock market." After a 20-year stretch of better-than-average returns, equities are likely to underperform in the coming years. He predicts annual equity returns of around 6 to 8 percent a year, well below their historic long-term average of more than 10 percent.

Savings edge. Moreover, Christine Fahlund, senior financial planner with T. Rowe Price, recently studied the probabilities of meeting retirement goals and discovered that saving more is far more effective in improving your odds of funding retirement than investing more aggressively.

But all is not lost. Young boomers have other assets at their disposal—such as real estate.

James Diamond, 48, has been buying real estate in recent years not for speculation but for income. Diamond, an estate planning attorney, purchased several rental properties in Southern California over the past two decades. When he leaves the workforce, he doesn't plan to sell those properties but rather to use their rent as supplemental income.

Dennis Poisson, 51, of Macomb Township, Mich., has a simpler plan in mind. While Poisson, a manager for General Motors in its design division, is eligible for a traditional pension, he says he and wife, Danielle, want to play it safe. Once they retire, in about a decade or so, their intent is to sell their 3,000-plus-square-foot home and downsize to a 1,500 square-foot condominium. "That's our insurance policy that we'll be able to travel and do all the things we like to do," he says.

But for many, if not most, the simplest option will be to work longer. A decade ago, with a bountiful stock market, the vast majority of Americans ages 45 to 54—83 percent—said they planned on retiring at 65 if not earlier. Today, with stocks trading below the highs they reached in 2000, a majority say they plan on leaving the workforce at 65 or older. One in 10 young boomers says he or she never plans to retire.

Part of this is tied to the current state of young boomers' finances. But it also has to do with the different views that young boomers have about work and retirement than those of their parents.

A recent Merrill Lynch survey of boomers found that only 17 percent want to retire for good. A majority want to either work part time or to cycle back between work and leisure. "What many boomers are beginning to realize is that maybe a life of complete and total leisure is first of all unaffordable," says Ken Dychtwald, chief executive of Age Wave, a consulting firm that focuses on boomer and retiree behavior. "And secondly, they are finding out that it may not be as satisfying as we once believed."

For young boomers, this attitude is a major asset, as working longer—whether part time or in another capacity—for even two more years can drastically improve a retirement plan.

A study by Hewitt Associates last year, for example, found that workers ages 50 to 54 at large U.S. firms—many with rich retirement plans—were on track to replace nearly 89 percent of their income if they retired at 65. This figure includes not just 401(k) balances but proceeds from pension plans and Social Security.

However, delay retirement to 67, and they would be able to replace more than 100 percent of their preretirement income.

This is why Patti Brennan, president of Key Financial, a financial planning firm in West Chester, Pa., says it is important for young boomers to plan for a so-called transitional phase between work and full retirement.

You can use this transitional phase to test the waters for retirement. The last thing you want to do, says Brennan, is step out of the workforce and begin tapping your nest egg just as a big bear market approaches.

Back to work. This transitional phase can also be used to build up additional savings by working longer. This is what the Eberts say they plan to do. After their youngest child finishes college, Margaret may shift from part-time work back to a full-time schedule while Paul might work well through his 60s to compensate for the years in which their retirement savings were diverted to college bills.

The good news is young boomers are by nature flexible. A recent survey by Principal Financial asked workers 45 to 54 what they would do if they found Social Security doesn't provide them the income they expected. The vast majority said they would either work longer or phase into retirement.

These are folks like David and Kim Scofield. The Ocala, Fla., couple spent years working on commission as sales agents in the tile and flooring industry. Because they weren't on a fixed salary, though, saving a regular amount of money each year was always a challenge, says Kim, 48.

Help Wanted

Surveys show that many young baby boomers plan to work beyond the traditional retirement age of 65. A majority say that even in retirement, they expect to work part time or to cycle back and forth between the workplace and leisure. Some want to do this just to stay active. Others need the money. But are there companies out there looking to hire 60- and 70-year-olds? In an effort to match up older Americans looking for work and companies looking for experienced hands, AARP has launched a new job page on its website. By clicking on www.aarp.org/featureemployers, you will find a list of 13 major companies that have job openings and have expressed an interest in recruiting older workers. Among them: **Home Depot, MetLife, Pitney Bowes, Universal Health Services,** and **Walgreens.** Emily Allen, director of AARP's workforce initiative, says that by October, 10 additional large employers should be added to the list.

Though she and husband, David, 53, always wanted to save 10 percent to 20 percent of their incomes, the reality is, they had less than $100,000 in their IRAs. "It's not very much money," she says. On top of that, they had amassed more than $25,000 in credit card debt.

Recently, the couple took a leap of faith and opened their own small business, which distributes tiles, matted rocks, and other flooring materials. Kim says the couple was able to more than double their income over the past year with the new business. As a result, they've been able to increase their IRA balances by more than 50 percent. But without a pension plan, the Scofields realize that they need to save more to make up for those lost years.

Kim says the couple plans to work well into their 60s, if not early 70s. Then, they may work part time while their son takes over the business. "We were in a situation, before the business, where we felt that we had to work the rest of our lives just to make ends meet," says Kim.

"We've been able to turn our finances around. But now, I'm having so much fun I don't even consider retiring." That may be just the attitude that young boomers need to make the new retirement model work.

Old. Smart. Productive.

Surprise! The graying of the workforce is better news than you think

Peter Coy

mma Shulman is a dynamo. The veteran social worker works up to 50 hours a week recruiting people for treatment at an Alzheimer's clinic at New York University School of Medicine. Her boss, psychiatrist Steven H. Ferris, dreads the day she decides to retire: "We'd definitely have to hire two or three people to replace her," he says. Complains Shulman: "One of my problems is excess energy, which drives me nuts."

Oh, one more thing about Emma Shulman. She's nearly 93 years old.

Shulman is more than one amazing woman. She just might be a harbinger of things to come as the leading edge of the 78 million-strong Baby Boom generation approaches its golden years. Of course, nobody's predicting that boomers will routinely work into their 90s. But Shulman—and better-known oldsters like investor Kirk Kerkorian, 87, and Federal Reserve Chairman Alan Greenspan, 79—are proof that productive, paying work does not have to end at 55, 60, or even 65.

Old. Smart. Productive. Rather than being an economic deadweight, the next generation of older Americans is likely to make a much bigger contribution to the economy than many of today's forecasts predict. Sure, most people slow down as they get older. But new research suggests that boomers will have the ability—and the desire—to work productively and innovatively well beyond today's normal retirement age. If society can tap their talents, employers will benefit, living standards will be higher, and the financing problems of Social Security and Medicare will be easier to solve. The logic is so powerful that it is likely to sweep aside many of the legal barriers and corporate practices that today keep older workers from achieving their full productive potential.

Internet Memory Tools

In coming years, more Americans reaching their 60s and 70s are going to want to work, at least part-time. Researchers are finding that far from wearing people down, work can actually help keep them mentally and physically fit. Many highly educated and well-paid workers—lawyers, physicians, architects—already work to advanced ages because their skills are valued. Boomers, with more education than any generation in history,

are likely to follow that pattern. And today's rapid obsolescence of knowledge can actually play to older workers' advantage: It used to be considered wasteful to train people near retirement. But if training has to be refreshed every year, then companies might as well retrain old employees as young ones.

"One of my problems is excess energy, which drives me nuts."

Equally important, high-level work is getting easier for the old. Thanks to medical advances, people are staying healthy, enabling them to work longer than before. Fewer jobs require physically demanding tasks such as heavy lifting. And technology—from memory-enhancing drugs to Internet search engines that serve as auxiliary memories—will help senior workers compensate for the effects of aging. "Assuming that the improved health trends continue, boomers should be able to work productively into their late 70s" if they choose to, says Elizabeth Zelinski, dean of the Leonard Davis School of Gerontology at the University of Southern California.

But realizing that potential requires that government and business discard the outdated rules, practices, and prejudices that prematurely retire people who would prefer to keep working. In many corporations, there's an unspoken assumption that older workers are much less capable than their younger counterparts. So in addition to ensuring older workers get their fair share of training, CEOs may also need to directly confront unintended age discrimination.

Society will also have to grapple with the tricky question of how to change the Social Security system to suit an aging but healthier population. A balanced approach might be to increase the Social Security retirement age at a more rapid clip while beefing up the Social Security disability program—which now covers 8 million disabled workers and dependents.

This optimistic vision of aging in America stands in sharp contrast to the conventional wisdom, which looks ahead with dread to the 60th birthday parties of the first boomers in 2006. Pessimistic pundits expect that boomers will retire in droves soon after hitting 60, as their predecessors did, while those who

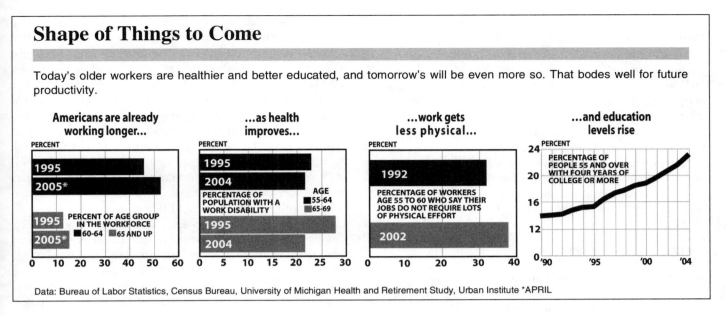

Shape of Things to Come

Today's older workers are healthier and better educated, and tomorrow's will be even more so. That bodes well for future productivity.

Americans are already working longer...

PERCENT

1995
2005*
1995
2005*

PERCENT OF AGE GROUP IN THE WORKFORCE
■ 60-64   ■ 65 AND UP

0 10 20 30 40 50 60

...as health improves...

PERCENT

1995
2004

PERCENTAGE OF POPULATION WITH A WORK DISABILITY

AGE
■ 55-64
■ 65-69

1995
2004

0 5 10 15 20 25 30

...work gets less physical...

PERCENT

1992

PERCENTAGE OF WORKERS AGE 55 TO 60 WHO SAY THEIR JOBS DO NOT REQUIRE LOTS OF PHYSICAL EFFORT

2002

0 10 20 30 40

...and education levels rise

PERCENT

PERCENTAGE OF PEOPLE 55 AND OVER WITH FOUR YEARS OF COLLEGE OR MORE

24
20
16
12
0
'90   '95   '00   '04

Data: Bureau of Labor Statistics, Census Bureau, University of Michigan Health and Retirement Study, Urban Institute *APRIL

do keep working will dial back to less challenging and less productive jobs. The fear is that boomers will finally heed Timothy Leary's call, dropping out (of the workforce) and turning on (the TV). "This explosion in the number of elderly Americans will place an unprecedented economic burden on working-age adults," investment banker Peter G. Peterson wrote last year in his latest book, *Running on Empty.*

But the burden won't be nearly so heavy if people's productive careers stretch out in synch with their extended lifetimes. How much could the economy benefit from people working longer and better?

An analysis by *BusinessWeek* finds that increased productivity of older Americans and higher labor-force participation could add 9% to gross domestic product by 2045, on top of what it otherwise would have been. (This assumes, for example, that over the next 40 years better health and technology reduce the productivity gap between older workers and their younger counterparts.) This 9% increase in gross domestic product would add more than $3 trillion a year, in today's dollars, to economic output.

The added growth would be a pure win for government finances, since a bigger economy with more productive workers yields higher tax revenues. And there's little doubt that encouraging people to work longer in step with longer life spans would do much to guarantee the solvency of Social Security.

The idea that citizens of a wealthy nation such as the U.S. would choose to work extra years is still a little new. For most of the 20th century, retirement ages fell as life spans grew. The trend seemed unstoppable: While in 1950, 46% of men 65 and older were in the labor force, by 1985 the fraction had plummeted to 16%. An influx of women into the labor force only partially offset the overall decline.

But starting in the mid-1980s, something highly unexpected began to happen: The trend reversed, and more older Americans chose to keep working. The upsurge accelerated even in the weak labor markets of recent years. The share of men 65 and over in the labor force is back up to almost 20%—the highest since the 1970s.

In part, of course, the latest uptick in working ages can be blamed on the stock market's drop from its 2000 peak, which dented retirement savings. Also, fewer workers have good defined-benefit pension plans, which would allow them to retire young. But financial need can't be the whole reason older Americans are working more. Federal Reserve surveys show that older families have been getting richer, not poorer. The average net worth of families headed by 55- to 64-year-olds soared by 74% from 1992 to 2001, after adjusting for inflation, and likely has gone up since then.

At least as important is that many institutional barriers to working longer have been removed. In 1986, in the name of equal rights, Congress banned mandatory retirement for all but a handful of workers, such as airline pilots. And 401(k) plans, which are gradually replacing defined-benefit plans, don't induce people to retire at a certain age.

Young As You Feel

Better yet, work doesn't feel like a burden to today's fit, older Americans. Many people over 60 don't think of themselves as old. A good example is Theodora Emiko "Teddy" Yoshikami, 61, who organizes cultural programs at New York's American Museum of Natural History. In her spare time, she whacks big drums in a Japanese percussion group. "People are always surprised to hear how old I am," says the former dancer.

The Baby Boom generation is even fitter for its age and more determined to stay active. Two-thirds of the people surveyed last year by the Employee Benefit Research Institute, a company-backed organization, said they expect to work for pay in retirement. A survey of boomers by AARP in January found that two in five workers age 50 to 65 were interested in a gradual, "phased" retirement instead of an abrupt cessation of work—and nearly 80% of those said that availability of phased retirement programs at work would encourage them to keep working longer. While it's likely that many boomers won't stick to those brave resolutions, the trend in work is clearly up.

Good health will help. The share of 65- to 69-year-olds with a disability affecting their ability to work fell from nearly 28% in 1995 to less than 22% last year. Advances in medicine are curing many of the problems that once forced older workers into retirement. For example, Genentech Inc. announced on May 23 that a drug undergoing trials for treatment of macular generation improves eyesight in the elderly. And better health is coinciding with less strenuous work, thanks to automation and the shrinkage of manufacturing. The share of workers 55 to 60 who said their jobs did not require lots of physical effort rose from 32% in 1992 to 38% in 2002, according to an Urban Institute study.

Trial and Error

Mental health appears to be improving as well. USC's Zelinski has discovered that heart disease, hypertension, and diabetes directly impair brain functioning—and she sees evidence that modern medicine is getting a better handle on those diseases. As a result, memory and other functions are improving among the elderly. Emma Shulman's boss at NYU Medical Center, Steven Ferris, expects further gains for older workers from the spreading use of memory-enhancing drugs and technological aids such as personal digital assistants and search engines. Says Ferris: "I remember my father with little scraps of paper to remember things. People don't have to do that anymore."

"Once I got gray hair, people actually listened to me. This is working really well"

Older workers who thrive tend to have skills that are prized in the workplace, even if they can't easily be measured by standard tests. What matters most, according to psychologist Regina Colonia-Willner, president of consultancy Practical Intelligence at Work Inc. in Boca Raton, Fla., is the ability to solve ill-defined business problems using rules of thumb that can't be put down on paper. Example: how to deal with a difficult boss. In a study of 200 banking executives, she found that the ones who exhibited the highest "practical intelligence" were as likely to be old as young—and the older among them excelled even though their scores on traditional intelligence tests were no better than average for their age. "Practical intelligence stays with you," says Colonia-Willner. "You don't lose it when you get older."

The rap that older workers are inflexible and uncreative is also overstated. Research by economists David W. Galenson of the University of Chicago and Bruce A. Weinberg of Ohio State University finds that the innovations of older people are more likely to be "experimental," vs. the break-the-mold "conceptual" innovations of younger types. The conceptual types tend to have a bolt from the blue, whereas the experimenters build new ideas from a lifetime of observation, trial, and error. Among the "experimental" innovators who produced some of their best work later in life:

painters Henri Matisse and Paul Cézanne, author Fyodor Dostoevsky, and architect Frank Lloyd Wright.

Some enlightened companies are catching on to all of this. They're hiring or retaining older workers with flexible work schedules and ample training. United Technologies Corp. spends more than $60 million a year on its Employee Scholar Program, which pays the costs of workers of any age who study in their spare time. At UTC's Hamilton Sundstrand facility in Miramar, Fla., 61-year-old lead mechanic Ed Perez is working on a bachelor's degree in legal studies. He finished an associate's degree in aviation-maintenance management two years ago and hopes to go to law school. "If I don't run out of time and UTC doesn't run out of money, I'll keep going," he says.

UTC Chairman and Chief Executive George David, at 63 a candidate himself for discounted movie tickets, argues that an educated worker like Perez is a better worker, regardless of age or area of study. What's more, the free education incentive tends to appeal to UTC's most skilled and motivated employees, so it's a way for the company to retain the people it most wants. Retention rates among "employee scholars" are about 20% higher than for regular U.S. workers.

Holding on to Experience

Consolidated Edison Inc., a New York power company with an aging workforce, is trying to hang on to its valuable older workers with benefits like an elder-care referral service and career-long training. It wants to retain the experience of workers like Frederick R. Simms, 67, an emergency field manager who has seen just about everything in his 49 years with the company, from water main breaks to the collapse of the World Trade Center. In a job where trust and rapport are vital, Simms is on a first-name basis with Fire Dept. officials and other emergency workers all over Manhattan. Con Ed recently sent him for a two-day "working people-smart" class. "I don't have the zip I used to have, but I'm good enough to work 16 hours if I had to today," says Simms, adding: "I know the company likes having me around."

It's common these days to find older workers on the sales floor of retailers like Home Depot Inc. and CVS Corp., but what's new is the growing presence of older workers in high-pay, high-productivity careers. MITRE Corp., a research and development outfit in Bedford, Mass., is worried about losing its expertise in fields such as radar, which is something of a lost art for young engineers. So it brings back retirees on what it calls a "part-time, on-call" basis. The Energy Dept.'s National Energy Technology Laboratory in Morgantown, W. Va., also recognizes the value of older workers with technical expertise. It has clung to chemical engineer Hugh D. Guthrie, 86, as a full-time technical adviser in part because he has ideas that younger engineers might never think of. Says Guthrie: "My experience gives me a perspective on questions, which may not always be right but nearly always will be different. The greatest service I provide is in stimulating the thinking of people involved in a project."

Unfortunately, many other companies haven't gotten the message. The Society for Human Resource Management, an association of personnel execs, says 59% of members surveyed don't actively recruit older workers and 65% don't do anything

Older and Wiser

Businesses often act as if older workers are a liability in an economy that prizes productivity, flexibility, and innovation. But research suggests that they are under-estimating these employees.

Two Kinds of Innovation

Creativity isn't just for the young. Economist David Galenson of the University of Chicago has identified two types of innovators. Break-the-mold **"conceptual" innovators** (like Vietnam Veterans Memorial designer Maya Lin), **do their best work when young.** In contrast, **"experimental" innovators** (novelist Fyodor Dostoevsky, sculptor Auguste Rodin) **do their best work at older ages,** drawing on a lifetime of observation, trial, and error.

Sound Bodies

University of Southern California gerontologist Elizabeth Zelinski has found that ailments such as **high blood pressure, diabetes, and heart disease are key factors depressing brain function among the elderly**. The ease with which we can treat these conditions now helps reduce the apparent cognitive handicap of older workers. In short, medicine is postponing mental decline.

Problem Solving

Conventional measures of mental function don't capture abilities important in business, such as accumulated knowledge or judgment. Psychologist Regina Colonia-Willner of Practical Intelligence at Work Inc. found that **managers who are successful at older ages are masters at solving ill-defined problems,** even though they do no better than other older workers on standard psychometric tests.

Compensation

Speed, reasoning, and memory decline steadily after age 20, while vocabulary increases to age 50. University of Virginia psychologist Timothy Salthouse found that **older workers make up for their shortfalls with clever coping strategies.** For example, older typists gain an edge by looking farther ahead in to-be-typed text during pauses, presumably to compensate for the slowdown in their ability to type words as read.
Data: *Business Week*

that older workers are getting a subtle message that training isn't for them.

Economists have found that businesses are missing an opportunity by giving less training to their older workers. Research shows that they tend to operate information technology more slowly but with fewer errors. Research on displaced workers who got retraining in community colleges in Washington State found that the pay gains were just as big for older workers who took training as for younger ones—indicating that the training they got took hold.

Will longer-working boomers block the advancement of younger workers? Maybe. But what worries employers more is the opposite—labor shortages that could emerge if boomers retire en masse and there aren't enough people to take their place. The Congressional Budget Office is forecasting that labor-force growth will slow by almost half over the next 10 years.

The U.S. takes better advantage of the potential of its older citizens than does most of Europe, where extremely early retirement is routine because of rich retirement benefits. Six in 10 Americans are still working at ages 55 to 64, vs. just four in 10 in the European Union.

Smart policy choices, such as the abolition of most mandatory retirement rules, have helped put the U.S. in a position to tap the ability and energy of older people. Since 2000, Social Security recipients have been allowed to receive their full benefits no matter how much they earn from working after age 65. The Internal Revenue Service has proposed rules, starting next year, to allow people 59½ and older to receive part of their pensions even while they are still working. Because people would not have to retire outright to get a pension, more are likely to remain on the job, experts predict. The proposed rules are a step in the right direction, although employer groups are complaining that there's too much red tape involved.

Creating Incentives

What more can be done to tap the productivity potential of older workers? The goal is to introduce more flexibility into pay and retirement systems, to create more options as workers age. Consultant Ken Dychtwald, author of **Age Wave,** recommends the example of Deloitte Consulting LLC, which lures highly valued older employees to stay by designating them "senior leaders" and giving them incentives such as flexible hours and work location, special projects, and opportunities for mentoring and research.

Another possibility is to allow companies to convert traditional defined-benefit pensions, which encourage retirement as early as age 55, to cash-balance plans, which have no built-in incentives to retire. Such conversions have been frozen since 1999 over legitimate age-discrimination concerns, though the Bush Administration has proposed legislation that would break the logjam. It's prudent to make sure that switching to cash-balance plans doesn't harm older workers, but such caution is also preserving a system that lures people into retiring when they still have much to contribute in the working world.

Perhaps the most controversial idea is to break the typical link between pay and seniority. As more people work into their

specific to retain older workers. The Bureau of Labor Statistics found in 1995, the last time it looked, that workers age 55 and up got only one-third as many hours of formal training as workers 45 to 54. Marian Stoltz-Loike, CEO of SeniorThinking LLC, a consultancy, says executives often aren't even aware

late 60s and 70s, pay should be adjusted to match how much people work and what they accomplish on the job.

It's also critical to rethink the role of Social Security in an economy where incomes—and life spans—are rising. In theory, Social Security should provide a secure safety net for those who are truly too old to work and lack savings, while encouraging the huge boomer generation to stay employed and productive for the good of themselves and the economy.

"The greatest service I provide is in stimulating the thinking of people involved in a project."

The logical conclusion: raise Social Security's normal retirement age incrementally to 70. From then on, peg further increases to gains in longevity. It's also essential to increase the age, now 62, at which people can first choose to take early retirement. Research suggests that many take the official early retirement age as a signal that it's O.K. to drop out of the workforce, even though they will get much smaller checks for the rest of their lifetimes. Raising the early retirement age would signal that 62 is too young for most people to quit in an era of marathon-running septuagenarians.

Increasing Social Security's early retirement age would be hard on workers with health problems, or whose jobs require more physical exertion. A possible solution is to liberalize the qualifications for Social Security's disability insurance program. The extra expense of disability payments to aging laborers would be far outweighed by the savings from raising the normal and early retirement ages in tandem.

There's no dispute that America is graying. But the solution to the demographic shift is staring us in the face. As Urban Institute senior fellow C. Eugene Steuerle told the House Ways & Means Committee in May: "People in their late 50s, 60s, and 70s have now become the largest underutilized pool of human resources in the economy." By working longer—and more productively—boomers will help the U.S. economy thrive even as their personal odometers keep clicking forward.

—With Diane Brady in New York

The Broken Promise

It was part of the American Dream, a pledge made by corporations to their workers: for your decades of toil, you will be assured of retirement benefits like a pension and health care. Now more and more companies are walking away from that promise, leaving millions of Americans at risk of an impoverished retirement. How can this be legal? A TIME investigation looks at how Congress let it happen and the widespread social insecurity it's causing

DONALD L. BARTLETT AND JAMES B. STEELE

The little shed behind Joy Whitehouse's modest home is filled with aluminum cans—soda cans, soup cans and vegetable cans—that she collects from neighbors or finds during her periodic expeditions along the roadside. Two times a month, she takes them to a recycler, who pays her as much as $30 for her harvest of castoffs. When your fixed income is $942 a month, an extra $30 here and there makes a big difference. After paying rent, utilities and insurance, Whitehouse is left with less than $40 a week to cover everything else. So the money from cans helps pay medical bills for the cancer and chronic lung disease she has been battling for years, as well as food expenses. "I eat a lot of soup," says the tiny, spirited 69-year-old, who lives in Majestic Meadows, a mobile-home park for senior citizens near Salt Lake City, Utah.

Whitehouse never envisioned spending her later years this way. She and her husband Alva Don raised four children. In the 1980s they lived in Montana, where he earned a good living as a long-haul truck driver for Pacific Intermountain Express. But in 1986 he was killed on the job in a highway accident attributed to faulty maintenance on his truck, as his company struggled to survive the cutthroat pricing of congressionally ordered deregulation. After her husband's death, Whitehouse knew the future would be tough, but she was confident in her economic survival. After all, the company had promised her a death benefit of $598 every two weeks for the rest of her life—a commitment she had in writing, one that was a matter of law.

She received the benefit payments until October 1990, when the check bounced. A corporate-takeover artist, later sent to prison for ripping off a pension fund and other financial improprieties, had stripped down the business and forced it into the U.S. bankruptcy court. There the obligation was erased, thanks to congressional legislation that gives employers the right to walk away from agreements with their employees. To support herself, Whitehouse had already sold the couple's Montana home and moved to the Salt Lake City area, where she had family and friends. With her savings running out, she applied early (at a reduced rate) for her husband's Social Security. She needed every penny. For health reasons, she couldn't work. She

had undergone a double mastectomy. An earlier cancer of the uterus had eaten away at her stomach muscle so that a metal plate and artificial bladder were installed. Her children and other relatives offered to help, but Whitehouse is fiercely self-sufficient. Friends and neighbors pitch in to fill her shed with aluminum. "You put your pride in your pocket, and you learn to help yourself," she says. "I save cans."

Through no fault of her own, Whitehouse had found herself thrust into the ranks of workers and their spouses—previously invisible but now fast growing—who believed the corporate promises about retirement and health care, often affirmed by the Federal Government: they would receive a guaranteed pension; they would have company-paid health insurance until they qualified for Medicare; they would receive company-paid supplemental medical insurance after turning 65; they would receive a fixed death benefit in the event of a fatal accident; and they would have a modest life-insurance policy.

They didn't get those things. And they won't.

Corporate promises are often not worth the paper they're printed on. Businesses in one industry after another are revoking long-standing commitments to their workers. It's the equivalent of your bank telling you that it needs the money you put into your savings account more than you do—and then keeping it. Result: a wholesale downsizing of the American Dream. It began in the 1980s with the elimination of middle-class, entry-level jobs in lower-paying industries—apparel, textiles and shoes, among others. More recently it spread to jobs that pay solid middle-class wages, starting with the steel industry, then airlines and now autos—with no end in sight.

That's why Whitehouse, as difficult as her situation is, is worried more about how her children and grandchildren will cope. And well she should. For while her story is the tale of millions of older Americans, it is also a window into the future for many millions more. A TIME investigation has concluded that long before today's working Americans reach retirement age, policy decisions by Congress favoring corporate and special interests over workers will drive millions of older Americans—a majority of them women—into poverty, push millions more to

Public vs. Private
Where Pensions Are Golden

By Donald L. Barlett, James B. Steele

All pensions and health-care plans are not created equal. At the same time millions of workers in private industry have lost the benefits they once thought they had for life, another group is doing quite nicely, secure in the knowledge that their benefits are protected forever—not by some government agency, but directly by you, the taxpayer.

They are public employees in state and local governments, ranging from teachers to cops. Most collect guaranteed pensions provided through state and local taxes and their own contributions and investment returns. Overall, 90% of public employees enjoy a defined-benefit pension, compared with only 20% (and falling) of the private work force.

Even though the commitment is there, the money isn't. A study by analysts at Barclays Global Investors in San Francisco estimates that public-employee pension funds in the U.S. are short $700 billion. That's more than all state and local governments collected last year in property, sales and corporate income taxes combined. As a result, many employees in the private sector will get hit with a double whammy: while their pensions erode, increasingly they will be hit with cuts in government services and forced to pay higher taxes to cover the pensions of public employees, the kind they can only dream about. In three-fourths of the states, public pensions even come with annual cost-of-living increases, a fringe benefit absent from private pensions.

Some public-employee pension plans are well managed and adequately funded. Most are not. A study of 64 state pension systems by Wilshire Associates, an investment advisory company, found that 54 of them were underfunded by a total of $175.4 billion. The situation is even worse at the municipal level. San Diego, which is on the brink of bankruptcy, is in the hole for $1.4 billion in pensions owed but not covered.

How could this happen? Politicians neglected to put money into pension plans, made poor investments, handed out extraordinarily generous retirement packages and gave special treatment to their fellow politicians. As San Diego city attorney Mike Aguirre put it, "What has happened is that the pension plan has somewhat become a personal-benefit slush fund for council members and senior officials." Not only did high-ranking San Diego officials give themselves preferential treatment for their pensions, they also distributed outsize benefits to city workers. A department director with 39 years of service collects $148,000 a year for life; an assistant port director with 31 years, $132,000. So far, the scandal has cost the mayor his job, six pension-fund trustees have been charged, city services are being slashed and investigations have been launched by the FBI, the SEC and the U.S. Attorney.

San Diego's excesses have attracted attention, but the city is hardly alone. The California Public Employees' Retirement System, better known as CalPERS, handed out a pension check last year for $272,200 to a retired university professor. A former water-district general manager collected $206,300.

CalPERS, by the way, invests in vulture funds formed by Wilbur Ross, the New York billionaire who specializes in buying bankrupt companies, slashing costs and then selling the firms for an oversize profit. Among the costs pared: pensions. In short, a public-employee pension fund makes money from the killing of private pensions.

Across the U.S., retirement plans in big cities and small ones are underwater. In Philadelphia, the city's three big pension funds were short $2.6 billion at the end of 2003. The police plan had enough assets to cover only 59% of promised retirement checks. That was after the city had sold $1.2 billion in pension-obligation bonds in 1999, the equivalent of paying your mortgage with a credit card. At the other end of the state, Pittsburgh was in even worse shape. In 2003, the police pension plan had enough assets to cover just 33% of promised retirement pay. That, too, was after Pittsburgh peddled $302 million in pension-obligation bonds between 1996 and 1998. In the end, taxpayers in both cities will have to pick up the tab. The place with the biggest problem is the state of Illinois, whose unfunded liability was estimated last year at $43.1 billion, or nearly double the state's budget.

And everywhere, the worst is yet to come: health-care obligations. A 2004 study by Workplace Economics Inc. found all 50 state-government employers offered health-care benefits for retirees under age 65. Many who work for state or local governments may retire in their 40s and collect a pension as well as receive subsidized health care. Although future pension costs are well known because contributions and estimates of potential liabilities must be accounted for, such is not the case with health care. Governmental entities pay the bills out of current revenue. As is the case with everyone else's, those bills are exploding. So, too, are future obligations, as the baby boomers prepare to leave their government jobs. This year New Jersey's State Health Benefits Program will cost taxpayers $1 billion for active workers and an additional $900 million for retirees, according to Fred Beaver, director of the Division of Pensions and Benefits. By 2010, the state will spend more on health care for retirees ($2.3 billion) than for active workers ($1.8 billion).

Come 2007, state and local taxpayers everywhere will get their first full picture of current and future health-care costs of public employees. That's when new accounting rules go into effect requiring governments to itemize health-care spending and forecast costs for coming years. The change in bookkeeping will either set off a wave of tax increases, reductions in government services or both. Lest anyone think state and local retirement-plan sponsors may emulate those in corporate America and simply walk away from the promised health-care benefits, think again. More than once, courts have ruled that health benefits promised to government workers (among them judges and legislators)—unlike those promised to workers in private industry—must be honored.

With reporting by Jeremy Caplan

the brink and turn retirement years into a time of need for everyone but the affluent. The transition is well under way, eroding efforts of the past three decades to eliminate poverty among the aging. From taxes to health care to pensions, Congress has enacted legislation that adds to the cost of retirement and eats away at dollars once earmarked for food and shelter. That reversal of fortunes is staggering, and even those already retired or near retirement will be squeezed by changing economic rules.

Congress's role has been pivotal. Lawmakers wrote bankruptcy regulations to allow corporations to scrap the health insurance they promised employees who retired early—sometimes voluntarily, quite often not. They wrote pension rules that encouraged corporations to underfund their retirement plans or switch to plans less favorable to employees. They denied workers the right to sue to enforce retirement promises. They have refused to overhaul America's health-care system, which has created the world's most expensive medical care without any comparable benefit. One by one, lawmakers have undermined or destroyed policies that once afforded at least the possibility of a livable existence to many seniors, while at the same time encouraging corporations to repudiate lifetime-benefit agreements. All this under the guise of ensuring workers that they are in charge of their own destiny—such as it is.

The process has accelerated dramatically this year. Two major U.S. airlines—Delta and Northwest—turned to bankruptcy court to cut costs and delay pension-fund contributions. This followed earlier bankruptcy filings by United Airlines and US-Airways, both of which jettisoned their guaranteed pension plans. Then on Oct. 8, the largest U.S. auto-parts maker, Delphi Corp., filed for bankruptcy protection, seeking to cut off medical and life-insurance benefits for its retirees. Delphi's pension funds are short $11 billion. To Elizabeth Warren, a Harvard law professor who specializes in bankruptcy, this is just going to get worse, as ever more companies see the value to their bottom line of "scraping off" employee obligations. "There's no business in America that isn't going to figure out a way to get rid of [these benefit promises]."

That may include the world's largest automaker—General Motors. Although GM chairman Rick Wagoner has insisted that "we don't consider bankruptcy to be a viable business strategy," some on Wall Street are skeptical, given the company's array of problems. Their view was reinforced when GM, the company that dominated the American economy through the 20th century, announced on Oct. 17 [2005] that it had reached a precedent-setting agreement with the United Auto Workers leadership to rescind $1 billion worth of health-care benefits for its retirees. If ratified by the union membership, the retrenchment will hasten the end to company-subsidized health care for all retirees. From 1988 to 2004, the share of employers with 200 or more workers offering retiree health insurance plunged, from 66% to 36%. The end result: a fresh and additional burden on retirees. Concluded a report by the Kaiser Family Foundation and Hewitt Associates: "For the majority of workers who retire before they turn age 65 and are eligible for Medicare, the coverage provided under employer plans is often difficult, if not impossible to find anywhere else." For retirees over 65, "employer plans remain the primary source of prescription drug coverage for seniors on

Medicare … This coverage is more generous than the standard prescription drug benefit that will be offered by Medicare plans beginning in 2006."

Perhaps the best yardstick to assess the outlook for the later years is the defined-benefit pension, long the gold standard for retirement because it guarantees a fixed income for life. The number of such plans offered by corporations has plunged from 112,200 in 1985 to 29,700 today. Since 1985, the number of active workers covered in the private sector declined from 22 million to 17 million. They are the last members of what once promised to be the U.S.'s golden retirement era, and they are fast disappearing. From 2001 to 2004, nearly 200 corporations in the FORTUNE 1000 killed or froze their defined-benefit plans. Most recently, Hewlett-Packard, long one of the most admired U.S. companies, pulled the plug on guaranteed pensions for new workers. An HP spokesman said the company had concluded that "pension plans are kind of a thing of the past." In that, HP was merely following the lead of business rival IBM and such other major companies as NCR Corp., Sears Holding Corp. and Motorola. The nation's largest employer, Wal-Mart, does not offer such pensions either. At the current pace, human-resources offices will turn out the lights in their defined-benefit section within a decade or so. At that point, individuals will assume all the risks for their retirement, just as they did 100 years ago.

The shift away from guaranteed pensions was encouraged by Congress, which structured the rules in a way that invites corporations to abandon their defined-benefit plans in favor of defined-contribution plans, increasingly 401(k)s, in which employees set aside a fixed sum of money toward retirement. Many companies also contribute; some don't. Whatever the case, the contributions will never be enough to match the certain and long-term income from a defined-benefit plan. What's more, once the money runs out, that's it. If people live longer than expected, get stuck with unanticipated expenses or suffer losses of other once promised benefits, they will have little besides their Social Security to sustain them.

The dawning perception among Americans that when it comes to retirement, you're on your own, baby, is surely a reason that President George Bush ran into so much opposition to his proposal to change Social Security from a risk-free plan into one with so-called private accounts. Critics of the 70-year-old system were determined to chip away at Social Security as part of a larger effort to promote what the Bush Administration calls an "ownership society." As Treasury Secretary John Snow told a congressional committee in February 2004: "I think we need to be concerned about pensions and the security that employees have in their pensions. And I think we need to encourage people to save and become part of an ownership society, which is very much a part of the President's vision for America."

Of course, it's much easier to own a piece of America when you have a pension like Snow's. When he stepped down as head of CSX Corp.—operator of the largest rail network in the eastern U.S.—to take over Treasury, Snow was given a lump-sum pension of $33.2 million. It was based on 44 years of employment at CSX. Unlike most ordinary people, who must work the actual years on which their pension is calculated, Snow was employed just 26 years. The additional 18 years of his CSX employment history were fictional, a gift from the company's board of directors.

Snow is not alone. The phantom employment record, as it might be called, is a common executive-retirement practice in corporate America—and one that is spelled out in corporate filings with the Securities and Exchange Commission (SEC). Drew Lewis, the Pennsylvania Republican and onetime head of the U.S. Department of Transportation, got a $1.5 million annual pension when he retired in 1996 as chairman and CEO of Union Pacific Corp. His pension was based on 30 years of service to the company, but he actually worked there only 11 years. The other 19 years of his employment history came courtesy of Union Pacific's board of directors, which included Vice President Dick Cheney. And then there's Leo Mullin, the former chairman and CEO of Delta Air Lines. Under Mullin's stewardship, Delta killed the defined-benefit pension of its nonunion workers and replaced it with a less generous plan. Now, little more than a year after he retired, the airline is in bankruptcy and can dump its pension obligations. But you need not fret about Mullin. On his way out the door, he picked up a $16 million retirement package. It's based on 28.5 years of employment with Delta, at least 21 years more than he worked at the airline.

How Savings Can Be Hijacked

At the same time corporate executives are paid retirement dollars for years they never worked, hapless employees lose supplemental retirement benefits for a lifetime of actual work. Just ask Betty Moss. She was one of thousands of workers at Polaroid Corp.—the Waltham, Mass., maker of instant cameras and film—who, beginning in 1988, gave up 8% of their salary to underwrite an employee stock-ownership plan, or ESOP. It was created to thwart a corporate takeover and "to provide a retirement benefit" to Polaroid employees to supplement their pension, the company pledged. Alas, it was not to be. Polaroid was slow to react to the digital revolution and began to lose money in the 1990s. From 1995 to 1998, the company racked up $359 million in losses. As its balance sheet deteriorated, so did the value of its stock, including shares in the ESOP. In October 2001, Polaroid sought bankruptcy protection from creditors.

By then, Polaroid's shares were virtually worthless, having plummeted from $60 in 1997 to less than the price of a Coke in October 2001. During that period, employees were forbidden to unload their stock, based on laws approved by Congress. But what employees weren't allowed to do at a higher price, the company-appointed trustee could do at the lowest possible price—without even seeking the workers' permission. Rather than wait for a possible return to profitability through restructuring, the trustee decided that it was "in the best interests" of the employees to sell the ESOP shares. They went for 9¢. In short order, a $300 million retirement nest egg put away by 6,000 Polaroid employees was wiped out. Many lost between $100,000 and $200,000.

Moss was one of the losers. Now 60, she spent 35 years at Polaroid, beginning as a file clerk out of high school, then working her way through college at night and eventually rising to be

senior regional operations manager in Atlanta. "It was the kind of place people dream of working at," she said. "I can honestly say I never dreaded going to work. It was just the sort of place where good things were always happening." One of those good things was supposed to be the ESOP, touted by the company as a plan that "forced employees to save for their retirement," as Moss recalled. "Everybody went for it. We had been so conditioned to believe what we were told was true."

Once Polaroid entered bankruptcy, Moss and her retired co-workers learned a bitter lesson—that they had no say in the security of benefits they had worked all their lives to accumulate. While the federal Pension Benefit Guaranty Corp. (PBGC) agreed to make good on most of their basic pensions, the rest of their benefits—notably the ESOP accounts, along with retirement health care and severance packages—were canceled. The retirees, generally well educated and financially savvy, organized to try to win back some of what they had lost by petitioning bankruptcy court, which would decide how to divide the company's assets among creditors. To no avail: Polaroid's management had already undercut the employees' effort. Rather than file for bankruptcy in Boston, near the corporate offices, the company took its petition to Wilmington, Del., and a bankruptcy court that had developed a reputation for favoring corporate managers. There, Polaroid's management contended that the company was in terrible financial shape and that the only option was to sell rather than reorganize. The retirees claimed that Polaroid executives were undervaluing the business so the company could ignore its obligations to retirees and sell out to private investors.

The bankruptcy judge ruled in favor of the company. In 2002 Polaroid was sold to One Equity Partners, an investment firm with a special interest in financially distressed businesses. (One Equity was a unit of Bank One Corp., now part of JPMorgan Chase.) Many retirees believed the purchase price of $255 million was only a fraction of the old Polaroid's value. Evidence supporting that view: the new owners financed their purchase, in part, with $138 million of Polaroid's own cash.

Employees did not leave bankruptcy court empty-handed. They all got something in the mail. Moss will never forget the day hers arrived. "I got a check for $47," she recalled. She had lost tens of thousands of dollars in ESOP contributions, health benefits and severance payments. Now she and the rest of Polaroid's other 6,000 retirees were being compensated with $47 checks. "You should have heard the jokes," she said. "How about we all meet at McDonald's and spend our $47?"

The $12.08 a share that Polaroid's new managers received was 134 times the 9¢ a share handed out to lifelong workers

Under a new management team headed by Jacques Nasser, former chairman of Ford Motor Co., Polaroid returned to profitability almost overnight. Little more than two years after the company emerged from bankruptcy, One Equity sold it to a Minnesota entrepreneur for $426 million in cash. The new managers, who had received stock in the post-bankruptcy Polaroid, walked away with millions of dollars. Nasser got $12.8 million for his 1 million shares. Other executives and directors were rewarded for their efforts. Rick Lazio, a four-term Republican from West Islip, N.Y., who effectively gave up his House seat for an unsuccessful Senate run against Hillary Rodham Clinton in 2000, collected $512,675 for a brief stint as a director. That amounted to nearly twice the $282,000 paid to all 6,000 retirees. The $12.08 a share that the new managers received for little more than two years of work was 134 times the 9¢ a share handed out earlier to lifelong workers.

Let's Break a Deal

Washington has a rich history of catering to special and corporate interests at the expense of ordinary citizens. Nowhere is this more evident than in legislation dealing with company pensions. It has been this way since 1964, when carmaker Studebaker Corp. collapsed after 60 years, junking the promised pensions of 4,000 workers not yet eligible for retirement, pensions the company had spelled out in brochures for years: "You may be a long way from retirement age now. Still, it's good to know that Studebaker is building up a fund for you, so that when you reach retirement age you can settle down on a farm, visit around the country or just take it easy, and know that you'll still be getting a regular monthly pension paid for entirely by the company."

Oops. There oughta be a law.

It took Congress 10 years to respond to the Studebaker pension abandonment by writing the Employee Retirement Income Security Act (ERISA) of 1974. It established minimum standards for retirement plans in private industry and created the PBGC to guarantee them. Then President Gerald Ford summed up the measure when he signed it into law that Labor Day: "This legislation will alleviate the fears and the anxiety of people who are on the production lines or in the mines or elsewhere, in that they now know that their investment in private pension funds will be better protected."

Perhaps for some, but far from all.

Another group that had no pension worries would turn out to be the biggest winners under the bill. Congress wrote the law so broadly that moneymen could dip into pension funds and remove cash set aside for workers' retirement. During the 1980s, that's exactly what a cast of corporate raiders, speculators, Wall Street buyout firms and company executives did with a vengeance. Throughout the decade, they walked away with an estimated $21 billion earmarked for workers' retirement pay. The raiders insisted that they took only excess assets that weren't needed. Among the pension buccaneers: Meshulam Riklis, a once flamboyant Beverly Hills, Calif., takeover artist who skimmed millions from several companies, including the McCrory Corp., the onetime retail fixture of Middle America that is now gone; and the late Victor Posner, the Miami Beach corporate raider who siphoned millions of dollars from more than half a dozen different companies, including Fischbach Corp., a New York electrical contractor that he drove to the edge of extinction. Those two raiders alone raked off about $100 million in workers' retirement dollars—all perfectly legal, thanks to

Congress. By the time all the billions of dollars were gone and the public outcry had grown too loud to ignore, Congress in 1990 belatedly rewrote the rules and imposed an excise tax on money removed from pension funds. The raids slowed to a trickle.

During those same years, the PBGC, which insures private pension plans, published an annual list of the 50 most underfunded of those plans. In shining a spotlight on those that had fallen behind in their contributions, the agency hoped to prod companies to keep current. Corporations hated the list. They maintained that the PBGC's methodology did not reflect the true financial condition of their pension plans. After all, as long as the stock market went up—and never down or sideways—the pension plans would be adequately funded. Congress liked that reasoning and, in 1994, reacting to corporate claims that the underfunded list caused needless anxiety among employees, voted to keep the data secret. When the PBGC killed its Top 50 list, David M. Strauss, then the agency's executive director, explained, "With full implementation of [the 1994 pension law], we now have better tools in place." PBGC officials were so bullish about those "better tools," including provisions to levy higher fees on companies ignoring obligations to their employees, they predicted that underfunded pension plans would be a thing of the past. As a story in the *Los Angeles Times* put it, "PBGC officials said the act nearly guarantees that large underfunded plans will strengthen and the chronic deficits suffered by the pension guaranty organization will be eliminated within 10 years."

Not even close; instead they accelerated at warp speed. In 1994 the deficit in PBGC plans was $31 billion. Today it's $450 billion, or $600 billion if one includes multiemployer plans of unionized employees who work for more than one business in such industries as construction.

Since the PBGC no longer publishes its Top 50 list, anyone looking for even remotely comparable information must sift through the voluminous filings of individual companies with the SEC or the Labor Department, where pension-plan finances are recorded, or turn to the reports of independent firms such as Standard & Poor's. The findings aren't reassuring. According to S&P, Sara Lee Corp. of Chicago, a global maker of food products, ended 2004 with a pension deficit of $1.5 billion. The company's pension plans held enough assets to cover 69.8% of promised retirement pay. Ford Motor Co.'s deficit came in at $12.3 billion. It could write retirement checks for 83% of money owed. ExxonMobil Corp. was down $11.5 billion, with enough money to issue retirement checks covering 61% of promised benefits. Exxon had extracted $1.6 billion from its pension plans in 1986 because they were deemed overfunded. The company explained then that "our shareholders would be better served" that way.

In reality, the deficits in many cases are worse than the published data suggest, which becomes evident when bankrupt corporations dump their pension plans on the PBGC. Time after time, the agency has discovered, the gap between retirement holdings and pensions owed was much wider than the companies reported to stockholders or employees. Thus LTV Corp., the giant Cleveland steelmaker, reported that its plan for hourly workers was about 80% funded, but when it was turned over to the PBGC, there were assets to cover only 52% of benefits—a shortfall of $1.6 billion to be assumed by the agency.

How can this be? Thanks to the way Congress writes the rules, pension accounting has a lot in common with Enron accounting, but with one exception: it's perfectly legal. By adjusting the arcane formulas used to calculate pension assets and obligations, corporate accountants can turn a drastically underfunded system into a financially healthy one, even inflate a company's profits and push up its stock price. Ethan Kra, chief actuary of Mercer Human Resources Consulting, once put it this way: "If you used the same accounting for the operations side [of a corporation] that is used on pension funds, you would be put in jail."

The old PBGC lists of deadbeat pension funds served another purpose. They were an early-warning sign of companies in trouble—a sign often ignored or denied by the companies themselves. "Somehow, if companies are making progress toward an objective that's consistent with [the PBGC's], then I think it's counterproductive to be exposed on this public listing," complained Gary Millenbruch, executive vice president of Bethlehem Steel, a perennial favorite on the Top 50.

Time proved Millenbruch wrong. The early warnings about Bethlehem's pension liabilities turned out to be right on target. Bethlehem Steel eventually filed for bankruptcy, and the PBGC took over its pension plans—which were short $3.7 billion. The company, once America's second largest steelmaker, no longer exists. In the Top 50 pension deadbeats of 1990, the PBGC reported that the funds of Pan Am Corp., operator of what was once the premier global airline, had only one-third of the assets needed to pay its promised pensions. Pan Am does not exist today.

Contrary to the assertions of company executives, PBGC officials and members of Congress, one company after another on the 1990 Top 50 disappeared. To be sure, many are still around. Like General Motors. That year, the PBGC reported a $1.9 billion deficit in GM's pension plans. Today, by GM's reckoning, the deficit is $10 billion. The PBGC estimates it at $31 billion. As for the pension-fund deficit, if GM or any other company can't come up with the money, the PBGC will cover retirement checks up to a fixed amount—$45,600 this year—or until the agency runs out of money. That's projected to occur around 2013. At that point, Congress will be forced to decide whether to bail out the agency at a cost of $100 billion or more. When judgment day comes, other economic forces will influence the decision. Medicare, which is in far worse shape than Social Security, already is in the red on a cash basis. In what promises to play out as a mean-spirited competition, Congress has laid the groundwork to pit individual citizens against one another, to fight over the budget scraps available for those and all other programs.

Who's Left Holding the Bag?

In the meantime, pension plans that companies are dumping are so short of assets that the PBGC's financial position is rapidly deteriorating. In 2000, the agency operated with a $10 billion sur-

plus. By 2004, the surplus had turned into a $23 billion deficit. By the end of this year, the shortfall may top $30 billion. As the Government Accountability Office put it earlier this year: "PBGC's accumulated deficit is too big, and plans simply do not have enough money in the system to back up the long-term promises many employers have made to their workers." To add to its woes, the agency has a record 350 active bankruptcy cases, according to Bradley D. Belt, executive director. Of those, Belt told Congress, "37 have underfunding claims of $100 million or more, including six in excess of $500 million."

Congress idly watched United Airlines and USAirways unload their pension obligations on the PBGC. Now Delta and Northwest are positioned to do the same. That increases the likelihood that other old-line carriers like American and Continental will be forced to do likewise. Northwest's CEO, Douglas Steenland, bluntly told the Senate Finance Committee last June, "Northwest has concluded that defined-benefit plans simply do not work for an industry that is as competitive and vulnerable from forces ranging from terrorism to international oil prices that are largely beyond its control, as is the airline industry." In that, he merely echoed Robert Crandall, former chief of American Airlines, who told another Senate committee in October 2004: "All the [older] legacy carriers must get rid of their defined-benefit pension plans." In all, the pension funds of those airlines are short $22 billion.

The sudden shift from annual pensions of a guaranteed amount for a lifetime to a lesser and uncertain amount for a limited period is taking its toll on workers. Robin Gilinger, 42, a United flight attendant for 14 years, sees a frightening financial picture. She has another 14 years to go before she can take early retirement. Under the old pension plan she would have received a monthly check of $2,184. Because of givebacks, that's down to $776—a poverty-level annual income of $9,312 by today's standards, even before inflation takes its toll over the coming years. And there is the distinct possibility it could be less than that. Her husband lost his pension in a corporate takeover.

Gilinger, who lives with her husband and 9-year-old daughter in Mount Laurel, N.J., is not planning on early retirement and certainly couldn't afford it in the current situation. But she has concerns reminiscent of Joy Whitehouse's experience. "It's scary. What if something happened to my husband or if I got disabled?" she asks. "Then I'm looking at nothing. Above all, what's frustrating is that we were told we were going to get our pension and we're not. The senior flight attendants, the ones who've worked 30 years, they're worried how they're going to survive." Each time the PBGC takes on another failed pension plan, it makes the pension-insurance program more expensive for the remaining businesses. That in turn prompts other companies to unload their plans. The PBGC receives no tax money. Its revenue comes from investment income and premiums that corporations pay on their insured workers. As a result, soundly managed companies with solid retirement plans are compelled to pick up the costs for plans in mismanaged companies as well as those that just want to unload their employee benefits. A proposal by the Bush Administration to overhaul the system, critics fear, would actually increase the likelihood that more companies will kill existing plans and that other companies considering establishment of a defined-benefit plan will choose a less expensive option. An analysis of 471 FORTUNE 1000 companies by Watson Wyatt Worldwide, a global consulting firm, concluded "healthy companies would see their total PBGC premiums increase 240% under the proposal, more than double the 113% increase for financially troubled employers."

Barring a reversal in government policies, the PBGC could require a multibillion-dollar taxpayer bailout. The last time that happened was during the 1980s and '90s, when another government insurer, the Federal Savings and Loan Insurance Corp., was unable to keep up with a thrift industry spinning out of control. The Federal Government eventually spent $124 billion. Unlike the FSLIC, which was backed by the U.S. government, the PBGC is not. That means an indifferent Congress could turn its back on the retirement crash. By the agency's estimate, that would translate into a 90% reduction in pensions it currently pays.

Where the 401(K) Falls Short

The universal replacement to the pension, by the consensus of the Bush Administration, Congress, Wall Street and corporate America, is the ubiquitous 401(k). As Bush explained at a gathering at Auburn University in Montgomery, Ala., earlier this year, "When I was young, I didn't know anything about 401(k)s because I don't think they existed. Defined-benefit plans were the main source of retirement. Now they've got what they call defined-contribution plans. Workers are taking aside some of their own money and watching it grow through safe and secure investments."

Tell that "safe and secure" part to the folks at Enron, who lost $1 billion in their 401(k)s. Or WorldCom employees, who also lost $1 billion. Or Kmart employees, who lost at least $100 million. Welcome to the 21st century version of Studebaker.

Truth to tell, the 401(k) was never intended as a retirement plan. It evolved out of a tax break that Congress awarded to corporate executives in 1978, allowing them to defer part of their salaries and cut their tax bills. At the time, federal income-tax rates were much higher for upper-income individuals—the top rate was 70%. (Today it's half that.) It wasn't until several years later that companies began to make 401(k)s available to most employees. Even then, the idea was to encourage saving and provide a tax shelter, not to substitute the plans for pensions. By 1985, assets in 401(k)s had risen to $91 billion, as more companies adopted plans. Still, the amount was only about one-tenth that in guaranteed pensions.

The 401(k) was never intended as a retirement plan. It evolved out of a tax break that Congress awarded to executives.

All that changed as corporations discovered they could improve their bottom lines by shifting workers out of costly defined-benefit plans and into much cheaper (for companies) and more risky (for workers) uninsured 401(k)s. In effect, employees took a hefty pay cut and barely seemed to notice. Lawmakers and supporters advocated the move by pointing to a changing economy in which employees switch jobs frequently. They maintained that because defined-benefit plans are based on length of service and an average of salaries over the last few years of work, they don't meet today's needs. But Congress could have revised the rules and made the plans portable over a working life, just like a 401(k), and retained the guarantee of a fixed retirement amount, just like corporations do for their executives.

As it is, 401(k) portability often impedes efforts to save for retirement. As today's job hoppers move from one employer to another, most succumb to the temptation to cash out their 401(k)s and spend the money, a practice hardly reflective of a serious retirement system. Today $2 trillion is invested in those accounts. But to understand why the 401(k) is no substitute for a defined-benefit pension, look beneath that big number. Earlier this year the airwaves crackled with announcements that the value of the average 401(k) had climbed to $61,000 in 2004. Noticeably absent from many accounts was any reference to the median value, a more accurate indicator of the health of America's retirement system. That number was $17,909, meaning half held less, half more. Nearly 1 in 4 accounts had a balance of less than $5,000.

So it is that in the end, all but the most affluent citizens will have two options. They can join Joy Whitehouse in the can-collection business, or they can follow in the footsteps of Betty Dizik of Fort Lauderdale, Fla., who is into her sixth decade as a working American. She has no choice. Dizik did not lose her pension. Like most Americans, she never had one, or a 401(k). After her husband died in 1968, she held a series of jobs managing apartments and self-storage facilities, tasks that brought her into contact with the public. "I like working with people," she said. But none of the jobs had a pension.

Hence the importance of her monthly Social Security check, which comes to less than $1,000. The benefit barely covers her medications for heart problems and diabetes, which she says can cost her as much as $800 a month. The new Medicare prescription-drug benefit, she estimates, will still leave her with substantial out-of-pocket expenses. To pay rent, utilities, gas for her car and other living expenses, Dizik has continued to work since she turned 65. For 10 years, she was with Broward County Meals on Wheels, which provides meals to seniors, some younger than she is. But three years ago, when she turned 75, driving 100 miles a day began exacting a toll.

Now she works at a nearby office of H&R Block, the tax-return service. "I do everything there," she says. "I am the receptionist. The cashier. I open the office, close the office. I'm the one who takes the money to the bank. I do taxes." A widow, she lives alone in an apartment building for seniors. Her four children help with the rent, but she is reluctant to accept anything more. "All my children are great, but I do not like to ask them for anything," she said. "I'm waiting for myself to get old, when I will need their help." For the time being, she says, "I'm going strong. I have to."

She doesn't have much hope that Washington will be able to help seniors like her. "They don't understand what it's like to worry: Are you going to be able to make it every month, to pay the telephone bill, the electric bill? How much are you going to have left over for food and other expenses?" Her key to getting by each month is forcing herself to live within a strict budget. "You learn to live very carefully," she said. Although Dizik really would like to retire, she can't. "I will be working the rest of my life." Soon, she will have lots of company.

Work/Retirement Choices and Lifestyle Patterns of Older Americans

HAROLD COX
Indiana State University
TERRANCE PARKS
Indiana State University

ANDRE HAMMONDS
Indiana State University
GURMEET SEKHON
Indiana State University

This study examined the work, retirement, and lifestyle choices of a sample of older Indiana residents. The six lifestyles examined in this study were:

1. *to continue to work full-time;*
2. *to continue to work part-time;*
3. *retire from work and become engaged in a variety of volunteer activities;*
4. *to retire from work and become involved in a variety of recreational and leisure activities;*
5. *to retire from work and later return to work part-time; and*
6. *to retire from work and later return to work full-time*

These findings indicate that health was not a critical factor in the older person's retirement decision, and that those who retired and engaged in volunteer or recreational activities were significantly more satisfied with their lives than those who continue to work. Those who retired and engaged in volunteer or recreational activities scored significantly higher on life satisfaction than those who had returned to work full or part-time. There was no significant difference between those who had retired and those who had continued working in terms of how they were viewed by their peers. Of those who retired and then returned to work, the most satisfied with their lives were the ones who returned to work in order to feel productive. Those least satisfied with their lives were the ones that returned to work because they needed money.

Introduction

There are basically six different choices of lifestyles from which older Americans choose when they reach retirement age. The can (1) continue to work full-time, (2) reduce work commitments but continue to work part-time, (3) retire from work and become engaged in a variety of volunteer activities that provide needed services but for which they will receive no economic compensation or (4) retire from work and become involved in a variety of recreational and leisure activities, (5) retire from work and later return to work part-time, (6) retire from work and return to work full-time.

There are a multitude of life experiences and retirement patterns that may ultimately lead older persons to choose among the diverse ways of occupying themselves during their later years. Some enjoy their work as well as the income, status, privilege, and power that go with full-time employment and never intend to retire. Some retire intending to engage in recreational and leisure activities on a full-time basis only to find this lifestyle less satisfying than they imagined and ultimately return to work. The need to feel productive and actively involved in life is often a critical factor inducing some retirees to return to work. Some retirees who have become widowed, divorced, or never married find themselves too socially isolated in retirement. They return to work either full-time or part-time because their job brings them into contact with a variety of people, and therefore they are less isolated. Thus, there are a variety of reasons why older persons may continue to work or to become active volunteers during their later years. On the other hand, many persons retire, dedicate themselves to recreation and leisure activities, and are most satisfied doing so.

The purpose of this study was to determine which of these six groups were better off in terms of their health, life satisfaction, retirement adjustment and the respect they received from their peers.

A second factor, which will be examined in this study, is the advisability for both government and industry of encouraging older workers to remain in the labor force longer. Changes in Social Security regulations after the year 2000 are going to gradually increase the age of eligibility for Social Security payment from 62 to 64 for early retirement and from 65 to 67 for full retirement benefits. Will changes in the age of eligibility for retirement income derived from Social Security regulations be good or bad for older Americans?

Review of Literature

Work

The meanings of such diverse activities as work, leisure, and retirement to a member of a social system are often quite complex. Paradoxically, the relevance of work and leisure activities for an individual is often intertwined in his or her thinking. Consequently, the concept of work or occupation has been difficult for sociologists to precisely define.

For some time sociologists have struggled to come up with an adequate definition of work. Dubin (1956), for example, defined work as continuous employment in the production of goods and services for remuneration. This definition ignores the fact that there are necessary tasks in society carried out by persons who receive no immediate pay. Mothers, fathers, housewives, and students do not receive pay for their valued activities.

Hall (1975) attempts to incorporate both the economic and social aspects of work in his definition: "An occupation is the social role performed by adult members of society that directly and/or indirectly yields social and financial consequences and that constitutes a major focus in the life of an adult." Similarly Bryant (1972) tries to include both the economic and social aspects of work life in his definition of labor: "Labor is any socially integrating activity which is connected with human subsistence." By *integrating activity* Bryant means sanctioned activity that presupposes, creates, and recreates social relationships. The last two definitions seem to take a broader view of work in the individual's total life. Moreover, they could include the work done by mothers, fathers, housewives, and students. The advantage of definitions that attach strong importance to the meaning and social aspects of a work role is that they recognize the importance of roles for which there is no, or very little, economic reward. The homemaker, while not receiving pay, may contribute considerably to a spouse's career and success. College students in the period of anticipatory socialization and preparation for an occupational role may not be receiving any economic benefits, but their efforts are crucial to their future career.

The most appropriate definitions of work, therefore, seem to be those that emphasize the social and role aspects of an occupation, which an individual reacts to and is shaped by, whether or not he or she is financially rewarded for assuming these roles. From the perspective of sociology, one's work life and the roles one assumes during the workday will, in time, shape one's self-concept, identity, and feelings about oneself, and therefore strongly affect one's personality and behavior. Moreover, from this perspective, the individual's choice of occupations is probably strongly affected by the desire to establish, maintain, and display a desired identity.

Individual Motivation to Work

Vroom (1964) has attempted to delineate the components of work motivation. The first component is wages and all the economic rewards associated with the fringe benefits of the job. People desire these rewards, which therefore serve as a strong incentive to work. Iams (1985), in a study of the post-retirement work patterns of women, found that unmarried women were very likely to work at least part-time after retirement if their monthly income was below $500. Hardy (1991) found that 80 percent of the retirees who later re-entered the labor force stated that money was the main reason they returned to work. The economic inducement to work is apparently a strong one.

A second inducement to work is the expenditure of physical and mental energy. People seem to need to expend energy in some meaningful way, and work provides this opportunity. Vroom (1964) notes that animals will often engage in spontaneous activity as a consequence of activity deprivation.

A third motivation, according to Vroom, is the production of goods and services. This inducement is directly related to the intrinsic satisfaction the individual derives from successful manipulation of the environment.

A fourth motivation is social interaction. Most work roles involve interaction with customers, clients, or members of identifiable work groups as part of the expected behavior of their occupants.

The final motivation Vroom mentions is social status. An individual's occupation is perhaps the best single determinant of his or her status in the community.

These various motivations for work undoubtedly assume different configurations for different people and occupational groups. Social interaction may be the most important for some, while economic considerations may be most important for others. For still others the intrinsic satisfaction derived from the production of goods and services may be all-important. Thus, the research by industrial sociologists has indicated that there are diverse reasons why individuals are motivated to work.

The critical questions for gerontologists is whether the same psychological and social factors that thrust people into work patterns for the major part of their adult life can channel them into leisure activities during their retirement years. Can people find the same satisfaction, feeling of worth, and identity in leisure activities that they did in work-related activities? Streib and Schneider (1971) think they can. They argue that the husband, wife, grandmother, and grandfather's roles may expand and become more salient in the retirement years. Simultaneously, public service and community roles become possible because of the flexibility of the retiree's time. They believe that the changing activities and roles, which accompany retirement, need not lead to a loss of self-respect or active involvement in the mainstream of life.

Retirement Trends

Demographic and economic trends in American society have resulted in an ever-increasing number of retired Americans. Streib and Schneider (1971) observed that for retirement to become an institutionalized social pattern in any society, certain conditions must be met. There must be a large group of people who live long enough to retire, the economy must be sufficiently productive to support segments of the population that are not included in the work force, and there must be some well-established forms of pension or insurance programs to support people during their retirement years.

There has been a rapid growth in both the number and percentage of the American population 65 and above since 1900.

Table 1 Civilian Labor Force Participation Rates: Actual and Projected*

	Men			Women		
Year	45–54	55–64	65 and over	45–54	55–64	65 and over
1950	95.8	86.9	45.8	37.9	27.0	9.7
1960	95.7	86.8	33.1	49.8	32.2	10.8
1970	94.2	83.0	26.8	54.4	43.0	9.7
1980	91.2	72.3	19.1	59.9	41.5	8.1
1986	91.0	67.3	16.0	65.9	42.3	7.4
1990*	90.7	65.1	14.1	69.0	42.8	7.0
2000*	90.1	63.2	9.9	75.4	45.8	5.4

SOURCE: For the rates from 1950–1970: U. S. Department of Labor (1980:224). For the rates from 1980–2000: Bureau of Labor Statistics (unpublished data).

*Values are projections from the Bureau of Labor Statistics middle growth path.

In 1900, there were 3.1 million Americans 65 and over, which constituted four percent of the population. Currently, approximately 31 million Americans are in this age category, which makes up 12.5 percent of the population. While the number and proportion of the population over 65 have been increasing steadily, the proportion of those who remain in the work force has decreased steadily. In 1900, nearly two thirds of those 65 worked. Sammartino (1979) reports that by 1947 this figure had declined to 47.8 percent. By 1987 only 16.5 percent of those 65 and older were still in the work force. In the past 20 years the decline in labor force participation in later years has extended into the 55–64 year old age group. Clark (1988) observed that between 1960 and 1970 the labor force participation of men (55–64) dropped from 86.8% to 83%. By 1990 the labor force participation rate of men in this age group (55–64) had dropped to 65.1% (see Table 1). Table 1 indicates that the labor force participation rates of women 55–64 rose from 27% to 43% from 1950 to 1970 but has remained relatively stable since 1970. Thus, while the labor force participation rate of 55-years and -older women has remained relatively stable since 1970, the labor force participation rate of women 45–54 has grown from 54.4% in 1970 to 69% in 1990. It would appear from these figures that, while younger women are in increasing numbers entering the labor force, women 55 and above are following the same path as their male counterparts and choosing to retire early.

Similarly, there appears to be a somewhat greater convergence in the work and retirement patterns of men and women when comparing 1900 with 1970. The earlier pattern of work histories seemed to be for men to enter the work force earlier and retire later; women tended to enter later and retire earlier. Current trends indicate that women are entering the work force earlier and working longer.

Men, on the other hand, enter the work force later and retire earlier. Thus, the work histories of men and women are becoming very similar, although men as a group still have longer work histories than women. Today, more women are both entering the labor force and also remaining in the labor force throughout their adult lives.

The trend for both men and women for the past 30 years has been for larger numbers to choose to claim Social Security benefits prior to age 65. Allen and Brotman (1981) point out that in 1968, 48 percent of all new Social Security payment awards to men were to claimants under 65; by 1978 this figure had increased to 61 percent. In 1968, 65 percent of all new Social Security awards to women were to claimants under 65; in 1978, the figure was 72 percent.

Simultaneously, fewer persons are choosing to remain in the labor force beyond the age of 65. Soldo and Agree (1988) report that 62 percent of the men and 72 percent of the women who received Social Security benefits in 1986 had retired prior to age 65 and therefore were receiving reduced benefits. The General Accounting Office reports that almost two-thirds of those receiving private retirement benefits in 1985 stopped working prior to age 65. Of those who do remain in the labor force after age 65, Soldo and Agree (1988) report that 47 percent of the men and 59 percent of the women held part-time positions.

Quinn and Burkhauser (1990) report that probably the most critical factor in the decision to retire early is adequate retirement income. They found that between 1975 and 1990 the proportion of workers covered by two pension plans had risen from 21 percent to 40 percent. Moreover, Gall, Evans, and Howard (1997) report a number of studies that found that those with higher incomes, or at least adequate finances, were more satisfied with their life in retirement (Fillenbau, George, and Palmore 1985; Seccombe and Lee 1986; Crowley 1990; Dorfman 1992).

There is a multiplicity of problems confronting the individual at retirement: the lowering of income; the loss of status, privilege, and power associated with one's position in the occupational hierarchy; a major reorganization of life activities, since the nine-to-five workday becomes meaningless; a changing definition of self, since most individuals over time shape their identity and personality in line with the demands of their major occupational roles; considerable social isolation if new activities are not found to replace work-related activities; and a search for a new identity, new meaning, and new values in one's life. Obviously, the major reorganization of one's life that must take place at retirement is a potential source of adjustment problems. Critical to the adjustment is the degree to which one's identity and personality structure was attached to the work role. For those individuals whose work identity is central to their self-concept and gives them the greatest satisfaction, retirement will represent somewhat of a crisis. For others, retirement should not represent a serious problem.

Work and Retirement Patterns in Later Life

Beck (1983) identified three different work and retirement patterns of older persons which include:

1. the fully retired
2. the partially retired
3. the formerly retired

What could be added to Beck's pattern are "the never retired."

There are a number of different studies and authors who have attempted to identify the critical factor determining who will or will not work during their later years. Beck (1983) found that individuals with high job autonomy and high demand jobs were most likely to return to work after formal retirement. Those with the greatest financial need—service workers and laborers—were less likely to return to work despite financial limitations. Beck concludes that income was the critical factor in the motivation of workers who were very poor to return to work. Those in other income categories were less likely to return to work because of actual financial benefits as much as for other factors.

A number of other studies tended to support Beck's analysis of work and retirement patterns. Tillenbaum (1971) found that those with higher levels of education were more likely to continue working beyond age 65 or to return to work after retiring if they chose to do so. Quinn (1980) found the self-employed were much more likely to work beyond retirement age. Streib and Schneider (1971) found that white collar workers were significantly more likely than blue collar workers to return to work. They found no relationship between income and post-retirement work. Howell (1988) reports that those who formally retire and engage in no substantial work during the next three years are more likely to have been unemployed before retirement and to have lower incomes after retirement. They are also more likely to be nonwhite urban dwellers in poor health.

The past research has indicated then that those who either continue to work after retirement age or return to work after retiring are most likely to:

1. have stable employment patterns throughout their adult life;
2. be in white collar occupations;
3. have higher incomes;
4. have a higher number of years of education;
5. be self-employed.

Those least likely to either work after retirement age or return to work after retirement age:

1. those who experienced periods of unemployment throughout their adult life;
2. those in blue collar occupations;
3. those with low incomes;
4. those who have a lower number of years of education;
5. those who are of minority status (Tillenbaum 1971; Quinn 1980; Howell 1988).

These findings support the idea that many people who continue to work after retirement do so for other than financial reasons. If work was stable and both social and psychologically meaningful to the individual, he/she is much more likely to be found working during the retirement years.

As a rule, retirees do not return to jobs with low autonomy, poor working conditions, and difficult physical labor. Those who most need to continue working during the retirement years for financial reasons are least likely to be able to do so. This is most probably related to their inability to find gainful employment.

Volunteer Work in Retirement

Social integration refers to the individual being actively involved in a variety of groups and organization and thus integrated into the web of community activity. The active older person is likely to be involved in a variety of groups ranging from family to social clubs to church and community organizations. While work and career often place the individual in disparate groups and organizations throughout much of his/her adult life, active engagement in voluntary organizations is likely to keep the individual socially involved during their retirement years.

Moen, Dempster-McClain, and Williams (1992) report that studies as early as 1956 reporting that older persons participating in volunteer work on an intermittent basis and belonging to clubs and organizations were positively related to various measures of health. They concluded that occupying multiple roles in the community was positively related to good health.

A number of studies have found a positive relationship between social integration (in the form of multiple roles) and health in later life (Berkman and Breslow 1983; House, Landes, and Umberson 1988; Moen et al.; Williams 1992).

The researchers were unable to determine if multiple roles lead to improved health or if healthy people were more likely to engage in multiple roles. Moen et al. (1992), however, once again found that being a member of a club or organization appeared to be a critical factor in the current health of the individual, after previous health had been controlled. Paid work over the life course, while positively related to multiple roles in later life, was negatively related to measures of health. However, any volunteer activity at any time during adult life appears to promote multiple role occupancy, social integration, and health in later life.

Mobert (1983) observes that church affiliation itself was not considered a volunteer group or activity; however, membership in groups sponsored by the church such as choir, Old Timers, etc. was considered a volunteer activity. Moreover, church members generally remain active participants in church-related activities long after dropping participation from other voluntary associations (Gray and Moberg 1977). Markides (1983) and Ortega, Crutchfield, and Rusling (1983) argue that the church serves as a focal point for individual and community integration of the elderly and that this is crucial to their sense of well-being. Both of these studies found that church attendance was significantly correlated with life satisfaction.

Productivity in Later Life

Older workers who remain in the work force have been found to be just as productive as younger workers. An industrial survey conducted by Parker (1982) found that older workers were most often regarded as superior to younger workers. Adjectives used by employers to describe older workers were responsible, reliable, conscientious, tolerant, reasonable, and loyal. Older workers have greater stability, they miss work less frequently, change jobs less frequently, and are more dedicated and loyal to the employing organization. Welford (1988) found that performance on production jobs tends to increase with age.

While this is true, employers generally offer incentive plans to encourage older workers to retire early. Older workers are generally higher on salary schedules, have accumulated more vacation time and fringe benefits. Thus, many employers see younger workers as cheaper. The fact that they are untested does not seem critical to the employer.

Fyock in discussing the early retirement policies of the 1970's states that:

> Employers liked it because it enabled them to hire and promote younger, more recently trained and lower paid workers. The public liked it because it didn't appear to cost anything and because at age 62 or earlier they could expect to retire; older workers for obvious reasons loved it. (Fyock 1991:422)

Fyock (1991) warns however that we currently have an aging work force and that in the near future employers may find it to their advantage to encourage older workers to remain in the work force longer. She believes that employers often find that retirement appeals to their best, instead of the most expendable, employee.

Projected job growth coupled with a declining number of younger workers has raised concern about possible labor shortages. If these projections prove accurate and labor shortages do develop, the answer to the problem would seem to be the retention of older workers—the very workers employers are currently encouraging to retire. Dennis (1986), Sheppard (1990), and Fyock (1991) all argue that an aging labor force can be a source of opportunity for employers. The smart employers, they believe, will be the ones who know how to take advantage of the opportunity.

McShulski (1997) reports the need for a "soft landing" program which eases older workers out of the labor force on a very gradual basis. Encouraging retiring employees to work a reduced number of hours and handle more limited duties for less pay, helps both the company and the employee. Future retirees can impart relevant job information to their coworkers and teach less experienced employees about specific tasks and customer needs. Thus, working for reduced hours and more limited responsibilities results in a gradual transition to retirement, which is good for the company and the employee according to McShulski.

Retirement Policies and Older Workers

Industrialized societies traditionally have low fertility rates and long life expectancy, resulting in an ever-growing number and percentage of our population that is over 65. Thus, industrialized nations very early began to shift social welfare programs from younger persons to older persons. Many economists are questioning the willingness of society to continue to support an ever-growing number of older persons through public-funded retirement incomes.

Initially, in 1935 when Social Security was passed, both management and labor were anxious to get older persons out of the labor force. Management believed that older workers were too expensive since they were high on salary schedules and had accumulated considerable fringe benefits. Labor unions believed that removing older workers would create jobs for younger workers. The public was happy since they were given economic help in support of their older family members and ultimately they looked forward to being able to retire themselves.

The post-WWII era saw major expansions in Social Security programs. Social Security was extended to cover nearly all wage earners and self-employed persons. The permissible retirement age was lowered to 62, and a national disability income program was added to Social Security. A legal interpretation of the Taft-Hartley Act resulted in private pension plans becoming legitimate items of collective bargaining. The result was that private pension plans have grown substantially from 1950 to present. As a result of these and related activities, a retirement norm has emerged in America. Most people now plan to retire and to live some part of their life out of the labor force.

Congress, with the passage of new Social Security legislation in 1983, began, for the first time, to question the desirability of removing seniors from the labor force. Concern about the financial solvency of the Social Security program led Congress and the President to increase Social Security taxes, to increase taxes on earned income of older persons, to tax Social Security benefits, and to raise the eligible age of Social Security benefits after the year 2000.

Retirement age will go up very gradually during the first quarter of the next century. Early retirement will be increased from 62 to 64 years of age. Full retirement will be increased from 65 to 67. Reduction in pension benefits for those who retire early will go up from 20% to 30% of their full retirement income. Those who stay at work after 65 will get a pension boost of 8% for each extra year of work instead of today's 3%.

The changes in Social Security benefits are clearly designed to encourage people to work longer and retire later. The question that remains, given the trend toward younger retirements, is will these changes really keep older workers in the work force longer or merely mean that more retirees will earn less and therefore more will fall below the poverty line.

Economists and labor planners have never been able to establish the fact that for every older worker who retires, a job is created for a younger worker. Changing technologies and the creation of new jobs have at different times created a greater or lesser demand for more workers. Morris (1986) states that:

> *If financial and social policy disincentives to employment could be reduced there is no prior reason to believe that the economy would be unable to expand gradually to accommodate more retired persons especially in part-time, self-employed, and service capacities (Morris 1986:291).*

Morris (1986) argues that half of the Social Security recipients abruptly leave the labor force and the other half engage in some short-term labor force participation after they retire.

The critical question raised by Congress in changing Social Security benefits in 1983 is can government policies change the age at which people choose to retire. If the older person is to be encouraged to remain in the labor force longer, both the individual worker and the business/industrial community must be convinced of the advantages of keeping older persons in the labor force longer. There seems to be no question that older persons

Table 2 One-Way Analysis of Variance: Mean Perceived Health Scores for Older Workers and Retirees

	MEAN	N=329
Work Full-Time	3.4706	51
Work Part-Time	3.2970	101
Retired/Engaged in Volunteer Activities	3.2867	143
Retired/Engaged Leisure Act.	3.2647	34

SOURCE	D.F.	SUM OF SQUARES	MEAN SQUARES	F-RATIO PROBABILITY	F
Between Groups	3	1.4682	.4891	.9956	.3951
Within Groups	325	159.6574	.4913		
TOTAL	328	161.1246			

can be productive members of the labor force beyond the retirement age if they have the opportunity and choose to do so.

Hypothesis

1. Those working full-time or part-time will be in better health than those who have retired.
2. Those people who have retired will score higher on measures of life satisfaction than those working full or part-time.
3. Those retirees engaged in volunteer or leisure activities will score higher on measures of life satisfaction than those returning to work.
4. Those people working full-time or part-time during their later years will be more highly regarded by their peers.

Methodology

The questionnaire utilized in this study included the standard demographic variables, as well as measures of attitude toward retirement, the respondent's perceived state of health, life satisfaction, retirement adjustment, and his/her perceived status among friends.

The questionnaire was mailed to 597 members of the Older Hoosiers Federation and 200 Green Thumb workers in Indiana. The Older Hoosiers Federation is a volunteer groups of senior citizens who lobby for or against various state and federal legislation which they perceive would affect older Americans. They are primarily retired Americans over the age of 55. The Green Thumb workers are persons 55 and older who work on various parks, roads, and community projects. They are employed by the federal government in community service projects in order to raise their income above the poverty level. A limitation of this study is that the sample was an available sample and not a random sample. It was the best available sample that the researchers could find at this time. There were 342 valid returns, which represented 42.91% of those surveyed.

Findings

The first hypothesis stated that those persons working full or part-time will be in better health than those who are retired. This hypothesis was not supported by the data. As Table 2 indicates, calculating the mean score on the subjects' perceived state of health for those working full-time, those working part-time, those retired and engaged in volunteer activities, and those retired and engaged in leisure activities and then performing a one-way analysis of variance resulted in a finding of no significant difference in the means of the four groups. While past studies of when people retire have indicated that perceived health and subjects' belief that they have adequate income to retire are often identified as the critical variables in the decision of when to retire, that would not appear to be the case with this sample. There were no significant differences in the perceived state of health for those subjects who were working in comparison to those subjects who were retired (Table 2).

Hypothesis Two stated that those persons who have retired will score higher on measures of life satisfaction than those who are working full or part-time. The mean scores on life satisfaction were calculated for those working full-time, those working part-time, those retired and engaged in volunteer activity, and those retired and engaged in leisure activity. The data indicated that those retired and engaged in volunteer activities and those retired and engaged in leisure activity scored significantly higher on measures of life satisfaction than those working either full or part-time (Table 3). The hypothesis was supported by the data (Table 3).

Hypothesis Three stated that those retirees engaged in volunteer or leisure activities will score higher on measures of life satisfaction than those who retired and then returned to work on a full-time or part-time basis. Mean life satisfaction scores were calculated for those who had retired and then returned to work full-time, those who had retired and then returned to work part-time, those who had retired and were engaged in volunteer activities, and those who had retired and were engaged in leisure activities. Those retired and engaged in volunteer or leisure activity scored significantly higher on life satisfaction than those

Table 3 One-Way Analysis of Variance: Mean Life Satisfaction Score for Older Workers and Retirees

	MEAN	N=318	
Work Full-Time	7.6372	49	
Work Part-Time	7.1875	96	
Retired/Engaged in Volunteer Activities	7.9928	139	
Retired/Engaged in Leisure Activities	8.0000	34	

SOURCE	D.F.	SUM OF SQUARES	MEAN SQUARES	F-RATIO	F PROBABILITY
Between Groups	3	40.4064	13.4688	8.2667	.0015
Within Groups	314	803.0056	2.5573		
TOTAL	317	843.4119			

Table 4 One-Way Analysis of Variance: Mean Life Satisfaction Scores for Older Workers and Retirees

	MEAN	N=268	
Returned to Work Full-Time	2.2000	5	
Returned to Work Part-Time	2.0333	90	
Retired/Engaged in Volunteer Activities	2.3885	139	
Retired/Engaged in Leisure Activities	2.2941	34	

SOURCE	D.F.	SUM OF SQUARES	MEAN SQUARES	F-RATIO	F PROBABILITY
Between Groups	3	6.9659	2.3220	5.9067	.0006
Within Groups	264	103.7804	.3931		
TOTAL	267	110.7463			

who had retired and returned to work full or part-time. As Table 4 indicates there were only five people in this sample who had retired and returned to work full-time. Returning to work full-time was rare in this sample of people.

Hypothesis Four stated that those retirees who returned to work full or part-time will be more respected by their peers than those who have retired and engaged in volunteer or leisure activities.

In terms of their perceived respect by friends, those retired and returning to work full-time scored highest with a mean of 3.0. Those who retired and were engaged in volunteer activities scored second with a mean of 2.86. Those who retired and were engaged in leisure activities scored third with a mean of 2.76. Those who had retired and returned to work part-time perceived they were least respected by their friends with a score of 2.68. While the analysis of variance did not find significant differences in these means at the .05 level of significance, they were significant at the .07 level of significance. Since the .05 level of significance is the normal level of acceptance of the significance of difference between groups, this hypothesis was not supported by the data (Table 5).

In order to clarify how the retirees' decision to return to work would affect their life satisfaction, an additional calculation was done. One question asked those who had returned to work was why

they had done so. The choices to this question were: I needed the money, I needed to do something that makes me feel productive, and I was lonely and bored and work gave me something interesting to do. Mean scores and measures of life satisfaction were calculated for each of these three groups (Table 6). The highest mean score was for the group who returned to work in order to feel productive, and their score was 8.27. The second highest mean score was for those who had returned to work because they were lonely and bored, and their score was 7.26. The lowest mean score on life satisfaction was 6.7 for those who had been forced to return to work because they needed the money (Table 6). Thus, most of the people that returned to work did so because they needed the money, but they were the least satisfied with their lives.

Conclusion

The data from this study indicate that those who retire and engage in volunteer or recreational activities score higher on measures of life satisfaction than those that never retired. Of those that retired and then returned to work, those that did so because they wanted to feel productive scored highest on life satisfaction. Those that

Table 5 One Way Analysis of Variance: Mean Scores for Perceived Respect of Older Workers and Retirees by Their Peers

	MEAN	N=277
Returned to Work Full-Time	3.00006	4
Returned to Work Part-Time	2.6869	99
Retired/Engaged in Volunteer Activities	2.8643	140
Retired/Engaged in Leisure Activities	2.7647	34

SOURCE	D.F.	SUM OF SQUARES	MEAN SQUARES	F RATIO	F PROBABILITY
Between Groups	3	2.0236	.6745	2.4254	.0657
Within Groups	272	75.8326	.2778		
TOTAL	276	77.8556			

Table 6. One Way Analysis of Variance: Mean Scores on Life Satisfaction Based on the Reasons Individuals Returned to Work

	MEAN	N=130
Needed the money	6.7027	74
Wanted to feel productive	8.2703	37
Lonely & bored	7.2632	19

SOURCE	D.F.	SUM OF SQUARES	MEAN SQUARES	F RATIO	F PROBABILITY
Between Groups	2	60.6360	30.3180	10.7420	.0000
Within Groups	127	358.4410	2.8224		
TOTAL	129	419.0769			

returned to work because they needed the money scored lowest on life satisfaction.

These findings would suggest that if the goal of the federal government is to keep older people in the labor force longer, some means must be found by which the older workers are kept at jobs in which they feel productive and needed. For the business community to continue, primarily for economic reasons, to encourage older workers to retire from highly skilled jobs in which they are more productive than younger workers does not seem desirable.

One possible solution to this problem might be for the federal government to give a tax incentive to businesses employing older workers so that the economic advantage business sees for retiring older workers and employing younger ones would diminish.

A major break in the cost of employing older workers in business would be for the federal government to develop a national health insurance program. One of the major costs to the employer of older workers is the amount of money they must put into health insurance for them. For the federal government to assume this cost would be a major reduction in the business cost of continuing to employ older workers.

Perhaps businesses could continue to utilize the talents of older workers by developing reduced and flexible work schedules which would pay them a lower salary but keep them involved in critical tasks for the industry, as suggested by McShulski (1997).

Since the trend of the last thirty years has been for an ever increasing number of workers to retire prior to age 65, perhaps the government's attempts to keep people in the workforce longer by increasing the age at which they can draw a Social Security check will not be successful. It is possible that through private savings, private investment programs, and pension programs financed by their employers, older workers will continue to retire prior to age 65.

On the other hand, improving technology may mean that business and industry will need fewer employees to produce the nations' good and services, and therefore they will continue to encourage their workers to retire at younger ages.

The complexity and unpredictability of the factors involved makes predicting future employment and retirement patterns for older Americans at best hazardous and at worst impossible. Observing the results of economic and political pressures placed on both business and government by an ever increasing number of the baby boom generation arriving at retirement age in the next 25 years should prove interesting.

References

Allen, Carole and Herman Brotman. 1981. *Chartbook on Aging.* Washington, D. C.: Administration on Aging.

Beck, S. 1983. "Determinants of Returning to Work after Retirement." Final Report for Grant No. 1R23AG035:65–101, Kansas City, MO.

Berkman, Lisa F. and Lister Breslow. 1983. *Health and Ways of Living: The Alameda Country Study.* New York: Oxford University Press.

Clark, Robert. 1988. "The Future of Work and Retirement." *Research on Aging* 10:169–193.

Clifton, Bryant. 1972. *The Social Dimensions of Work.* Upper Saddle River, NJ: Prentice Hall.

Crowley, J. E. 1990. "Longitudinal Effects of Retirement on Men's Well-Being and Health." Journal *of Business and Psychology* 1:95–113.

Dennis, Helen. 1986. *Fourteen Steps to Managing an Aging Work Force,* edited by Helen Dennis, Lexington, MA: Lexington Books.

Dorfman, L. T. 1992. "Academics and the Transition to Retirement." *Educational Gerontology* 18:343–363.

Dubin, Robert. 1956. "Industrial Workers' Word: A Study of the Central Life Interests of Industrial Workers." *Social Problems* 3:131–142.

Fillenbau, G. G., L. K. George, and E. B. Palmore. 1985. "Determinants and Consequences of Retirement." *Journal of Gerontology* 39:364–371.

Fyock, Catherine. 1991. "American Work Force Is Coming of Age." *The Gerontologist* 31:422–425.

Gall, Terry, David Evans, and John Howard. May 1997. "The Retirement Adjustment Process; Changes in Well-Being of Male Retirees Across Time." *The Journal of Gerontology* 52B(3):110–117.

Gray, Robert M. and David O. Moberg. 1977. *The Church and the Older Person,* revised edition. Grand Rapids, MI: Ermanns

Hall, Richard. 1975. *Occupations and the Social Structure.* Englewood Cliffs, NJ: Prentice Hall.

Hardy, Melissa. 1991. "Employment After Retirement." *Research on Aging* 13(3):267–288.

House, James S., Karl R. Landes, and Debra Umberson. 1988. "Social Relationships and Health." *Science* 241:540–545.

Howell, Nancy Morrow. 1988. "Life Span Determinants of Work in Retirement Years." *International Journal of Aging and Human Development* 27(2):125–140.

Iams, Howard M. 1985 "New Social Security Beneficiary Women." Correlates of work paper read at the 1985 meeting of the American Sociological Association.

Markides, Kyrakos S. 1983. "Aging, Religiosity and Adjustment: A Longitudinal Analysis." *Journal of Gerontology* 38:621–625.

McShulski, Elaine. 1997. "Ease Employer and Employee Retirement Adjustment with 'Soft Landing' Program." *HR Magazine,* Alexandria: 30–32.

Mobert, David D. 1983. "Compartmentalization and Parochialism in Religion and Voluntary Action Research." *Review of Religious Research* 22(4):318–321.

Moen, Phyllis, Donna Dempster-McClain, and Robin Williams. 1992. "Successful Aging: A Life Course Perspective on Women's Multiple Roles and Health." *American Journal of Sociology* 97(6):1612–1633.

Morris, Malcolm. 1986. "Work and Retirement in an Aging Society." *Daedalus* 115:269–293.

Ortega, Suzanne T., Robert D. Crutchfield, and William A. Rusling. 1983. "Race Differences in Elderly Personal Well-Being, Friendship, Family and Church." *Research on Aging* 5(1):101–118.

Parker, Stanley. 1982. *Works and Retirement.* London: Allen & Unwin Publishers.

Quinn, Joseph and Richard Burkhauser. *1990 Handbook of Aging and the Social Sciences,* edited by Richard Beinstock and Linda K. Gorge. Academic Press.

Quinn, J. F. 1980. *Retirement Patterns of Self-Employed Workers in Retirement Policy on an Aging Society,* R. L. Clark ed., Durham, NC:. Duke University Press.

Soldo, Beth J. and Emily M. Agree. 1988. *Population Bulletin* 43(3). Population Reference Bureau.

Sammartino, Frank. 1979. "Early Retirement." in *Monographs of Aging,* No. 1, Madison: Joyce MacBeth Institute on Aging and Adult Life, University of Wisconsin.

Seccombe, K. and G. R. Lee. 1986. "Gender Differences in Retirement Satisfaction and Its Antecedents." *Research on Aging* 8:426–440.

Sheppard, Harold. 1990. *The Future of Older Workers.* International Exchange Center on Gerontology, University of South Florida, Tampa. FL.

Streib, G. F. and C. J. Schneider. 1971. *Retirement in American Society.* Cornell University Press, Ithaca, NY.

Tillenbaum, G. C. 1971. "The Working Retired." *Journal of Gerontology* 26:1:82–89. U. S. Department of Labor, Civilian Labor Force Participation Rates: Actual and Projected 1980.

Vroom, Victor. 1964. *Work & Motivation.* New York: John Wiley.

Welford, A. T. 1988. "Preventing Adverse Changes of Work with Age." *American Journal of Aging and Human Development* 4:283–291.

From *Journal of Applied Sociology,* by Harold Cox, Terrance Parks, Andre Hammonds and Gurmeet Sekhon, pp. 131-149. Copyright © 2001 by Society for Applied Sociology. Reprinted by permission.

UNIT 6

The Experience of Dying

Unit Selections

Key Points to Consider

- Oregon is a state that has made euthanasia (assisted suicide) legal. Why are so many of the seriously ill older persons there choosing to end their lives by refusing to eat rather than euthanasia?

- What are the steps a person goes through in the grieving process?

- Should dying patients be told the truth about their impending death, or should the information be withheld? Defend your answer.

- What are the six mind frames toward death that a person might adopt after being informed of their impending death?

Student Website

www.mhcls.com/online

Internet References

Further information regarding these websites may be found in this book's preface or online.

Agency for Health Care Policy and Research
http://www.ahcpr.gov

Growth House, Inc.
http://www.growthhouse.org/

Hospice Foundation of America
http://www.HospiceFoundation.org

Hospice HotLinks
http://www.hospiceweb.com/links.htm

Modern science has allowed individuals to have some control over the conception of their children and has provided people with the ability to prolong life. However, life and death still defy scientific explanation or reason. The world can be divided into two categories: sacred and secular. The sacred (that which is usually embodied in the religion of a culture) is used to explain all the forces of nature and the environment that can neither be understood nor controlled. On the other hand, the secular (defined as "of or relating to the world") is used to explain all the aspects of the world that can be understood or controlled. Through scientific invention, more and more of the natural world can be controlled. It still seems highly doubtful, however, that science will ever be able to provide an acceptable explanation of the meaning of death. In this domain, religion may always prevail. Death is universally feared. Sometimes it is more bearable for those who believe in a life after death. Here, religion offers a solution to this dilemma. In the words of anthropologist Bronislaw Malinowski (1884–1942):

> Religion steps in, selecting the positive creed, the comforting view, the culturally valuable belief in immortality, in the spirit of the body, and in the continuance of life after death. (Bronislaw Malinowski, *Magic, Science and Religion and Other Essays*, Glencoe, Illinois: Free Press, 1948)

The fear of death leads people to develop defense mechanisms in order to insulate themselves psychologically from the reality of their own death. The individual knows that someday he or she must die, but this event is nearly always thought to be likely to occur in the far distant future. The individual does not think of himself or herself as dying tomorrow or the next day, but rather years from now. In this way, people are able to control their anxiety about death.

Losing a close friend or relative brings people dangerously close to the reality of death. Individuals come face to face with the fact that there is always an end to life. Latent fears surface. During times of mourning, people grieve not only for the dead, but also for themselves, and for the finiteness of life.

The readings in this section address bereavement, grief, arguments for and against euthanasia, and adjustments to the stages of dying. Janet McConnaughey, in "More Hospice Pa-

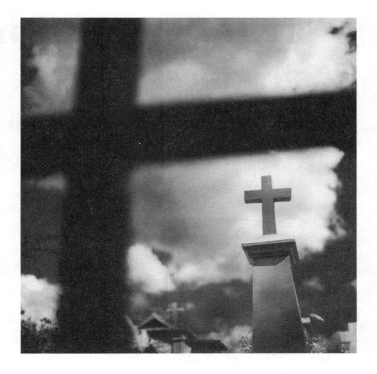

tients Forgoing Sustenance," points out that in the state of Oregon, twice as many hospice patients choose to end their lives by refusing to eat as choose to die by physician-assisted suicide. The reasons for this decision are examined. In "The Grieving Process," the authors list and describe the stages of grief that the individual will experience following the death of a loved one.

"Start the Conversation" explains what the dying person will experience physically and emotionally. Moreover, the inevitable caregiving choices that must be made are clearly outlined. In "Mind Frames Towards Dying and Factors Motivating Their Adoption by Terminally Ill Elders," the author describes the six different mind frames the person can hold regarding their own death once they recognize that they are terminally ill.

More Hospice Patients Forgoing Sustenance

Oregon study shows more ending lives by not eating, drinking.

JANET MCCONNAUGHEY

A surprising number of terminally ill hospice patients choose to speed their deaths by refusing food and drink, a study in Oregon suggests.

In fact the survey of hospice nurses found that patients pick this means of ending life–which is legal everywhere in the United States—twice as often as physician assisted suicide, which is legal only in Oregon.

The study further found that these patients are not depressed and typically die tranquilly, within two weeks.

The patients said they were ready to die, their quality of life was poor or they were afraid it would become so, and they saw no point in going on. They also wanted to die at home—where nearly all hospice care is given—and control the circumstances of their death, the nurses reported.

Nearly three-quarters of Oregon's 429 hospice nurses returned the survey. One-third of those who did said at least one of their patients had deliberately hastened death by stopping food and fluids during the previous four years.

That was only a tiny fraction of the 10,000-plus people who die under hospice care each year in Oregon. But Dr. Linda Ganzini, who directed the study, said the figure at first seemed too high to believe.

"I went back to my research assistant and said, 'Can we check this? Can we have these codes right?'" said Ganzini, who works at Oregon Health and Science University and the Portland Veterans Affairs Medical Center, and is on the board of the American Hospice Association.

After all, when she went through the medical journals, she found only three case studies about patients who had made this choice. A fourth report, from St. Christopher's Hospice in England, said that only two patients had done so in 30 years.

As striking as the numbers themselves is the fact that the nurses rated the overall quality of those deaths as "8" on a scale in which zero was "very bad" and 9 was "very good." Three-quarters of those scores were 7 or above, according to the study in Thursday's New England Journal of Medicine.

In all, 102 of the 307 nurses who answered her survey had worked with patients who ended their lives this way. At least 16 other patients stopped eating and drinking but later resumed doing so.

Over the same four years, 55 other terminally ill patients had used Oregon's assisted suicide law to get their doctors to prescribe a lethal dose of narcotics.

Other hospice professionals said that although having patients decide to refuse food and drink is far from an everyday occurrence, they found Ganzini's results completely believable. Dr. William Lamers of Malibu, Calif., medical consultant to Hospice Foundation of America, estimated that he had treated 50 such patients over 30 years of hospice practice.

"It is not an uncommon thing for people to talk about it—not uncommon for them to say, 'I'm not hungry. I don't want to eat any more, I just want to go,'" Lamers said.

The Grieving Process

MICHAEL R. LEMING
St. Olaf College

GEORGE E. DICKINSON
College of Charleston

G rief is a very powerful emotion that is often triggered or stimulated by death. Thomas Attig makes an important distinction between grief and the grieving process. Although grief is an emotion that engenders feelings of helplessness and passivity, the process of grieving is a more complex coping process that presents challenges and opportunities for the griever and requires energy to be invested, tasks to be undertaken, and choices to be made (Attig, 1991).

Most people believe that grieving is a disease-like and debilitating process that renders the individual passive and helpless. According to Attig (1991, p. 389):

> It is misleading and dangerous to mistake grief for the whole of the experience of the bereaved. It is misleading because the experience is far more complex, entailing diverse emotional, physical, intellectual, spiritual, and social impacts. It is dangerous because it is precisely this aspect of the experience of the bereaved that is potentially the most frustrating and debilitating.

Death ascribes to the griever a passive social position in the bereavement role. Grief is an emotion over which the individual has no control. However, understanding that grieving is an active coping process can restore to the griever a sense of autonomy in which the process is permeated with choice and there are many areas over which the griever does have some control.

Coping with Grief

The grieving process, like the dying process, is essentially a series of behaviors and attitudes related to coping with the stressful situation of a change in the status of a relationship. Many individuals have attempted to understand coping with dying as a series of universal, mutually exclusive, and linear stages. Not all people, however, will progress through the stages in the same manner.

Seven behaviors and feelings that are part of the coping process are identified by Robert Kavanaugh (1972): shock and denial, disorganization, volatile emotions, guilt, loss and loneliness, relief, and reestablishment. It is not difficult to see similarities between these behaviors and Kübler-Ross's five

stages (denial, anger, bargaining, depression, and acceptance) of the dying process. According to Kavanaugh (1972, p. 23), "these seven stages do not subscribe to the logic of the head as much as to the irrational tugs of the heart—the logic of need and permission."

Shock and Denial

Even when a significant other is expected to die, at the time of death there is often a sense in which the death is not real. For most of us our first response is, "No, this can't be true." With time, our experience of shock diminishes, but we find new ways to deny the reality of death.

Some believe that denial is dysfunctional behavior for those in bereavement. However, denial not only is a common experience among the newly bereaved but also serves positive functions in the process of adaptation. The main function of denial is to provide the bereaved with a "temporary safe place" from the ugly realities of a social world that offers only loneliness and pain.

With time, the meaning of loss tends to expand, and it may be impossible for one to deal with all of the social meanings of death at once. For example, if a man's wife dies, not only does he lose his spouse, but also his best friend, his sexual partner, the mother of his children, a source of income, and so on. Denial can protect an individual from some of the magnitude of this social loss, which may be unbearable at times. With denial, one can work through different aspects of loss over time.

Disorganization

Disorganization is the stage in the bereavement process in which one may feel totally out of touch with the reality of everyday life. Some go through the 2- to 3-day time period just before the funeral as if on "automatic pilot" or "in a daze." Nothing normal "makes sense," and they may feel that life has no inherent meaning. For some, death is perceived as preferable to life, which appears to be devoid of meaning.

This emotional response is also a normal experience for the newly bereaved. Confusion is normal for those whose social world has been disorganized through death. When Michael

Leming's father died, his mother lost not only all of those things that one loses with a death of a spouse, but also her care-giving role—a social role and master status that had defined her identity in the 5 years that her husband lived with cancer. It is only natural to experience confusion and social disorganization when one's social identity has been destroyed.

Volatile Reactions

Whenever one's identity and social order face the possibility of destruction, there is a natural tendency to feel angry, frustrated, helpless, and/or hurt. The volatile reactions of terror, hatred, resentment, and jealousy are often experienced as emotional manifestations of these feelings. Grieving humans are sometimes more successful at masking their feelings in socially acceptable behaviors than other animals, whose instincts cause them to go into a fit of rage when their order is threatened by external forces. However apparently dissimilar, the internal emotional experience is similar.

In working with bereaved persons over the past 20 years, Michael Leming has observed that the following become objects of volatile grief reactions: God, medical personnel, funeral directors, other family members, in-laws, friends who have not experienced death in their families, and/or even the person who has died. Mild-mannered individuals may become raging and resentful persons when grieving. Some of these people have experienced physical symptoms such as migraine headaches, ulcers, neuropathy, and colitis as a result of living with these intense emotions.

The expression of anger seems more natural for men than expressing other feelings (Golden, 2000). Expressing anger requires taking a stand. This is quite different from the mechanics of sadness, where an open and vulnerable stance is more common. Men may find their grief through anger. Rage may suddenly become tears, as deep feelings trigger other deep feelings. This process is reversed with women, notes Golden. Many times a woman will be in tears, crying and crying, and state that she is angry.

As noted earlier, a person's anger during grief can range from being angry with the person who died to being angry with God, and all points in between. Golden's mentor, Father William Wendt, shared the story of his visits with a widow and his working with her on her grief. He noticed that many times when he arrived she was driving her car up and down the driveway. One day he asked her what she was doing. She proceeded to tell him that she had a ritual she used in dealing with her grief. She would come home, go to the living room, and get her recently deceased husband's ashes out of the urn on the mantle. She would take a very small amount and place them on the driveway. She then said, "It helps me to run over the son of a bitch every day." He concluded the story by saying, "Now that is good grief." It was "good" grief because it was this woman's way of connecting to and expressing the anger component of her grief.

Guilt

Guilt is similar to the emotional reactions discussed earlier. Guilt is anger and resentment turned in on oneself and often results in self-deprecation and depression. It typically manifests itself in statements like "If only I had . . . " "I should have . . . ," "I could have done it differently…," and "Maybe I did the wrong thing." Guilt is a normal part of the bereavement process.

From a sociological perspective, guilt can become a social mechanism to resolve the **dissonance** that people feel when unable to explain why someone else's loved one has died. Rather than view death as something that can happen at any time to anyone, people can **blame the victim** of bereavement and believe that the victim of bereavement was in some way responsible for the death— "If the individual had been a better parent, the child might not have been hit by the car," or "If I had been married to that person, I might also have committed suicide," or "No wonder that individual died of a heart attack, the spouse's cooking would give anyone high cholesterol." Therefore, bereaved persons are sometimes encouraged to feel guilt because they are subtly sanctioned by others' reactions.

Loss and Loneliness

Feelings of loss and loneliness creep in as denial subsides. The full experience of the loss does not hit all at once. It becomes more evident as bereaved individuals resume a social life without their loved one. They realize how much they needed and depended upon their significant other. Social situations in which we expected them always to be present seem different now that they are gone. Holiday celebrations are also diminished by their absence. In fact, for some, most of life takes on a "something's missing" feeling. This feeling was captured in the 1960s love song "End of the World."

> Why does the world go on turning?
>
> Why must the sea rush to shore?
>
> Don't they know it's the end of the world
>
> Cause you don't love me anymore?

Loss and loneliness are often transformed into depression and sadness, fed by feelings of self-pity. According to Kavanaugh (1972, p. 118), this effect is magnified by the fact that the dead loved one grows out of focus in memory— "an elf becomes a giant, a sinner becomes a saint because the grieving heart needs giants and saints to fill an expanding void." Even a formerly undesirable spouse, such as an alcoholic, is missed in a way that few can understand unless their own hearts are involved. This is a time in the grieving process when anybody is better than nobody, and being alone only adds to the curse of loss and loneliness (Kavanaugh, 1972).

Those who try to escape this experience will either turn to denial in an attempt to reject their feelings of loss or try to find surrogates-new friends at a bar, a quick remarriage, or a new pet. This escape can never be permanent, however, because loss and loneliness are a necessary part of the bereavement experience. According to Kavanaugh (1972, p. 119), the "ultimate goal in conquering loneliness" is to build a new independence or to find a new and equally viable relationship.

Relief

The experience of relief in the midst of the bereavement process may seem odd for some and add to their feelings of guilt. Michael Leming observed a friend's relief 6 months after her husband died. This older friend was the wife of a minister, and her whole life before he died was his ministry. With time, as she built a new world of social involvements and relationships of which he was not a part, she discovered a new independent person in herself whom she perceived was a better person than she had ever before been.

Relief can give rise to feelings of guilt. However, according to Kavanaugh (1972, p. 121): "The feeling of relief does not imply any criticism for the love we lost. Instead, it is a reflection of our need for ever deeper love, our quest for someone or something always better, our search for the infinite, that best and perfect love religious people name as God."

Reestablishment

As one moves toward reestablishment of a life without the deceased, it is obvious that the process involves extensive adjustment and time, especially if the relationship was meaningful. It is likely that one may have feelings of loneliness, guilt, and disorganization at the same time and that just when one may experience a sense of relief, something will happen to trigger a denial of the death.

What facilitates bereavement and adjustment is fully experiencing each of these feelings as normal and realizing that it is hope (holding the grieving person together in fantasy at first) that will provide the promise of a new life filled with order, purpose, and meaning.

Reestablishment occurs gradually, and often we realize it has been achieved long after it has occurred. In some ways it is similar to Dorothy's realization at the end of *The Wizard of* Oz— she had always possessed the magic that could return her to Kansas. And, like Dorothy, we have to experience our loss before we really appreciate the joy of investing our lives again in new relationships.

Four Tasks of Mourning

In 1982 J. William Worden published *Grief Counseling and Grief Therapy,* which summarized the research conclusions of a National Institutes of Health study called the Omega Project (occasionally referred to as the Harvard Bereavement Study). Two of the more significant findings of this research, displaying the active nature of the grieving process, are that mourning is necessary for all persons who have experienced a loss through death and that four tasks of mourning must be accomplished before mourning can be completed and reestablishment can take place.

According to Worden (1982), unfinished grief tasks can impair further growth and development of the individual. Furthermore, the necessity of these tasks suggests that those in bereavement must attend to "grief work" because successful grief resolution is not automatic, as Kavanaugh's (1972) stages might imply. Each bereaved person must accomplish four necessary tasks: (1) accept the reality of the loss, (2) experience the pain of grief, (3) adjust to an environment in which the deceased person is missing, and (4) withdraw emotional energy and reinvest it in another relationship (Worden, 1982).

Accept the Reality of the Loss

Especially in situations when death is unexpected and/or the deceased lived far away, it is difficult to conceptualize the reality of the loss. The first task of mourning is to overcome the natural denial response and realize that the person is dead and will not return.

Bereaved persons can facilitate the actualization of death in many ways. The traditional ways are to view the body, attend the funeral and committal services, and visit the place of final disposition. The following is a partial list of additional activities that can assist in making death real for grieving persons.

1. View the body at the place of death before preparation by the funeral director.
2. Talk about the deceased person and the circumstances surrounding the death.
3. View photographs and personal effects of the deceased person.
4. Distribute the possessions of the deceased person among relatives and friends.

Experience the Pain of Grief

Part of coming to grips with the reality of death is experiencing the emotional and physical pain caused by the loss. Many people in the denial stage of grieving attempt to avoid pain by choosing to reject the emotions and feelings that they are experiencing. As discussed by Erich Lindemann (1944), some do this by avoiding places and circumstances that remind them of the deceased. Michael Leming knows one widow who quit playing golf and quit eating at a particular restaurant because these were activities that she had enjoyed with her husband. Another widow found it extremely painful to be with her dead husband's twin, even though he and her sister-in-law were her most supportive friends.

Worden (1982, pp. 13–14) cites the following case study to illustrate the performance of this task of mourning:

> One young woman minimized her loss by believing her brother was *out* of his dark place and into a better place after his suicide. This might not have been true, but it kept her from feeling her intense anger at him for leaving her. In treatment, when she first allowed herself to feel anger, she said, "I'm angry with his behavior and not him!" Finally she was able to acknowledge this anger directly.

The problem with the avoidance strategy is that people cannot escape the pain associated with mourning. According to Bowlby (cited by Worden, 1982, p. 14), "Sooner or later, some of those who avoid all conscious grieving, break down—usually with some form of depression." Tears can afford cleansing for wounds created by loss, and fully experiencing the pain ultimately provides wonderful relief to those who suffer while eliminating long-term chronic grief.

Assume New Social Roles

The third task, practical in nature, requires the griever to take on some of the social roles performed by the deceased person or to find others who will. According to Worden (1982), to abort this task is to become helpless by refusing to develop the skills necessary in daily living and by ultimately withdrawing from life.

An acquaintance of Michael Leming's refused to adjust to the social environment in which she found herself after the death of her husband. He was her business partner, as well as her best and only friend. After 30 years of marriage, they had no children, and she had no close relatives. She had never learned to drive a car. Her entire social world had been controlled by her former husband. Three weeks after his funeral she went into the basement and committed suicide.

The alternative to withdrawing is assuming new social roles by taking on additional responsibilities. Extended families who always gathered at Grandma's house for Thanksgiving will be tempted to have a number of small Thanksgiving dinners at different places after her death. The members of this family may believe that "no one can take Grandma's place." Although this may be true, members of the extended family will grieve better if someone else is willing to do Grandma's work, enabling the entire family to come together for Thanksgiving. Not to do so will cause double pain—the family will not gather, and Grandma will still be missed.

Reinvest in New Relationships

The final task of mourning is a difficult one for many because they feel disloyal or unfaithful in withdrawing emotional energy from their dead loved one. One of Michael Leming's family members once said that she could never love another man after her husband died. His twice-widowed aunt responded, "I once felt like that, but I now consider myself to be fortunate to have been married to two of the best men in the world."

Other people find themselves unable to reinvest in new relationships because they are unwilling to experience again the pain caused by loss. The quotation from John Brantner provides perspective on this problem: "Only people who avoid love can avoid grief. The point is to learn from it and remain vulnerable to love."

However, those who are able to withdraw emotional energy and reinvest it in other relationships find the possibility of a newly established social life. Kavanaugh (1972, pp. 122-123) depicts this situation well with the following description:

> At this point fantasies fade into constructive efforts to reach out and build anew. The phone is answered more quickly, the door as well, and meetings seem important, invitations are treasured and any social gathering becomes an opportunity rather than a curse. Mementos of the past are put away for occasional family gatherings. New clothes and new places promise dreams instead of only fears. Old friends are important for encouragement and permission to rebuild one's life. New friends can offer realistic opportunities for coming out from under the grieving mantle. With newly acquired friends, one is not a widow, widower, or survivor—just a person. Life begins again at the point of new friendships. All the rest is of yesterday, buried, unimportant to the now and tomorrow.

Start the Conversation

The Modern Maturity guide to end-of-life care

The Body Speaks

Physically, dying means that "the body's various physiological systems, such as the circulatory, respiratory, and digestive systems, are no longer able to support the demands required to stay alive," says Barney Spivack, M.D., director of Geriatric Medicine for the Stamford (Connecticut) Health System. "When there is no meaningful chance for recovery, the physician should discuss realistic goals of care with the patient and family, which may include letting nature take its course. Lacking that direction," he says, "physicians differ in their perception of when enough is enough. We use our best judgment, taking into account the situation, the information available at the time, consultation with another doctor, or guidance from an ethics committee."

Without instructions from the patient or family, a doctor's obligation to a terminally ill person is to provide life-sustaining treatment. When a decision to "let nature take its course" has been made, the doctor will remove the treatment, based on the patient's needs. Early on, the patient or surrogate may choose to stop interventions such as antibiotics, dialysis, resuscitation, and defibrillation. Caregivers may want to offer food and fluids, but those can cause choking and the pooling of dangerous fluids in the lungs. A dying patient does not desire or need nourishment; without it he or she goes into a deep sleep and dies in days to weeks. A breathing machine would be the last support: It is uncomfortable for the patient, and may be disconnected when the patient or family finds that it is merely prolonging the dying process.

The Best Defense Against Pain

Pain-management activists are fervently trying to reeducate physicians about the importance and safety of making patients comfortable. "In medical school 30 years ago, we worried a lot about creating addicts," says Philadelphia internist Nicholas Scharff. "Now we know that addiction is not a problem: People who are in pain take pain medication as long as they need it, and then they stop." Spivack says, "We have new formulations and delivery systems, so a dying patient should never have unmet pain needs."

In 1999, the Joint Commission on Accreditation of Healthcare Organizations issued stern new guidelines about easing pain in both terminal and nonterminal patients. The movement intends to take pain seriously: to measure and treat it as the fifth

In Search of a Good Death

If we think about death at all, we say that we want to go quickly, in our sleep, or, perhaps, while fly-fishing. But in fact only 10 percent of us die suddenly. The more common process is a slow decline with episodes of organ or system failure. Most of us want to die at home; most of us won't. All of us hope to die without pain; many of us will be kept alive, in pain, beyond a time when we would choose to call a halt. Yet very few of us take steps ahead of time to spell out what kind of physical and emotional care we will want at the end.

The new movement to improve the end of life is pioneering ways to make available to each of us a good death—as we each define it. One goal of the movement is to bring death through the cultural process that childbirth has achieved; from an unconscious, solitary act in a cold hospital room to a situation in which one is buffered by pillows, pictures, music, loved ones, and the solaces of home. But as in the childbirth movement, the real goal is choice—here, to have the death you want. Much of death's sting can be averted by planning in advance, knowing the facts, and knowing what options we all have. Here, we have gathered new and relevant information to help us all make a difference for the people we are taking care of, and ultimately, for ourselves.

vital sign in hospitals, along with blood pressure, pulse, temperature, and respiration.

The best defense against pain, says Spivack, is a combination of education and assertiveness. "Don't be afraid to speak up," he says. "If your doctor isn't listening, talk to the nurses. They see more and usually have a good sense of what's happening." Hospice workers, too, are experts on physical comfort, and a good doctor will respond to a hospice worker's recommendations. "The best situation for pain management," says Scharff, "is at home with a family caregiver being guided by a hospice program."

The downsides to pain medication are, first, that narcotics given to a fragile body may have a double effect: The drug may ease the pain, but it may cause respiratory depression and possibly death. Second, pain medication may induce grogginess or unconsciousness when a patient wants to be alert. "Most people seem to be much more willing to tolerate pain than mental confusion," says senior research scientist M. Powell Lawton,

Ph.D., of the Philadelphia Geriatric Center. Dying patients may choose to be alert one day for visitors, and asleep the next to cope with pain. Studies show that when patients control their own pain medication, they use less.

Final Symptoms

Depression This condition is not an inevitable part of dying but can and should be treated. In fact, untreated depression can prevent pain medications from working effectively, and antidepressant medication can help relieve pain. A dying patient should be kept in the best possible emotional state for the final stage of life. A combination of medications and psychotherapy works best to treat depression.

Anorexia In the last few days of life, anorexia—an unwillingness or inability to eat—often sets in. "It has a protective effect, releasing endorphins in the system and contributing to a greater feeling of well-being," says Spivack. "Force-feeding a dying patient could make him uncomfortable and cause choking."

Dehydration Most people want to drink little or nothing in their last days. Again, this is a protective mechanism, triggering a release of helpful endorphins.

Drowsiness and Unarousable Sleep In spite of a coma-like state, says Spivack, "presume that the patient hears everything that is being said in the room."

Agitation and Restlessness, Moaning and Groaning The features of "terminal delirium" occur when the patient's level of consciousness is markedly decreased; there is no significant likelihood that any pain sensation can reach consciousness. Family members and other caregivers may interpret what they see as "the patient is in pain" but as these signs arise at a point very close to death, terminal delirium should be suspected.

The Ultimate Emotional Challenge

A dying person is grieving the loss of control over life, of body image, of normal physical functions, mobility and strength, freedom and independence, security, and the illusion of immortality. He is also grieving the loss of an earthly future, and reorienting himself to an unknowable destiny.

At the same time, an emotionally healthy dying person will be trying to satisfy his survival drive by adapting to this new phase, making the most of life at the moment, calling in loved ones, examining and appreciating his own joys and accomplishments. Not all dying people are depressed; many embrace death easily.

Facing the Fact

Doctors are usually the ones to inform a patient that he or she is dying, and the end-of-life movement is training physicians to bring empathy to that conversation in place of medspeak and time estimates. The more sensitive doctor will first ask how the patient feels things are going. "The patient may say, 'Well, I

Hospice: The Comfort Team

Hospice is really a bundle of services. It organizes a team of people to help patients and their families, most often in the patient's home but also in hospice residences, nursing homes, and hospitals:

- Registered nurses who check medication and the patient's condition, communicate with the patient's doctor, and educate caregivers.
- Medical services by the patient's physician and a hospice's medical director, limited to pain medication and other comfort care.
- Medical supplies and equipment.
- Drugs for pain relief and symptom control.
- Home-care aides for personal care, homemakers for light housekeeping.
- Continuous care in the home as needed on a short-term basis.
- Trained volunteers for support services.
- Physical, occupational, and speech therapists to help patients adapt to new disabilities.
- Temporary hospitalization during a crisis.
- Counselors and social workers who provide emotional and spiritual support to the patient and family.
- Respite care—brief noncrisis hospitalization to provide relief for family caregivers for up to five days.
- Bereavement support for the family, including counseling, referral to support groups, and periodic check-ins during the first year after the death.

Hospice Residences Still rare, but a growing phenomenon. They provide all these services on-site. They're for patients without family caregivers; with frail, elderly spouses; and for families who cannot provide at-home care because of other commitments. At the moment, Medicare covers only hospice services; the patient must pay for room and board. In many states Medicaid also covers hospice services (see How Much Will It Cost?). Keep in mind that not all residences are certified, bonded, or licensed; and not all are covered by Medicare.

Getting In A physician can recommend hospice for a patient who is terminally ill and probably has less than six months to live. The aim of hospice is to help people cope with an illness, not to cure it. All patients entering hospice waive their rights to curative treatments, though only for conditions relating to their terminal illness. "If you break a leg, of course you'll be treated for that," says Karen Woods, executive director of the Hospice Association of America. No one is forced to accept a hospice referral, and patients may leave and opt for curative care at any time. Hospice programs are listed in the Yellow Pages. For more information, see Resources.

don't think I'm getting better,' and I would say, 'I think you're right,' " says internist Nicholas Scharff.

At this point, a doctor might ask if the patient wants to hear more now or later, in broad strokes or in detail. Some people will

Survival Kit for Caregivers

A study published in the March 21, 2000, issue of **Annals of Internal Medicine** shows that caregivers of the dying are twice as likely to have depressive symptoms as the dying themselves.

No wonder. Caring for a dying parent, says social worker Roni Lang, "brings a fierce tangle of emotions. That part of us that is a child must grow up." Parallel struggles occur when caring for a spouse, a child, another relative, or a friend. Caregivers may also experience sibling rivalry, income loss, isolation, fatigue, burnout, and resentment.

To deal with these difficult stresses, Lang suggests that caregivers:

- Set limits in advance. How far am I willing to go? What level of care is needed? Who can I get to help? Resist the temptation to let the illness always take center stage, or to be drawn into guilt-inducing conversations with people who think you should be doing more.
- Join a caregiver support group, either disease-related like the Alzheimer's Association or Gilda's Club, or a more general support group like The Well Spouse Foundation. Ask the social services department at your hospital for advice. Telephone support and online chat rooms also exist (see Resources).
- Acknowledge anger and express it constructively by keeping a journal or talking to an understanding friend or family member. Anger is a normal reaction to powerlessness.
- When people offer to help, give them a specific assignment. And then, take time to do what energizes you and make a point of rewarding yourself.
- Remember that people who are critically ill are self-absorbed. If your empathy fails you and you lose patience, make amends and forgive yourself.

need to first process the emotional blow with tears and anger before learning about the course of their disease in the future.

"Accept and understand whatever reaction the patient has," says Roni Lang, director of the Geriatric Assessment Program for the Stamford (Connecticut) Health System, and a social worker who is a longtime veteran of such conversations. "Don't be too quick with the tissue. That sends a message that it's not okay to be upset. It's okay for the patient to be however she is."

Getting to Acceptance

Some patients keep hoping that they will get better. Denial is one of the mind's miracles, a way to ward off painful realities until consciousness can deal with them. Denial may not be a problem for the dying person, but it can create difficulties for the family. The dying person could be leaving a lot of tough decisions, stress, and confusion behind. The classic stages of grief outlined by Elisabeth Kübler-Ross—denial, anger, bargaining, depression, and acceptance—are often used to describe post-death grieving, but were in fact delineated for the process of accepting impending

loss. We now know that these states may not progress in order. "Most people oscillate between anger and sadness, embracing the prospect of death and unrealistic episodes of optimism," says Lang. Still, she says, "don't place demands on them to accept their death. This is not a time to proselytize." It is enough for the family to accept the coming loss, and if necessary, introduce the idea of an advance directive and health-care proxy, approaching it as a "just in case" idea. When one member of the family cannot accept death, and insists that doctors do more, says Lang, "that's the worst nightmare. I would call a meeting, hear all views without interrupting, and get the conversation around to what the patient would want. You may need another person to come in, perhaps the doctor, to help 'hear' the voice of the patient."

What Are You Afraid Of?

The most important question for doctors and caregivers to ask a dying person is, What are you afraid of? "Fear aggravates pain," says Lang, "and pain aggravates fear." Fear of pain, says Spivack, is one of the most common problems, and can be dealt with rationally. Many people do not know, for example, that pain in dying is not inevitable. Other typical fears are of being separated from loved ones, from home, from work; fear of being a burden, losing control, being dependent, and leaving things undone. Voicing fear helps lessen it, and pin-pointing fear helps a caregiver know how to respond.

How to Be With a Dying Person

Our usual instinct is to avoid everything about death, including the people moving most rapidly toward it. But, Spivack says, "In all my years of working with dying people, I've never heard one say 'I want to die alone.' " Dying people are greatly comforted by company; the benefit far outweighs the awkwardness of the visit. Lang offers these suggestions for visitors:

- Be close. Sit at eye level, and don't be afraid to touch. Let the dying person set the pace for the conversation. Allow for silence. Your presence alone is valuable.
- Don't contradict a patient who says he's going to die. Acceptance is okay. Allow for anger, guilt, and fear, without trying to "fix" it. Just listen and empathize.
- Give the patient as much decision-making power as possible, as long as possible. Allow for talk about unfinished business. Ask: "Who can I contact for you?"
- Encourage happy reminiscences. It's okay to laugh.
- Never pass up the chance to express love or say good-bye. But if you don't get the chance, remember that not everything is worked through. Do the best you can.

Taking Control Now

Sixty years ago, before the invention of dialysis, defibrillators, and ventilators, the failure of vital organs automatically meant death. There were few choices to be made to end suffering, and when there were—the fatal dose of morphine, for example—these decisions were made privately by family and doctors who knew each other well. Since the 1950s, medical technology has been capable of extending lives, but also of prolonging dying. In 1967, an organization called Choice in Dying (now the Partnership for Caring: America's Voices for the Dying; see Resources) designed the first advance directive—a document that allows you to designate under what conditions you would want life-sustaining treatment to be continued or terminated. But the idea did not gain popular understanding until 1976, when the parents of Karen Ann Quinlan won a long legal battle to disconnect her from respiratory support as she lay for months in a vegetative state. Some 75 percent of Americans are in favor of advance directives, although only 30–35 percent actually write them.

Designing the Care You Want

There are two kinds of advance directives, and you may use one or both. A Living Will details what kind of life-sustaining treatment you want or don't want, in the event of an illness when death is imminent. A durable power of attorney for health care appoints someone to be your decision-maker if you can't speak for yourself. This person is also called a surrogate, attorney-in-fact, or health-care proxy. An advance directive such as Five Wishes covers both.

Most experts agree that a Living Will alone is not sufficient. "You don't need to write specific instructions about different kinds of life support, as you don't yet know any of the facts of your situation, and they may change," says Charles Sabatino, assistant director of the American Bar Association's Commission on Legal Problems of the Elderly.

The proxy, Sabatino says, is far more important. "It means someone you trust will find out all the options and make a decision consistent with what you would want." In most states, you may write your own advance directive, though some states require a specific form, available at hospital admitting offices or at the state department of health.

When Should You Draw Up a Directive?

Without an advance directive, a hospital staff is legally bound to do everything to keep you alive as long as possible, until you or a family member decides otherwise. So advance directives are best written before emergency status or a terminal diagnosis. Some people write them at the same time they make a will. The process begins with discussions between you and your family and doctor. If anybody is reluctant to discuss the subject, Sabatino suggests starting the conversation with a story. "Remember what happened to Bob Jones and what his family went through? I want us to be different...." You can use existing tools—a booklet or questionnaire (see Resources)—to keep the conversation moving. Get your doctor's commitment to support your wishes. "If you're asking for something that is against your doctor's conscience" (such as prescribing a lethal dose of pain medication or removing life support at a time he considers premature), Sabatino says, "he may have an obligation to transfer

you to another doctor." And make sure the person you name as surrogate agrees to act for you and understands your wishes.

Filing, Storing, Safekeeping...

An estimated 35 percent of advance directives cannot be found when needed.

- Give a copy to your surrogate, your doctor, your hospital, and other family members. Tell them where to find the original in the house—not in a safe deposit box where it might not be found until after death.
- Some people carry a copy in their wallet or glove compartment of their car.
- Be aware that if you have more than one home and you split your time in several regions of the country, you should be registering your wishes with a hospital in each region, and consider naming more than one proxy.
- You may register your Living Will and health-care proxy online at uslivingwillregistry.com (or call 800-548-9455). The free, privately funded confidential service will instantly fax a copy to a hospital when the hospital requests one. It will also remind you to update it: You may want to choose a new surrogate, accommodate medical advances, or change your idea of when "enough is enough." M. Powell Lawton, who is doing a study on how people anticipate the terminal life stages, has discovered that "people adapt relatively well to states of poor health. The idea that life is still worth living continues to readjust itself."

Assisted Suicide: The Reality

While advance directives allow for the termination of life-sustaining treatment, assisted suicide means supplying the patient with a prescription for life-ending medication. A doctor writes the prescription for the medication; the patient takes the fatal dose him- or herself. Physician-assisted suicide is legal only in Oregon (and under consideration in Maine) but only with rigorous preconditions. Of the approximately 30,000 people who died in Oregon in 1999, only 33 received permission to have a lethal dose of medication and only 26 of those actually died of the medication. Surrogates may request an end to life support, but to assist in a suicide puts one at risk for charges of homicide.

Good Care: Can You Afford It?

The ordinary person is only one serious illness away from poverty," says Joanne Lynn, M.D., director of the Arlington, Virginia, Center to Improve Care of the Dying. An ethicist, hospice physician, and health-services researcher, she is one of the founding members of the end-of-life-care movement. "On the whole, hospitalization and the cost of suppressing symptoms is very easy to afford," says Lynn. Medicare and Medicaid will help cover that kind of acute medical care. But what is harder to afford is at-home medication, monitoring, daily help with eating and walking, and all the care that will go on for the rest of the patient's life.

Five Wishes

Five Wishes is a questionnaire that guides people in making essential decisions about the care they want at the end of their life. About a million people have filled out the eight-page form in the past two years. This advance directive is legally valid in 34 states and the District of Columbia. (The other 16 require a specific state-mandated form.)

The document was designed by lawyer Jim Towey, founder of Aging With Dignity, a nonprofit organization that advocates for the needs of elders and their caregivers. Towey, who was legal counsel to Mother Teresa, visited her Home for the Dying in Calcutta in the 1980s. He was struck that in that haven in the Third World, "the dying people's hands were held, their pain was managed, and they weren't alone. In the First World, you see a lot of medical technology, but people die in pain, and alone." Towey talked to MODERN MATURITY about his directive and what it means.

What are the five wishes? Who do I want to make care decisions for me when I can't? What kind of medical treatment do I want toward the end? What would help me feel comfortable while I am dying? How do I want people to treat me? What do I want my loved ones to know about me and my feelings after I'm gone?

Why is it so vital to make advance decisions now? Medical technology has extended longevity, which is good, but it can prolong the dying process in ways that are almost cruel. Medical schools are still concentrating on curing, not caring for the dying. We can have a dignified season in our life, or die alone in pain with futile interventions. Most people only discover they have options when checking into the hospital, and often they no longer have the capacity to choose. This leaves the family members with a guessing game and, frequently, guilt.

What's the ideal way to use this document? First you do a little soul searching about what you want. Then discuss it with people you trust, in the livingroom instead of the waiting room—before a crisis. Just say, "I want a choice about how I spend my last days," talk about your choices, and pick someone to be your health-care surrogate.

What makes the Five Wishes directive unique? It's easy to use and understand, not written in the language of doctors or lawyers. It also allows people to discuss comfort dignity, and forgivness, not just medical concerns. When my father filled it out, he said he wanted his favorite afghan blanket in his bed. It made a huge difference to me that, as he was dying, he had his wishes fulfilled.

For a copy of Five Wishes in English or Spanish, send a $5 check or money order to Aging With Dignity, PO Box 1661, Tallahassee, FL 32302. For more information, visit www.agingwithdignity. org.

"When people are dying," Lynn says, "an increasing proportion of their overall care does not need to be done by doctors. But when policymakers say the care is nonmedical, then it's second class, it's not important, and nobody will pay for it."

Bottom line, Medicare pays for about 57 percent of the cost of medical care for Medicare beneficiaries. Another 11 percent is paid by Medicaid, 20 percent by the patient, 10 percent from private insurance, and the rest from other sources, such as charitable organizations.

Medi-what?

This public-plus-private network of funding sources for end-of-life care is complex, and who pays for how much of what is determined by diagnosis, age, site of care, and income. Besides the private health insurance that many of us have from our employers, other sources of funding may enter the picture when patients are terminally ill.

- **Medicare** A federal insurance program that covers health-care services for people 65 and over, some disabled people, and those with end-stage kidney disease. Medicare Part A covers inpatient care in hospitals, nursing homes, hospice, and some home health care. For most people, the Part A premium is free. Part B covers doctor fees, tests, and other outpatient medical services. Although Part B is optional, most people choose to enroll through their local Social Security office and pay the monthly premium ($45.50). Medicare beneficiaries share in the cost of care through deductibles and co-insurance. What Medicare does not cover at all is outpatient medication, long-term nonacute care, and support services.

- **Medicaid** A state and federally funded program that covers health-care services for people with income or assets below certain levels, which vary from state to state.

- **Medigap** Private insurance policies covering the gaps in Medicare, such as deductibles and co-payments, and in some cases additional health-care services, medical supplies, and outpatient prescription drugs.

Many of the services not paid for by Medicare can be covered by private long-term-care insurance. About 50 percent of us over the age of 65 will need long-term care at home or in a nursing home, and this insurance is an extra bit of protection for people with major assets to protect. It pays for skilled nursing care as well as non-health services, such as help with dressing, eating, and bathing. You select a dollar amount of coverage per day (for example, $100 in a nursing home, or $50 for at-home care), and a coverage period (for example, three years—the average nursing-home stay is 2.7 years). Depending on your age and the benefits you choose, the insurance can cost anywhere from around $500 to more than $8,000 a year. People with pre-existing conditions such as Alzheimer's or MS are usually not eligible.

How Much Will It Cost?

Where you get end-of-life care will affect the cost and who pays for it.

- **Hospital** Dying in a hospital costs about $1,000 a day. After a $766 deductible (per benefit period), Medicare reimburses the hospital a fixed rate per day, which varies by region and diagnosis. After the first 60 days in a hospital, a patient will pay a daily deductible ($194) that goes up (to $388) after 90 days. The patient is responsible for all costs for each day beyond 150 days. Medicaid and some private insurance, either through an employer or a Medigap plan, often help cover these costs.

- **Nursing home** About $1,000 a week. Medicare covers up to 100 days of skilled nursing care after a three-day hospitalization, and most medication costs during that time. For days 21–100, your daily co-insurance of $97 is usually covered by private insurance—if you have it. For nursing-home care not covered by Medicare, you must use your private assets, or Medicaid if your assets run out, which happens to approximately one-third of nursing-home residents. Long-term-care insurance may also cover some of the costs.

- **Hospice care** About $100 a day for in-home care. Medicare covers hospice care to patients who have a life expectancy of less than six months. (See Hospice: The Comfort Team.) Such care may be provided at home, in a hospice facility, a hospital, or a nursing-home. Patients may be asked to pay up to $5 for each prescription and a 5 percent co-pay for in-patient respite care, which is a short hospital stay to relieve caregivers. Medicaid covers hospice care in all but six states, even for those without Medicare.

  About 60 percent of full-time employees of medium and large firms also have coverage for hospice services, but the benefits vary widely.

- **Home care without hospice services** Medicare Part A pays the full cost of medical home health care for up to 100 visits following a hospital stay of at least three days. Medicare Part B covers home health-care visits beyond those 100 visits or without a hospital stay. To qualify, the patient must be homebound, require skilled nursing care or physical or speech therapy, be under a physician's care, and use services from a Medicare-participating home-health agency. Note that this coverage is for medical care only; hired help for personal nonmedical services, such as that often required by Alzheimer's patients, is not covered by Medicare. It is covered by Medicaid in some states.

  A major financial disadvantage of dying at home without hospice is that Medicare does not cover out-patient prescription drugs, even those for pain. Medicaid does cover these drugs, but often with restrictions on their price and quantity. Private insurance can fill the gap to some extent. Long-term-care insurance may cover payments to family caregivers who have to stop work to care for a dying patient, but this type of coverage is very rare.

Resources
Medical Care

For information about pain relief and symptom management:
Supportive Care of the Dying (503-215-5053; care-ofdying.org).

For a comprehensive guide to living with the medical, emotional, and spiritual aspects of dying:
Handbook for Mortals by Joanne Lynn and Joan Harrold, Oxford University Press.

For a 24-hour hotline offering counseling, pain management, downloadable advance directives, and more:
The Partnership for Caring (800-989-9455; www.partnershipforcaring.org).

Emotional Care

To find mental-health counselors with an emphasis on lifespan human development and spiritual discussion:
American Counseling Association (800-347-6647; counseling.org).

For disease-related support groups and general resources for caregivers:
Caregiver Survival Resources (caregiver911.com).

For AARP's online caregiver support chatroom, access **America Online** every Wednesday night, 8:30–9:30 EST (keyword: AARP).

Education and advocacy for family caregivers:
National Family Caregivers Association (800-896-3650; nfcacares.org).

For the booklet,
Understanding the Grief Process (D16832, EEO143C), e-mail order with title and numbers to member@aarp.org or send postcard to AARP Fulfillment, 601 E St NW, Washington DC 20049. Please allow two to four weeks for delivery.

To find a volunteer to help with supportive services to the frail and their caregivers:
National Federation of Interfaith Volunteer Caregivers (816-931-5442; nfivc.org).

For information on support to partners of the chronically ill and/or the disabled:
The Well Spouse Foundation (800-838-0879; www.wellspouse.org).

Legal Help

AARP members are entitled to a free half-hour of legal advice with a lawyer from **AARP's Legal Services Network**. (800-424-3410; www.aarp.org/lsn).

For **Planning for Incapacity,** *a guide to advance directives in your state,* send $5 to Legal Counsel for the Elderly, Inc., PO Box 96474, Washington DC 20090-6474. Make out check to LCE Inc.

For a **Caring Conversations** *booklet on advance-directive discussion:*
Midwest Bioethics Center (816-221-1100; midbio.org).

For information on care at the end of life, online discussion groups, conferences:
Last Acts Campaign (800-844-7616; lastacts.org).

Hospice

To learn about end-of-life care options and grief issues through videotapes, books, newsletters, and brochures:

Hospice Foundation of America (800-854-3402; hospice-foundation.org).

For information on hospice programs, FAQs, and general facts about hospice:

National Hospice and Palliative Care Organization (800-658-8898; nhpco.org).

For **All About Hospice: A Consumer's Guide** (202-546-4759; www.hospice-america.org).

Financial Help

For **Organizing Your Future**, *a simple guide to end-of-life financial decisions*, send $5 to Legal Counsel for the Elderly, Inc., PO Box 96474, Washington DC 20090-6474. Make out check to LCE Inc.

For **Medicare and You 2000** *and a* **2000 Guide to Health Insurance for People With Medicare** (800-MEDICARE [633-4227]; medicare.gov).

To find your State Agency on Aging: **Administration on Aging, U.S. Department of Health and Human Services** (800-677-1116; aoa.dhhs.gov).

General

For information on end-of-life planning and bereavement: (www.aarp.org/endoflife/).

For health professionals and others who want to start conversations on end-of-life issues in their community:

Discussion Guide: On Our Own Terms: Moyers on Dying, based on the PBS series, airing September 10–13. The guide provides essays, instructions, and contacts. From PBS, www.pbs.org/onourownterms Or send a postcard request to On Our Own Terms Discussion Guide, Thirteen/WNET New York, PO Box 245, Little Falls, NJ 07424-9766.

Funded with a grant from The Robert Wood Johnson Foundation, Princeton, N.J. *Editor* Amy Gross; *Writer* Louise Lague; *Designer* David Herbick

Mind Frames Towards Dying and Factors Motivating Their Adoption by Terminally Ill Elders

Objectives. This study was designed to advance the understanding of the physical and psychosocial factors that motivate terminally ill elders not only to consider a hastened death but also *not* to consider such a death.

Methods. I conducted face-to-face in-depth qualitative interviews with 96 terminally ill elders. An inductive approach was taken to locating themes and patterns regarding factors motivating terminally ill elders to consider or not to consider hastening death.

Results. Six mind frames towards dying emerged: (a) neither ready nor accepting; (b) not ready but accepting; (c) ready and accepting; (d) ready, accepting, and wishing death would come; (e) considering a hastened death but having no specific plan; and (f) considering a hastened death with a specific plan. From the data emerged approaches towards dying and accompanying emotions characterizing each mind frame, as well as factors motivating their adoption by elders. The results showed that psychosocial factors served more often than physical factors as motivators.

Discussion. The results demonstrate the importance of assessing the mind frame adopted by a terminally ill elder and his or her level of satisfaction with it. Terminally ill elders may experience a higher quality dying process when a traditional medical care approach is replaced by a holistic approach that addresses physical, spiritual, emotional, and social needs.

TRACY A. SCHROEPFER

School of Social Work, University of Wisconsin, Madison.

A national mandate has been put forth to improve the comfort or palliative care provided to terminally ill individuals. This mandate is particularly relevant to Americans older than age 65, whose numbers have tripled in the 20th century and who have experienced a significant increase in their life expectancy (Hetzel & Smith, 2001). Elders now experience the greatest number of deaths in the United States (Arias, 2003), deaths that are often of poor quality. Research has shown that American elders experience severe pain in their dying process (Bernabei et al., 1998; SUPPORT Investigators, 1997), are undermedicated for their pain (Bernabei et al.; Cleeland et al., 1994), receive health care at odds with their end-of-life preferences (SUPPORT Investigators), experience psychosocial suffering (Chochinov et al., 2002; Pessin, Rosenfeld, & Breitbart, 2002), and experience existential suffering (Black & Rubinstein, 2004). These poor-quality dying experiences have contributed to the demand for the legalization of physician-assisted death, a demand that has raised ethical concerns and has led to research on the number of individuals requesting this option and the factors motivating them to do so. Knowledge of these factors serves to inform and guide health care practitioners in their quest to improve palliative care. It can also be argued, however, that knowledge of the factors that contribute to a quality dying process such that terminally ill individuals are motivated *not* to consider a hastened death is also essential to providing quality palliative care. This latter avenue of research has received little, if any, attention. The purpose of this article is to advance the understanding of physical and psychosocial factors that motivate terminally ill elders not only to consider a hastened death but also not to consider such a death.

Current Findings Regarding the Consideration to Hasten Death

Two types of studies emerge from a review of the literature on the consideration to hasten death: retrospective and prospective. Retrospective studies ask physicians, nurses, social workers, or survivors of the deceased to write case studies or answer surveys concerning the motivating factors cited by now-deceased patients who had considered or requested physician-assisted death prior to their death. Prospective studies interview a mix of individuals with a terminal illness (an illness likely to result in death) and people who have been defined as terminally ill (having fewer than six months to live) and ask whether they have considered hastening their death and, if so, their reasons for doing so.

Retrospective case study results have found that psychosocial factors play a more significant role than physical factors as motivators of a hastened death. Health care professionals have reported psychosocial factors that include a decreased ability to participate in activities that made life enjoyable (Chin, Hedberg, Higginson, & Fleming, 1999; Oregon Department of Human Services [ODHS], 2000, 2001, 2002, 2003), fear of future pain (Chin et al.; ODHS, 2000, 2001, 2002, 2003; Volker, 2001) or of uncontrollable symptoms, loss of meaning in life (Meier et al., 1998), the feeling that one is a burden (Back, Wallace, Starks, & Pearlman, 1996; Meier et al.; ODHS, 2001, 2002, 2003), loss of dignity (Back et al.; Meier et al.), loss of autonomy (Chin et al.; ODHS, 2000, 2001, 2002, 2003), loss of control over bodily functions (Back et al.; Chin et al.; ODHS, 2000, 2001, 2002, 2003) and over manner of death (ODHS, 2000; Volker), and loss of control in general (Back et al.). These studies reported neither depression nor religiosity, factors often discussed in relation to hastening death, as significant factors. Only two studies (Back et al.; Meier et al.) reported evidence of pain as a motivator.

Two retrospective studies that employed a quantitative approach also found that psychosocial factors were key motivators of the consideration to hasten death; they did not find pain to be a significant factor (Ganzini et al., 2002; Jacobson et al., 1995). Hospice nurses and social workers reported that a desire to control the circumstances of death, the wish to die at home, the feeling that living was pointless, and a loss of dignity were most often discussed by patients desiring a hastened death (Ganzini et al.).

Quantitative prospective studies support the importance of psychosocial factors and provide evidence of the role physical factors play in the consideration to hasten death. These studies found that patients with a terminal illness or who were terminally ill were not likely to attend church (Breitbart et al., 1996) or to be religious (Breitbart et al.; Emanuel, Fairclough, Daniels, & Clarridge, 1996), had few social supports (Breitbart et al.), experienced a low quality of social support (Arnold, 2004; Breitbartet al., 1996; Chochinov et al., 1995), and perceived their caregiving needs as high (Emanuel, Fairclough, & Emanuel, 2000). Emotionally, these patients reported a higher level of anxiety, a lower level of hope (Arnold) and a higher level of depression (Arnold; Breitbart et al.; Chochinov et al., 1995; Emanuel et al.) than did those individuals not considering a hastened death. Results regarding the role of pain were mixed. Three studies found that pain was not significantly related to the consideration to hasten death (Breitbart et al.; Chochinov et al., 1995; Emanuel et al., 1996), but two later studies found it to be a significant predictor (Arnold; Emanuel et al., 2000). These prospective studies did not measure loss of control.

The only qualitative study on the consideration to hasten death that could be located was conducted by Lavery, Boyle, Dickens, Maclean, and Singer (2001) on patients with HIV-l or AIDS. According to this study, two major themes developed from discussions with participants considering a hastened death. The first theme involved a sense of disintegration, which resulted from the multiple symptoms and loss of bodily functions that eventually led participants to a dependency on others and a loss of dignity. The second theme, loss of community, reflected the lack of contact these individuals had with others. Participants also reported that the result of experiencing disintegration and loss of community was a perceived loss of self.

Much can be learned from these studies that can be used to guide health care practitioners in their quest to improve end-of-life care. Loss of self, dignity, and autonomy; loss of control over bodily functions and manner of death; lack of enjoyment and meaning in life; lower quantity and quality of social support; lack of hope; and higher levels of anxiety and depression are all key psychosocial factors that motivate some terminally ill individuals to consider hastening their death. Although pain was a significant predictor of hastening death in only two studies, fear of future pain or uncontrollable suffering surfaced as a key factor in most studies. Clearly, some individuals who are not suffering in the present fear they will be suffering at some point in the future.

Addressing Current Limitations

Although current empirical evidence regarding the factors that motivate terminally ill individuals to consider hastening their death has provided insight into this issue, three major limitations exist that need to be addressed. First, the considerable research on hastening death described in the preceding section was conducted retrospectively (either with physicians or survivors) or prospectively (with patients who had a terminal illness). Studies conducted with physicians or survivors result in second-hand information that may not provide an accurate record of patients' motivating factors. Although prospective studies do provide firsthand information, they too are problematic. Some patients with a terminal illness may be in the early stages of their illness and so are being asked to speculate about whether they would consider hastening death before death becomes imminent; in the later stages of their illness, their feelings may change. Prospective studies that include only terminally ill individuals are the most likely to provide the information necessary to understand the motivating factors for considering a hastened death.

Second, the main approach taken in research on considering a hastened death has been to measure quantitatively factors presumed to be key motivators, such as pain and depression. This approach has provided important information and should be continued. However, due to the current lack of information on the motivating factors for considering a hastened death, it may also be useful to step back and take a more open-ended approach to this research. The qualitative method is not constrained by what has been hypothesized; it allows for the exploration of the individual's reasoning regarding his or her consideration to hasten or not to hasten death, and it allows one to discover the unknown. As evidenced in the literature review above, this method has rarely been used. Continuing to limit research in this manner may result in crucial factors remaining undetected, unaddressed, and not well understood.

Third, the lack of attention given to studying the factors that motivate terminally ill individuals not to consider hastening their death may limit the understanding of factors key to a quality dying experience. The current approach of focusing on the factors motivating the consideration to hasten death assumes that such information provides all the knowledge necessary for improving palliative care. Extending this approach to include asking individuals what it is about their dying process that keeps them from considering a hastened death can also serve to inform palliative care.

The current study addresses each of these three limitations. I used a prospective qualitative approach, sampled only elders who had fewer than six months to live, and examined the factors motivating the consideration not to hasten death in addition to factors motivating the consideration to hasten death.

Methods
Sample

The selection criteria for the study were threefold. Respondents had to (a) be 50 years of age or older; (b) be deemed mentally competent by their physician, nurse, or social worker; and (c) have been given a prognosis by a physician of 6 months or less to live. I initially set the age selection criterion at 60 years or older in order to coincide with typical age definitions of elders. Six months into the study, however, I lowered the criterion to 50 years or older in order to obtain a sufficient number of male participants so that I could examine gender differences.

I used purposive sampling. I contacted hospices, hospital-based inpatient palliative care programs, and hospital-based outpatient clinics caring for the terminally ill throughout Michigan in hopes of obtaining a population that varied with regard to race, education, and occupation. Of the 17 programs contacted, 10 agreed to participate: 2 palliative care programs, 2 hospital outpatient clinics, and 6 hospices. Ninety-six terminally ill elders were approached by either a social worker or a nurse regarding the study, and all agreed to participate.

Participating elders ranged in age from 51 to 98 (*M* = 73.5). The majority of elders were White (84.4%), 15.6% were Black, and a little more than half were married (52.1%). Elders were quite varied in their religious preferences: Catholic (19.8%), Methodist (14.6%), Baptist (15.6%), other Protestant religions (35.4%), Jewish (2.1%), and no religious preference (12.5%). Most elders had some form of cancer (49.0%); others were diagnosed with end-stage renal disease (26.0%) or heart disease (15.6%). A small percentage (9.4%) of elders was dying of respiratory, neurological, or other diseases.

Data Collection

In face-to-face interviews, I asked respondents if they had given serious thought to hastening their death since finding out they had a serious illness that may shorten their life. If they answered no, I asked about their reasons for not considering a hastened death. If they answered yes, I asked how they were considering hastening their death and whether they were still thinking about doing so. If they were no longer considering doing so, I asked about their rea-

sons for having once considered hastening their death, and their reasons for no longer thinking this way. If they were still considering a hastened death, I asked their reasons for thinking about doing so. All interviews were audiotaped and transcribed.

When answering these questions, respondents did not appear to construct their reality as they went along or to do so within the boundaries of hastening or not hastening death. Most respondents raised the topic on their own and began describing their mind frame towards dying prior to being asked questions regarding considering a hastened death. Although some respondents did not raise the topic and, when asked, dismissed any thought of hastening their death, their responses regarding why they would not do so were immediate and very indepth. I had the sense that they had already given the issue much thought and were simply sharing those thoughts with me.

Data Analysis

I analyzed the content of answers for themes regarding respondents' reasons for considering or not considering a hastened death: Content analysis involved "identifying" and "categorizing" the main themes and patterns found in the data (Patton, 1990, p. 381). I took an inductive method in locating these themes and patterns. That is, I did not determine the themes and patterns prior to the analysis; rather, they emerged from repeated readings of the transcripts (Patton). I used this approach to identify respondents who were considering a hastened death and those who were not considering one, as well as the psychosocial and physical factors motivating their considerations. As a reliability check, a hospice social worker independently coded the thematic areas identified, and we reached complete agreement.

Results

As was previously discussed, studies on the consideration to hasten death have traditionally assumed that terminally ill individuals face their dying in one of two ways: not considering a hastened death or considering a hastened death. I initially approached the present study operating under these same assumptions. Content analysis of the qualitative data revealed, however, that this dichotomous approach is an over-simplification of an elder's potential mind frame towards dying. No label in the death and dying literature appeared adequate to describe what evolved in the qualitative analyses, and so I chose the term *mind frame* to refer to the overall attitude or orientation an elder had adopted towards his or her dying. Six distinct mind frames towards dying emerged: (a) neither ready nor accepting; (b) not ready but accepting; (c) ready and accepting; (d) ready, accepting, and wishing death would come; (e) considering a hastened death but having no specific plan; and (f) considering a hastened death with a specific plan. Figure 1 illustrates how these six mind frames fall within the two traditional categories. Table 1 provides descriptive information regarding the elders who adopted each mind frame. I did not gather information regarding the approach or mind frame respondents had taken to previous life crises or whether past experiences influenced their current mind frame towards dying.

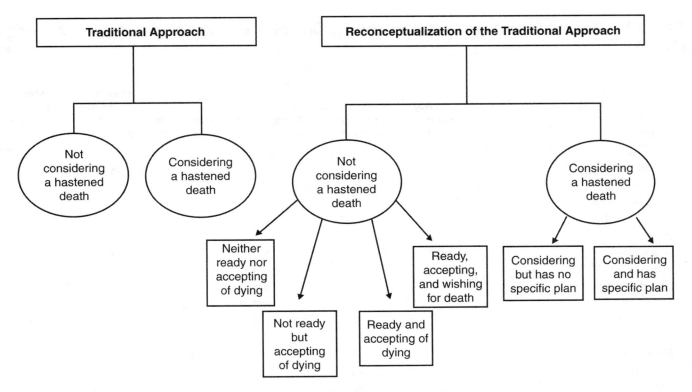

Figure 1 Traditional approach to research on considering a hastened death and a new conceptualization.

Approach Towards Dying, Accompanying Emotions, and Motivating Factors

Each mind frame towards dying that emerged from the interviews was distinguished by an approach towards dying, personal characteristics, accompanying emotions, and factors motivating the elder to adopt a particular mind frame. Motivating factors emerged from responses to the questions about the elders' reasons for either not considering or considering a hastened death. The approaches, personal characteristics, emotions, and motivating factors characterizing each mind frame are summarized in the following sections.

It is important to note that respondents did not appear to shift from one mind frame to another during their interviews. Although 15 respondents spoke of having transitioned earlier in their dying process from another mind frame (this topic will be discussed in another article), neither they nor the other respondents appeared to shift from one mind frame to another during the interview. I did not determine the reasons for this consistency; however, one could speculate that the factors motivating their adoption of a mind frame did not change during the interview process and so neither did the mind frame itself.

Mind Frame 1: Neither Ready Nor Accepting

Approach towards dying. —Thirty-three elders (34%) spoke strongly about not being ready to die or willing to accept that death was imminent. Two approaches towards dying characterized this mind frame: fighting to live, and hoping or believing science would find a cure.

The predominant approach that emerged among these elders was that of fighting to live and not giving in to the disease. One 74-year-old divorced woman stated adamantly, "And I'm not ready, and I'll tell you why. They can say four months; I'm going to live longer than that." A 51-year-old man who stated emphatically, "I figure, I don't really have to die if I don't want to and I'm not going to," talked about his wife's determination and how he had adopted her attitude.

The second approach towards dying centered on the belief and hope that science would find a cure and that the elders would survive their illness. A 63-year-old elder said, "They're going to find a cure for everything I've got, and I'm going to be able to live a lot longer." This woman spoke with quiet resolve throughout the interview, as did the other respondents who spoke of a cure being found for their illness.

Personal characteristics. —Respondents adopting this mind frame towards dying had a mean age of 69 and had, on average, less than a high school education. They were predominantly women (52%), White (79%), married (67%), and of the Protestant faith (70%).

Accompanying emotions. —Elders who had adopted this mind frame spoke adamantly about their feelings and appeared to possess a strong will to live. They were dismissive of any questions or thoughts regarding dying. When discussing the issue of dying, they were not tearful; rather, they often showed anger or derisive humor. These elders did not view any aspect of dying as positive.

Table 1 Demographics of Elders Adopting One of Six Mind Frames Towards Dying (*N* = 96)

Demographic	Not-Ready nor Accepting of Dying (34%)	Not Ready but Accepting of Dying (25%)	Ready and Accepting of Dying (16%)	Wishing for Death (6%)	Hasten Death, No Specific Plan (9%)	Hasten Death, Specific Plan (9%)
Age, in years (*M*)	69.3	71.9	81.3	83.2	73.8	74.0
Education, in years (*M*)	11.6	11.5	12.3	11.5	13.6	14.4
Gender (%)						
Female (*n* = 54)	51.5	58.3	66.7	50.0	44.4	66.7
Male (*n* = 42)	48.5	41.7	33.3	50.0	55.6	33.3
Race (%)						
Black (*n* = 15)	21.2	20.8	6.7	0.0	11.1	11.1
White (*n* = 81)	78.8	79.2	93.3	100.0	88.9	88.9
Marital status (%)						
Married (*n* = 50)	66.7	45.8	26.7	50.0	44.4	66.7
Not married (*n* = 46)	33.3	54.2	73.3	50.0	55.6	33.3
Religion (%)						
None (*n* = 12)	15.2	12.5	13.3	16.7	0.0	11.1
Catholic (*n* = 19)	15.2	25.0	33.3	16.7	11.1	11.1
Protestant (*n* = 63)	69.7	62.5	53.3	66.7	88.9	55.6
Jewish (*n* = 2)	0.0	0.0	0.0	0.0	0.0	22.0
Primary diagnosis (%)						
Cancer (*n* = 47)	54.5	54.2	46.7	16.7	55.6	33.3
End-stage renal disease (*n* = 25)	36.4	25.0	20.0	16.7	0.0	33.3
Heart disease (*n* = 15)	6.1	16.7	26.7	66.7	11.1	0.0
Other diseases (*n* = 9)	3.0	4.2	6.7	0.0	33.3	33.3

Factors motivating lack of readiness regarding dying. —Elders discussed being with family, enjoying life, and having unfinished business as the factors motivating their lack of readiness regarding dying. Family was the factor discussed most often, and many elders became tearful when talking about leaving family behind. They enjoyed being with their family and watching their children and grandchildren grow up. Some elders felt their family members still needed their help and so wanted to stay alive to melders who were also not ready to die was motivated by their religious beliefs or a fear of death. Most of the women and only a few men, regardless of age or race, believed that God wanted them to fight to live as long as possible: "See, I believe the good Lord is healing me . . . I'm going through a healing process now, and He's healing me every day. And as long as I feel good and have a positive attitude, that's the way it's going to be. And I really believe that I will be healed sooner or later."

Several men and one woman spoke of fearing the unknown, being alone in the grave, and being afraid that loved ones would forget them after they die. An 81-year-old widower depicted these fears clearly: "There's no future in dying. And, uh, you have to stay all alone in the grave and everything. . . If you die, uh, isn't nobody going to care anyway. They're going to forget you in less than two months." The future pictured by these elders at the time of the interview did not include their death.

Mind Frame 2: Not Ready But Accepting

Approach towards dying. —Of the 96 persons interviewed, 24 elders (25%) indicated they were not ready to die but that they had accepted the fact that they were dying. The main approach towards dying expressed by these 24 elders was the recognition that death is natural. Although they spoke of not being ready for death, they did accept death as a natural part of life and were matter-of-fact in their approach. One 73-year-old married woman stated, "Like I say, I don't want to die, but when that time comes, if that's it, that's it." A 74-year-old never-married man took a similar approach: "Oh, I don't think much about it [dying]. I just don't, uh, dwell on that too much. It's, oh, it's just something that, it happens to everybody. It's inevitable."

Personal characteristics. —Respondents who had adopted this mind frame had a mean age of 72 and had slightly less than a high school education. Almost two thirds were women (58%), slightly more than half were not married (54%), 79% were White, and 63% were Protestant.

Accompanying emotions. —Elders who had adopted Mind Frame 2 appeared less adamant about their approach towards dying than did elders who had adopted Mind Frame 1. They were calm when talking about their approaching death and did not appear to be in a hurry to move on to other topics.

Factors motivating lack of readiness regarding dying. —As with elders who had adopted Mind Frame 1, family and unfinished business were mentioned as motivators for lack of readiness on the part of elders who had adopted Mind Frame 2. Most elders reported that they did not want to hasten their death because they were enjoying their life. This enjoyment of life included being with family and still having the ability to take an active role in their lives.

When elders who had adopted Mind Frame 2 spoke of families, the nature of the family ties differed from those of elders who had adopted Mind Frame 1. Only a few elders discussed how their loved ones still needed them. Instead, most spoke of how the instrumental and emotional support received from family members served as a motivator not to hasten the time they had left. A 73-year-old married man stated, "They [family] care about me and will, will walk that extra mile for me." In addition, these elders were concerned about how emotionally difficult their death would be on their families. A 71-year-old married woman stated with sadness, "I guess it's going to be harder on them than on me because I won't be here . . . They've got all the mourning to do and everything."

Unfinished business, a factor reported by elders who had adopted Mind Frame 1, was also reported by elders who had adopted Mind Frame 2. The difference, however, was that unfinished business was discussed in terms of a sense of purpose or responsibility. As one 74-year-old never-married man noted, "I have taken it upon myself to decorate the graves on Memorial Day. And that's quite a job, by the way. Somebody has to decorate the family graves, and I've sort of assumed that responsibility for myself."

Factors motivating acceptance of dying. —Religious beliefs, which motivated elders who had adopted Mind Frame 1 not to be accepting of their dying, were a factor cited by elders who had adopted Mind Frame 2 regarding their acceptance of dying. The beliefs of both groups of elders centered on God's will regarding their acceptance of dying, but the two groups differed in their view of what was God's will Elders who were neither ready nor accepting of their dying defined God's will as for them to fight death. Elders who were not ready but who had accepted their dying reported that it was in God's power to decide the time of death. Although they did not feel ready to die, this latter group of elders accepted that time of death was God's will, not their decision to make, as expressed in the following statement made by a 71-year-old widow: "So I said, well, Lord, I'm just not ready to go, but if it's Your will, I will go."

Elders who had adopted Mind Frames 1 and 2 viewed death differently regarding the non-acceptance or acceptance of dying. Elders who were not accepting of their dying espoused a negative view of death that included fear of the unknown. In comparison, elders who were accepting of their dying took a matter-of-fact approach towards dying. They viewed death as inevitable and either reported not being fearful or spoke of their fear in a matter-of-fact way:

Everybody's scared of dying, I think. It's the inescapable fact. We don't . . . everybody wants to see the sun come up. There is a certain amount of fear attached, I think.

You know, even though we know that death is inevitable and it's going to happen to each and every one of us, we fear the unknown. Yeah. We fear the unknown.

Unlike elders who had adopted Mind Frame 1, the future these elders pictured did include their death.

Mind Frame 3: Ready and Accepting

Approach towards dying. —Fifteen elders (16%) indicated a readiness and acceptance regarding dying. Not only did these elders talk about not being afraid to die, many saw death as the avenue to a better place than they were in at the present. One 92-year-old widow said simply, "I'm not scared to die. I know there is a better place for me." Others spoke of their belief in the goodness of God and of reunions with deceased loved ones.

The majority of these elders viewed death as a natural part of life. Some talked about how happy they would be when death finally arrived and that they were simply waiting: "I'm going to be happy when I leave this earth. I guess it's kind of a selfish attitude, but I'll be out of my misery . . . All I'm doing is just passing time. I'm just waiting for the day."

Personal characteristics. —Respondents who had adopted this mind frame had a mean age of 81 and had, on average, a high school education. Two thirds of these respondents were women, three fourths were not married, 93% were White, and slightly more than half were Protestant.

Accompanying emotions. —Elders with this mind frame revealed two predominant emotions towards life and death. Some elders had found peace and were enjoying the time they had left. Others had not found peace, nor were they enjoying the time they had left. These individuals were simply waiting for death to come as they no longer felt they could justify their existence.

Factors motivating readiness for dying. —Enjoying life was reported by several elders when describing their readiness to die. Because it was measured in relation to the limited time the elders had remaining before dying, enjoyment of life differed between elders who had adopted Mind Frame 2 and those who had adopted Mind Frame 3. A 92-year-old widow who was ready and accepting of death stated with a smile, "Whatever God gives me, I'm willing to take."

Several elders talked about no longer enjoying life; that their lives were full of sadness; and that they felt useless, dependent, and burdensome to others. These individuals were simply waiting for death to come, as evidenced by the following 75-year-old widow's statement:

And, uh, so I'm ready to go any time. It's hard on the family, and I'm really not living. Even here [her son's house] with my family. I get up, and they're wonderful to me, and I'm so thankful I have a place to be. But, uh, they're trying too hard, and it's putting them out . . . They say it isn't, but you know it is. But like I say, I'm ready to cash in my chips.

A few elders discussed the openness they shared with family regarding their impending death and the loving manner in which their family responded to this openness. This openness appeared to allow them to ready themselves for death by being able to make plans and express feelings they needed to express before they died. For example, an 84-year-old widow stated, "Well, they [her sons] asked me . . . what kind of funeral do I want . . . We've always talked about death very openly, because we all know it's going to happen some day to one of us. So you might as well . . . be ready."

Other elders' readiness for death was explained in terms of their age. They had lived what they felt was a long time and so were taking their impending death in stride. One widow stated, "I just figure I'm 70 years old, and you kind of expect you got to die sometime, and you got to have some kind of a disease. You know, so I just kind of put it in my stride."

Factors motivating acceptance of dying. —Three motivating factors were discussed by elders who were accepting of their impending death: (a) the belief that one's time of death was God's decision and not their decision, (b) having no fear of death, and (c) the belief that dying may be better than living: The first two factors were also cited by elders who had adopted Mind Frame 2. In addition, elders who had adopted Mind Frame 3 reported being motivated by their belief that death would be better than their current state of living. One 80-year-old married woman said, "I feel, uh, that I've accepted it [dying], know what I'm saying? So, and there's worse things. Oh, yeah. There's worse things than dying. Sometimes it's worse living." Although her statement could be interpreted as a wish for death to come, when directly asked, she denied ever wishing for death.

Mind Frame 4: Ready, Accepting, and Wishing for Death

Approach towards dying. —When asked if they had seriously considered hastening death, six elders (6%) were adamant that they would not consider taking any action but that they did wish death would come soon. These individuals were similar to those who had adopted Mind Frame 3 except they explicitly spoke of wishing daily for death to come. Even though each talked about how difficult life was for them, all six elders were steadfast regarding not considering a hastened death. One 93-year-old widow stated, "I wish I could go to a better place, but I will not take my own life."

Personal characteristics. —Respondents who had adopted this mind frame had a mean age of 83 and had, on average, less than a high school education. Fifty percent of these respondents were women, 50% were married, 100% were White, and two thirds were Protestant.

Accompanying emotions. —Elders who had adopted Mind Frame 4 demonstrated different emotions than elders who had adopted Mind Frame 3. Elders who were ready and accepting appeared peaceful or were simply waiting for death to come. Elders who were also wishing for death, however, displayed conflicting emotions regarding living and dying. At times, they laughed nervously about their situation, and at other times they spoke with great sadness, often crying. Elders who had adopted

Mind Frames 3 and 4 did share feelings of uselessness and a sense that they could no longer justify their existence.

Factors motivating wish for death. —Half of these elders spoke only of psychosocial reasons for wishing death to come soon. Several elders were no longer enjoying life, and one 87-year-old woman reported feeling useless: "It's just the way I feel like it, you know, like I might as well go. What good am I anymore, you know."

Other elders also discussed physical motivators, including exhaustion and daily pain. A 90-year-old widow noted, "Sometimes I feel so rotten that I don't care anymore." Others, like this 93-year-old widow, expressed a fear of future suffering as a reason for wishing death to come: "My first husband, he suffered a long time. He had on those machines, and I used to say, 'God,' I said, 'don't let me go under those machines.'"

Factors motivating against the consideration to hasten death. —When these elders were asked why they had never moved beyond wishing for death to considering hastening it, two factors emerged. The first was the belief that the time of one's death was God's decision, as demonstrated by a married 84-year-old man's statement: "I leave that [dying] up to the good Lord, and He'll take you when He wants you." The other factor was family. Elders talked about the love and support of their family and friends, as well as wanting to protect them from the pain that their suicide would bring.

Mind Frame 5: Considering a Hastened Death But Having No Specific Plan

Approach towards dying. —The approach nine elders (9%) took towards dying was to consider hastening their death. However, although they were considering hastening their death, they had not developed a specific plan to actually do so.

Personal characteristics. —Respondents who had adopted this mind frame had a mean age of 74 and had, on average, some college education. Men outnumbered women, a slightly higher percentage were not married (57%), 90% were White, and the majority was Protestant (89%).

Accompanying emotions. —These elders demonstrated conflicting emotions regarding their desire to hasten death and their taking the next step to develop a specific plan to carry out that desire. Their voices resonated with the emotional pain involved in considering hastening their death and taking the necessary actions to make it happen. As was the case with individuals who had adopted Mind Frames 3 and 4, individuals who had adopted Mind Frame 5 felt they could not justify their existence.

Factors motivating the serious consideration of a hastened death. —The factors motivating these elders to consider a hastened death were mostly psychosocial in nature, as they were for those elders who had adopted Mind Frame 4. Eight of the nine elders who had adopted Mind Frame 5 reported psychosocial factors that included loneliness, not enjoying life, lack of hope, boredom, uselessness, and being a burden.

One 92-year-old man aptly expressed his lack of enjoyment in life: "I, if I could do away with myself, I would . . . I had to give up everything . . . golfing and bowling, sex life, riding my bike."

Physical factors served as motivators for four of the nine elders. Two of these individuals were suffering pain at the time of the interview. One 53-year-old married woman reported despondently, "I'm tired. I'm tired of the struggle and the fighting and the pain and all of that." A 75-year-old married man, who was one of two elders not currently experiencing pain but fearful of future suffering, stated sadly, "I, I fear some of the, uh, some of the physical stress that may come in the course of my dying. Nobody chooses to die little by little. At least, I can't visualize that."

Factors motivating the lack of a specific plan to hasten death.

—All nine elders who had adopted this mind frame were suffering emotionally and/or physically such that death was preferable to living, yet they had not developed a specific plan for hastening death. Although only a few elders stated this preference specifically, others echoed this sentiment but used different words. For example, one 72-year-old widower stated in a voice full of despair, "I just want to get it over with . . . Tomorrow is the same thing, the same thing." Discussions with these individuals revealed the physical limitations and psychosocial reasons preventing them from actually developing a plan to hasten their death.

Three elders were physically unable to hasten their death due to the limitations placed on them by their disease. For example, one man had multiple system atrophy and could only move his lips. These individuals would have required assistance to carry out any plan but either lacked family or friends who might have provided such assistance or, out of love and a sense of responsibility, would not ask them to do so.

The six elders who possessed the physical ability to carry out a plan without assistance had yet to develop one because of their family and friends. For example, two individuals were suffering from respiratory diseases that made breathing difficult, painful, and exhausting. One woman, who was presented at the interview, stated that she knew her terminally ill husband wanted to hasten his death but was vehemently opposed because she felt unable to cope without him. The other elder's spouse, who was not present at the interview, was unaware of his wife's desire to hasten death. The wife, however, knew that her husband was dependent on her emotionally and financially; this dependence kept her from developing a plan. Faced with the love and support they both gave to, and received from, others, these two elders could not make a plan.

Only one elder cited religious beliefs as her reason for not developing a specific plan. Although this 87-year-old widow felt that "there doesn't seem to be any hope for anything," and she refused to explain what her religious beliefs were, she felt strongly that these beliefs would not permit her to take the next step towards hastening her death.

Except for the respondent who felt that her religious beliefs would not allow her to make a specific plan to hasten her death, I felt the others would make a plan in the future should their circumstances change. The physical and psychosocial anguish expressed by these elders was very real. If someone had volunteered to assist them, or if their spouses had changed their mind regarding not wanting them to leave, I believe these elders would have sought the opportunity to develop a plan.

Mind Frame 6: Considering a Hastened Death With a Specific Plan

Approach towards dying. —The remaining nine elders (9%) were seriously considering hastening their death and had a specific plan of action. One 55-year-old married man had developed a suicide plan he could carry out on his own were his suffering to intensify. Three elderly women (aged 65, 70, and 79), two of whom were married, all had end-stage renal disease and planned to go off dialysis. They had discussed with their physicians stopping their dialysis treatment and their physicians told them they would support their decision and provide the necessary assistance. A 75-year-old married woman had contacted the Hemlock Society and had received their support. Two elderly women and two elderly men (aged 75, 91, 69, and 76, respectively) were considering physician-assisted death and had received verbal support from their physician, with whom they had a close relationship. One of the women stated, "I have considered, I do like this physician-assisted suicide. With the assistance of a doctor, so you won't have a, a, messy death . . . and they [doctors] have said that any time I'm going to want to, it's up to me. That's right. I'm very glad about it. Yeah."

Personal characteristics. —Respondents who had adopted this mind frame had a mean age of 74 and had, on average, some college education. Two thirds were women, two thirds were married, and 90% were White. Although more than half of these respondents were Protestants, all respondents of Jewish faith ($n = 2$) were in this category.

Accompanying emotions. —Some of these individuals were very emotional when speaking of hastening their death, whereas others had a matter-of-fact approach to the topic. Elders who had family or friends felt conflicting feelings when they spoke of the impact their plan might have on loved ones. Elders who had adopted Mind Frames 3, 4, 5, and 6 all shared feelings of uselessness and the sense that their existence could no longer be justified.

Factors motivating the serious consideration of a hastened death. —All nine elders reported psychosocial factors as playing a crucial role in their desire for a hastened death. Eight of the nine elders expressed feeling useless. The frustration of feeling useless was evident in a 70-year-old widow's inability to do the normal tasks of daily living: "I just can't do what I used to. Urn, I can't go out, I can't go to the store . . . I can't write a check for nothing. I, it's just a lot of things . . . Oh, I hate it" A 91-year-old widow talked about how she no longer felt useful to others: "There's not any good reason for me to go on living. Nobody really needs me . . . I'm really not serving any purpose. If you don't, aren't needed by anybody, you kind of have a different feeling about life."

Six elders felt life no longer brought any enjoyment. Each day was filled with the limitations of their illness and the misery it wrought on their lives. One 76-year-old man had reached the point in his illness where he had lost the ability to move his body or speak. He had always loved to socialize, travel, and work—all things he was no longer able to do. Not being able to communicate with others or get around like he used to had a profound negative impact on him.

In addition expressing psychosocial factors as motivators, two elders who were currently only experiencing mild physical discomfort feared they would suffer terribly as death drew near. One elder had heard on television and read in the newspaper about how painful dying had been for other Americans and feared the same fate. The other elder had witnessed his mother's suffering and was reminded daily of her terrible experiences.

The desire to hasten death was strong for the nine elders, and they all noted how having a plan provided a sense of control in case living became too unbearable. One 91-year-old widow was fueled by her desire for control over her body: "I just feel sometimes as though cancer is, uh, an opponent. And, it seems to me, it says to itself, 'I am in control of this body. This is mine, I will do whatever I want to with it'" She spoke with her long-time doctor about physician-assisted death, and he promised his support when she was ready. She felt that although the cancer now had the upper hand, she had the ultimate control through physician-assisted death.

Factors motivating against implementation of plan to hasten death. —Although all nine elders possessed a plan for hastening their death, they had not yet set an exact time for putting their plan into action. For some, physical limitations prevented them from carrying out their plan alone. For others, life was still bearable and they felt the need to protect their family from the taint and pain their suicide would bring. At that moment, the factors motivating elders not to move forward with their plan were proving stronger than the motivators for hastening death.

For some elders, physical limitations resulted in their not being able to carry out specific suicide plans. They had waited too long to put them into action and now were physically unable to do so. The anger and frustration felt by these individuals was expressed clearly by a 69-year-old married man who was suffering with amyotrophic lateral sclerosis: "... I can't pull the trigger. Too weak. I'd have to make a fixture and fasten it and have a string and pull my arm."

Although some elders had family who could assist and were supportive of their plan to hasten death, they could not bring themselves to accept their family's assistance. They did not want to place loved ones in this position and were hoping to find others who would do so; they also did not feel comfortable about approaching their physician.

For the elders who were physically able to carry out their plan, family also played a role in their not yet having executed the plan. These individuals talked about the emotional pain a hastened death would bring their loved ones. Feelings of protecting family members from this emotional pain were uppermost in their minds. One 55-year-old married man, whose son had killed himself, his wife, and his children, was reluctant to put his wife through his own suicide if possible:

And basically for one reason. Yeah, I'll tell you. We lost our son and his family back in '91 ... It was to do with drugs. And we don't know ... what happened, but supposedly he, he shot and killed his wife and the two-year-old son. And then himself, and they had a five-month-old baby that was suffocated ... We found them, which made it ten times worse. And because of that, I would never do that to my wife. I wouldn't do that.

For the other elders who also could go through with their plan without any assistance, life was still bearable. However, should the time come when they could no longer tolerate their lives, they indicated that their plan would be put into action.

All nine elders were experiencing critical junctures in their dying process. Either life had become unbearable due to their illness, or they feared it would be so in the future. The only solution they saw to address their physical and emotional pain was to hasten their death, and they were strong in their conviction to do so, if it became necessary.

Discussion

Prior studies on factors motivating terminally ill individuals to consider a hastened death assumed that they faced their dying by either considering or not considering a hastened death. This dichotomy was originally proposed for the present study; however, as the respondents' stories unfolded, it quickly became clear that these 96 terminally ill elders had mind frames towards dying that were much more complex. Instead of the simple consideration to hasten or not to hasten death, six mind frames towards dying emerged. Furthermore, elders with differing mind frames were struggling with various issues related to their dying. Elders not considering a hastened death reported grappling with issues of readiness and acceptance, whereas elders wishing for or considering a hastened death reported grappling with whether to take action.

Researchers can draw no conclusion from the data regarding whether elders' six mind frames fall along a continuum from neither ready nor accepting of dying to having a specific plan by which to hasten death. To consider these mind frames as a continuum implies that (a) these mind frames are stages terminally ill elders move through, and (b) one stage progresses to the next. The data support neither implication. Fifteen elders reported moving from one mind frame to another during their dying process, whereas others reported only having experienced one mind frame (this topic will be discussed in another article). Elders who reported changing their mind frame did not necessarily move sequentially consistent with the mind frames being a continuum or a series of stages. Although the cross-sectional data do not provide information on the issue of progression, they do provide insights into personal characteristics, approaches towards dying, and accompanying emotions that characterize each mind frame, as well as the factors that motivate its adoption by the elder.

Personal Characteristics

The elders who participated in this study did not enter into their dying process with a blank slate; rather, each brought with them values, beliefs, and experiences based on their age, education, gender, race, marital status, and religion (see Table 1). It was noted earlier that information was not gathered regarding the mind frame respondents had adopted in previous life crises, or whether past experiences influenced their current mind frame. Respondents' personal characteristics, however, serve to provide some of this information.

Age and race showed some patterns in relation to respondents' readiness for death. Respondents who were not ready to die, regardless of whether they did or did no accept death, were younger (71 and 69 years old, respectively), on average, than respondents who were ready and accepting (81 years old) or wishing for death (83 years old). It could be that age may reflect the timing of the death; that is, younger elders may feel that death is coming sooner than they had anticipated and so they are less ready for it. Race also revealed an important pattern, in that few Black respondents reported a readiness to die, and none wished for death. It is unclear why Black respondents might lack readiness, but it could be related to their spiritual beliefs.

Education, gender, marital status, and religion revealed some noteworthy patterns with regard to respondents who were considering a hastened death. Regardless of whether they did or did not have a specific plan, respondents who were considering a hastened death reported having at least some college education (14 and 13 years, respectively), whereas respondents who had adopted other mind frames reported having a high school education or less. Education may provide knowledge of end-of-life options as well as access to resources necessary to hasten one's death. It is also important to note that a higher percentage of women than men reported having a specific plan to hasten their death, although the reason for this pattern is not clear. For the most part, respondents who were married and who were considering a hastened death had a specific plan, whereas unmarried respondents who were considering a hastened death did not. Having a partner to assist with hastening death may make it easier to develop a specific plan and act on it. Finally, although Catholics reported a high level of acceptance of dying regardless of their level of readiness, both Jewish respondents possessed a specific plan to hasten death. Again, it is difficult to speculate about the reasons for this difference.

The patterns noted above provide support for delving more deeply into the role that a respondent's personal characteristics may play in the adoption of his or her mind frame. A mixed-method research approach would help gather information not only on which characteristics playa role in the adoption of mind frames but also on how they do so.

Importance of the Psychosocial Aspects of Dying

Family relationships; unfinished business; enjoying life; fear of dying; having lived a long time already; not enjoying life; feeling bored, lonely, useless, dependent, and burdensome to others; lack of hope; lack of control; religious beliefs; fear of future suffering; and physical suffering were all factors that motivated the elders interviewed for this study to adopt one of six mind frames. Many of these factors reflect what has been found in previous studies; however, the current study provides rich information on how the factors motivate the adoption of different mind frames towards dying. It is important to note that in the present study, as well as in the studies reviewed earlier in this article, psychosocial factors were mentioned as motivating factors more often than were physical factors. Physical suffering, however, is not a factor that can be ignored. In the current study, physical suffering was a motivating factor for 3 of the 6 respondents who were wishing for death to come and for 2 of the 9 respondents who were considering a hastened death but had no specific plan on how to bring it about. Although elders discussed psychosocial issues more often than physical ones, it may be that some of these issues were the result of physical limitations or problems brought on by their illness.

Complexity of Motivating Factors

The results of this study demonstrate that some motivating factors differed among elders with each of the six mind frames, and, even in the cases where some similarities existed, a closer look showed that these factors were not the same. Family is an excellent example of this. Family was a motivator for both elders who were neither ready nor accepting of dying (Mind Frame 1) and for elders who were not ready but who had accepted their dying (Mind Frame 2). Yet how family motivated these elders' lack of readiness differed. Elders who had adopted Mind Frame 1 cited the importance of *providing* emotional and instrumental support to their family. Elders who had adopted Mind Frame 2 spoke of *receiving* emotional and instrumental support from their family. Thus, it is not enough for health care practitioners to know that family is an important influence on readiness to die. It is also important to understand just how family ties affect the terminally ill elder's readiness for and acceptance of their death.

Religious belief is another example of how a factor can appear to be the same across mind frames and yet can motivate elders to adopt different mind frames. Elders who were neither ready nor accepting of dying spoke of how God wanted them to fight to stay alive and did not want them just to accept their dying. God was important in a quite different way for some elders who explained their acceptance of death as based on their belief that time of death was God's decision. The religious belief that God decides time of death also served to motivate some elders who wished for death but who were not seriously considering hastening it. These differences raise the issue of whether the respondent's religious beliefs were of long standing and had led him or her to adopt the views towards death that had been described in the interviews, or whether the beliefs developed after the respondent's diagnosis in order to support the mind frame the respondent needed to be in at that time. Either way, the religious beliefs held by some respondents gave them support for their mind frame.

These are only two examples of the complexity of the motivating factors that needs to be taken into consideration when health care professionals are working with terminally ill elders. For example, strong family ties or religious beliefs cannot always be assumed to operate in the same manner. Instead, professionals need to uncover the specific nature of such ties or beliefs.

Palliative Care Program and Practice Implications

The overarching implication to emerge from this study is the need to develop palliative care programs from a holistic rather than a primarily medical perspective. The elders participating in this study provided quite a bit of evidence as to the importance of addressing not only their physical needs, but their spiritual, emotional, and social needs as well. Developing a program that meets these needs has several underlying implications.

Once elders have been told they have fewer than six months to live, the main goal of palliative care programs becomes ensuring that they receive a quality dying process. The term *quality dying process* is ambiguous and so necessitates defining. The qualitative information provided by the 96 terminally ill elders interviewed for this study serves as a step towards such a definition.

For elders participating in the current study, a quality dying process meant recognizing that each had his or her own psychosocial, spiritual, and physical needs, and that whether or not these needs were met had an impact on the mind frame that elder adopted towards dying. If palliative care programs were to adopt the definition of a quality dying process as holistic and individualistic, it would be important to develop instruments that ensure a comprehensive assessment of each elder's mind frame; the psychosocial, physical, and spiritual factors that led to its adoption; and the elder's level of satisfaction with it. If the elder is satisfied, then such programs can emphasize to their practitioners the importance of respecting the elder's wishes, even if the practitioner does not agree with them. However, if the elder is not happy with his or her current mind frame, then the elder and practitioner can address the factors that may allow for transitioning to another mind frame. It is crucial that palliative care programs acknowledge the fluidity of movement between mind frames (as evidenced by 15 of the 96 respondents who reported previous transitioning), such that elders' psychosocial, spiritual, and physical needs are continually assessed as they move through the dying process.

In an attempt to ensure that each terminally ill elder has a quality dying process, I suggest the following guidelines for palliative care programs. First, the design of these programs may best be guided by the input of clergy, nurses, physicians, and social workers so that all aspects of care are considered. Second, once programs have been established, it may be beneficial for staff to work as a team in order to ensure that each terminally ill elder has all of his or her needs met. Third, in order to develop effective care plans, it may be helpful to develop evaluation instruments that assess the spiritual, emotional, social, and physical needs of the elder, as well as his or her current mind frame towards dying and the elder's level of satisfaction with that mind frame. It is important, however, to honor the el-

der's self-determination regarding his or her needs. This means that guidelines should be established that specify the need for practitioners to determine and honor what each elder feels are the most critical issues to be addressed. As was revealed in the current study, some terminally ill elders gave psychosocial issues higher priority than physical ones. Time is limited for these individuals, and it is important that elders be the ones to determine how their limited time is spent. Fourth, in the current study, sense of control served as a key motivating factor for not only considering a hastened death but also for developing a specific plan to carry it out. Although more research is necessary regarding the role sense of control plays in relation to a terminally ill elder's dying process, palliative care programs should include the assessment and fulfillment of control needs in their care plans. Finally, palliative care health professionals need to attend training sessions that allow them to explore their own values and beliefs regarding death. An increased self-awareness and comfort with dying and death could result in practitioners being more receptive to allowing terminally ill elders to express their fears and concerns honestly throughout the dying process.

Study Limitations and Research Implications

Although this study advanced knowledge on hastening death and had an unusually large sample size for a qualitative study, there were also limitations. First, the sampling technique used in this study was purposive, so the findings cannot be considered representative of the population of terminally ill elders. Second, the research design used for this study was cross-sectional and only captured the elders' mind frames at one point in time. I asked elders who were not currently considering a hastened death to recall whether they had ever considered hastening their death; in this way, I gained evidence regarding past mind frames. This evidence, however, was based on recall that could have been impacted by the elder's medication or current situation. I did not ask elders who were considering a hastened death about prior views regarding hastening death.

Therefore, I do not know whether they had been considering a hastened death since they were diagnosed as terminally ill or whether, at one time, they had not been considering a hastened death. The current evidence that terminally ill elders transition between mind frames is an important finding and one that would be best followed up by using a longitudinal research design.

Additional research on this topic using a random sample and a longitudinal research design may add support and clarification to the program and practice implications suggested by the current data. Qualitative studies focused on race/ethnicity, gender, social class differences, and sites of care are necessary in order to obtain information that will improve the care of terminally ill elders. In addition, future research on this topic should aim to develop a multidimensional assessment tool that not only captures elders' personal characteristics and their mind frames towards dying, but also assesses elders' spiritual, emotional, social, and physical needs.

Acknowledgments

Support for this article was provided by the John A Hartford Foundation Geriatric Social Work Doctoral Fellowship Program.

Address correspondence to Tracy A. Schroepfer, University of Wisconsin, Madison, School of Social Work, 1350 University Ave., Madison, WI 53706. E-mail: tschroepfer@wisc.edu

References

Arias, E., Anderson, R., Hsiang-Ching, K., Murphy, S., & Kochanek, K. (2003, September 18). Deaths: Final data for 2001. *National Vital Statistics Report, 52* (3), 1–116.

Arnold, E. (2004). Factors that influence consideration of hastening death among people with life-threatening illnesses. *Health & Social Work, 29* (1), 17–26.

Back, A., Wallace, J., Starks, H., & Pearlman, R. (1996). Physician-assisted suicide and euthanasia in Washington state: Patient requests and physician responses. *Journal of the American Medical Association, 275,* 919–925.

Bernabei, R., Gambassi, G., Lapane, K., Landi, G., Gatsonis, C., Dunlop, R., et al. (1998). Management of pain in elderly patients with cancer. *Journal of the American Medical Association, 279,* 1877–1882.

Black, H., & Rubinstein, R. L. (2004). Themes of suffering in later life. *Journal of Gerontology: Social Sciences, 59B,* SI7–S24.

Breitbart, W., Rosenfeld, B., & Passik, S. (1996). Interest in physician assisted suicide among ambulatory HIV-infected patients. *American Journal of Psychiatry, 153,* 238–242.

Chin, A., Hedberg, K., Higginson, G., & Fleming, D. (1999). Legalized physician-assisted suicide in Oregon: The first year's experience. *New England Journal of Medicine, 340,* 577–583.

Chochinov, H., Hack, T., Hassard, T., Kristjanson, L., McClement, S., & Harlos, M. (2002). Dignity in the terminally ill: A cross-sectional, cohort study. *Lancet, 360,* 2026–2030.

Chochinov, H., Wilson, K., Enns, M., Mowchun, N., Lander, S., Levitt, M., et al. (1995). Desire for death in the terminally ill. *American Journal of Psychiatry, 152,* 1185–1191.

Cleeland, C., Gonin, R., Hatfield, A., Edmonson, J., Blum, R., Stewart, J., & Pandya, K. (1994). Pain and its treatment in outpatients with metastatic cancer. *New England Journal of Medicine, 330,* 592–596.

Emanuel, E., Fairclough, D., Daniels, E., & Clarridge, B. (1996). Euthanasia and physician-assisted suicide: Attitudes and experiences of oncology patients, oncologists, and the public. *Lancet, 347,* 1805–1810.

Emanuel, E., Fairclough, D., & Emanuel, L. (2000). Attitudes and desires related to euthanasia and physician-assisted suicide among terminally ill patients and their caregivers. *Journal of the American Medical Association, 284,* 2460–2468.

Ganzini, L., Harvath, T., Jackson, A., Goy, E., Miller, L., & Delorit, M. (2002). Experiences of Oregon nurses and social workers with hospice patients who requested assistance with suicide. *New England Journal of Medicine, 347,* 582–588.

Hetzel, L., & Smith, A. (2001). *The 65 years and over population: 2000* (Census 2000 Brief No. C2KBR/01-10). Washington, DC: U.S. Census Bureau.

Jacobson, J., Kasworm, E., Battin, M., Botkin, J., Francis, L., & Green, D. (1995). Decedents' reported preferences for physician-assisted death: A survey of informants listed on death certificates in Utah. *Journal of Clinical Ethics, 6* (2), 149–157.

Lavery, J., Boyle, J., Dickens, B., Maclean, H., & Singer, P. (2001). Origins of the desire for euthanasia and assisted suicide in people with HIV-1 or AIDS: A qualitative study. *Lancet, 358,* 362–367.

Meier, E., Emmons, C., Wallenstein, S., Quill, T., Morrison, R., & Cassel, C. (1998). A national survey of physician-assisted suicide and euthanasia in the United States. *New England Journal of Medicine, 338,* 1193–1201.

Oregon Department of Human Services. (2000). *Oregon's death with dignity act: The second year's experience.* Portland: Oregon Health Division.

Oregon Department of Human Services. (2001). *Oregon's death with dignity act: Three years of legalized physician-assisted suicide.* Portland: Oregon Health Division.

Oregon Department of Human Services. (2002). *Fourth annual report on Oregon's death with dignity act.* Portland: Oregon Health Division.

Oregon Department of Human Services. (2003). *Fifth annual report on Oregon's death with dignity act.* Portland: Oregon Health Division.

Patton, M. (1990). *Qualitative evaluation and research methods* (2nd ed.). Newbury Park, CA: Sage.

Pessin, H., Rosenfeld, B., & Breitbart, W. (2002). Assessing psychological distress near the end of life. *American Behavioral Scientist, 46,* 357–372.

SUPPORT Investigators. (1997). Perceptions by family members of the dying: Experiences of older and seriously ill patients. *Annals of Internal Medicine, 126,* 97–106.

Volker, D. (2001). Oncology nurses' experiences with requests for assisted dying from terminally ill patients with cancer. *Oncology Nursing Forum, 28* (1), 39–49.

UNIT 7

Living Environment in Later Life

Unit Selections

Key Points to Consider

- How does Bill Thomas propose changing the nursing home so that people don't think of it as just a place where people go to die?

- What are the advantages to old persons that move into continuing care communities?

- What are the things family members should investigate and consider before placing a loved one in a nursing home?

- How was Beacon Hill turned into a place where older persons could live for their entire life?

Student Website

www.mhcls.com/online

Internet References

Further information regarding these websites may be found in this book's preface or online.

American Association of Homes and Services for the Aging
http://www.aahsa.org

Center for Demographic Studies
http://cds.duke.edu

Guide to Retirement Living Online
http://www.retirement-living.com

The United States Department of Housing and Urban Development
http://www.hud.gov

Unit 4 noted that old age is often a period of shrinking life space. This concept is crucial to an understanding of the living environments of older Americans. When older people retire, they may find that they travel less frequently and over shorter distances because they no longer work and most neighborhoods have stores, gas stations, and churches in close proximity. As the retirement years roll by, older people may feel less in control of their environments due to a decline in their hearing and vision as well as other health problems. As the aging process continues, the elderly are likely to restrict their mobility to the areas where they feel most secure. This usually means that an increasing amount of time is spent at home. Estimates show that individuals age 65 and over spend 80 to 90 percent of their lives in their home environments. Of all the other age groups, only small children are as house- and neighborhood-bound.

The house, neighborhood, and community environments are, therefore, more crucial to the elderly than to any other adult age group. The interaction with others that they experience within their homes and neighborhoods can be either stimulating or foreboding, pleasant or threatening. Across the country, older Americans find themselves living in a variety of circumstances, ranging from desirable to undesirable.

Approximately 70 percent of the elderly live in a family setting, usually a husband-wife household; 20 percent live alone or with nonrelatives; and the remaining number live in institutions such as nursing homes. Although only about 5 percent of the elderly will be living in nursing homes at any one time, 25 percent of people 65 and over will spend some time in a nursing home setting. The longer one lives, the more likely he or she is to end up in a total-care institution. Because most older Americans would prefer to live independently in their own homes for as long as possible, their relocation—to other houses, apartments, or nursing homes—is often accompanied by a considerable amount of trauma and unrest. Because the aged tend to be less mobile and more neighborhood-bound than any other age group makes their living environment most crucial to their sense of well-being.

Articles in this section focus on some of the alternatives available to the aged: from family care to assisted living to nursing homes. In "(Not) the Same Old Story," Chuck Salter reviews recommendations from gerontologist Bill Thomas for changing

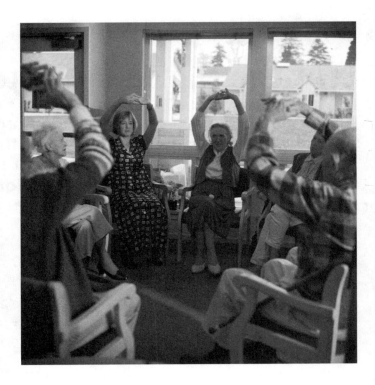

nursing homes to make them livable and enjoyable to the residents. In "A Home for the Rest of Your Life," Jane Bennett Clark describes continuing care communities where you may initially move into your own apartment, later move into an assisted living area, and, if necessary, ultimately move into a nursing home. In "Nursing Homes: Business As Usual," *Consumer Reports* examined the quality of care in nursing homes and came up with suggestions for how an individual might choose the best nursing home for a family member. In "Declaration of Independents," Barbara Basler tells how Beacon Hill in Boston turned itself from a residential neighborhood into a non-profit association which provides services to its residents on a 24-hour-a-day basis.

The Big Fix

Not the Same Old Story

Eden Alternative is a change-minded organization determined to save a critically ill patient: long-term care for the elderly. The nursing-home industry should be about living, argues founder Bill Thomas, not about dying. Here's his prescription—and lessons for changing any industry.

CHUCK SALTER

In 1999, after writing a book about improving long-term care for the elderly, Bill Thomas did what authors do: He hit the road for a promotional tour. He appeared on radio and television. He also met with public officials, offering his perspective as a gerontologist—a doctor who specializes in treating the elderly—on what was wrong with nursing homes: They were utterly devoid of hope, love, humor, meaning—the very stuff of life. He gave lectures on the changes he had in mind, which included adding pets, plants, and children to nursing-home life. But at each stop, he also demonstrated why this is no ordinary book and this was no ordinary tour—and why he is certainly no ordinary doctor.

"Does anyone want to leave his home and go live in a nursing home? That's why we're turning the industry upside down."

Thomas, now 42, didn't write a prosaic account of the principles behind Eden Alternative, the nonprofit organization that he and his wife, Jude, operate out of their farm in Sherburne, New York. Instead, he told a story, a fantastic tale interweaving fact and fiction. *Learning from Hannah: Secrets for a Life Worth Living* (VanderWyk & Burnham, 1999) is a novel that doesn't call itself a novel. It begins with Thomas and his wife completing a book about the medical aspects of aging and then taking a much-needed vacation. While sailing south from San Juan toward the island of Montserrat, they get caught in a storm that leaves them shipwrecked. For nearly a year, they live in a mysterious place called Kallimos, where they learn the ways of a society in which the elderly play a vibrant role in the community. Instead of living apart from younger generations, the oldest inhabitants are embraced by them. The wisdom and experience of the elderly are valued as a resource. When Thomas and wife eventually return home, the lessons from Hannah, the old woman who mentored them, become the inspiration and foundation for Eden Alternative.

It wasn't enough for Thomas to communicate his vision for better long-term care through an imaginative book. He also developed a one-man show based on the tale. In the summer of 1999, the Harvard-educated doctor turned novelist turned actor launched the Eden Across America Tour, traveling by private bus to 27 cities in 31 days with his wife, their five children, and his parents. It's not hard to imagine Thomas on stage; he's alternately funny, exuberant, and sincere, offering glimpses of a natural theatricality. After a performance at a medical school in the Midwest, he wrote in his online journal, "I had the strange sense that the ghosts of medical professors past were looking on us and clucking their tongues. I didn't care."

For Thomas, the Eden Across America Tour never ended. It can't. Not if he's going to fix long-term care in this country. For all practical purposes, he says, the industry is broken. "Does anyone want to leave his home and go live in a nursing home?" he asks. "Does anyone want to put a parent, spouse, or loved one there? That's why we're turning the industry upside down."

It's an audacious mission and a truly big fix—one that requires more than just fresh ideas. It demands an unorthodox approach to mobilizing and motivating a wide range of forces, many of which have little incentive to change. "You need to have people go a little nuts about what you want to do," Thomas says. On its own, the industry isn't going to do an about-face and overhaul its core ideas. And individual nursing homes are often too overwhelmed by the day-to-day demands of caring for residents in a heavily regulated field to try anything new. Hoping to prod people into going a little nuts about radical reform, Thomas appeals to their imaginations and their hearts. Hence the book, the tour, and the play. "A lot of innovators don't focus enough on the story that they're telling," he says. "But the story is the only thing that ever gets people to change. It captures your passion and conviction and inspires others to feel the same way."

> ### "Some homes think that Eden and the operation of the facility are two separate things. But Eden is all over. It affects everything you do."

It's no accident that Eden Alternative evokes another story: that of the Garden of Eden. A garden is the central metaphor behind Thomas's vision. "Human beings aren't meant to live in institutions," he says, "but that's what most nursing homes are: big, impersonal, cold institutions that don't treat people the way they want to be treated. People are meant to live in a garden, a place where they can grow and thrive as human beings."

So far, about 300 nursing homes in the United States (as well as a handful in Europe and Australia) have been "Edenized." Which is to say that these institutions have been deinstitutionalized and turned into warm, nurturing human habitats. The results have proven not only good for residents but also good for business. Impressed by the improved quality of care, residents' health, and staff retention, several states have begun offering Eden grants—using the fines that more backward-looking facilities pay for violating regulations.

Typically, an Eden nursing home is divided into neighborhoods, with a staff that knows the residents personally—their background and interests as well as their medications. There's all sorts of activity: children playing, dogs and cats visiting rooms, birds chirping. The institution becomes a close-knit community teeming with life.

The transformation, however, is often arduous. Creating an Eden home involves major organizational and cultural change, because the facility has to think differently about care, priorities, and old habits. For instance, the residents have more input into how the facility operates, as do the staff members who work closest with them—a shift that often proves difficult for traditional-minded administrators.

> ### "Caring for the elderly is not simply about health care or medicine or technology… It's about creating the right environment and caring relationships that sustain an older adult in his last years." says Bill Thomas.

"Out of all the people we've talked to about creating Eden homes, no one says, 'This is a horrible idea,'" says Jude Thomas, who conducts Eden workshops with her husband. "But some people think that all they have to do is bring in a dog, and everything will be better. It won't be. This is an entirely different philosophy. It's a total change."

Voices in the Garden (Part I) *Jane Lough, administrator, Toomsboro Nursing Center, Toomsboro, Georgia: "This one lady, Mrs. Miller, dressed nicely every day and got her hair done once a week for the first year and a half she was here. Then she went into the hospital for pneumonia, and when she came*

How Does Your Garden Grow?

Through Eden Alternative, Bill Thomas is making a difference in long-term care for the elderly. He's turning institutions into places where residents actually enjoy living. Here's how he's fixing things.

Have a good story to tell. Stories help people understand your ideas. Through your passion, stories inspire others to get on board and make your vision a reality. "You need a mythic, heroic story that people will respond to," Thomas says. "Ours is about creating gardens for our elders where they can thrive. That's something that people want for their mothers and fathers."

Watch your language. Eden has a vocabulary all its own, most of which grew (pun intended) out of its defining metaphor of cultivating gardens. Eden practitioners know what they mean by "warming the soil" and "experiencing a frost." It may sound goofy, but it's a way of changing the conversation within an organization.

Don't mistake tokens for real change. The most visible component of Eden is the animals that reside in nursing homes. But "fur and feathers," says Thomas, aren't a shortcut to transformation. Unless you change the culture and philosophy, the facility won't be different. It will still be an institution—but with pets. Big deal.

Make innovation a group activity. Thomas doesn't claim to have all the answers for improving nursing homes. The Eden program gives a framework and some ideas, but individual facilities decide which changes are best to make. Administrators share ideas through Eden's Web site and at get-togethers. Thomas has the same "open source" philosophy about the Greenhouse Project, which involves building homes for small groups of elders. He's sharing his ideas online and letting others build on them. "You can't do it alone," he says.

Expect setbacks. Failure is an inevitable part of the change process. So you'd better be prepared for it, or you won't be able to bounce back. Understand that people are going to get scared and revert back to doing things the old way. Forgive them and move forward—and expect it to happen again. "Frost always comes," says Thomas. "We've never been wrong on that one."

back, she wouldn't get out of bed. She gave up. So I got her a blue parakeet named Mercy, and we put the cage on an IV pole next to her bed. She would feed it crackers and sing to it. After three or four months, she got up, got her hair done, and started going everywhere with Mercy. She'd tell people she loved that bird."

Mission: Overcoming the Three Plagues

After graduating from Harvard Medical School, Bill Thomas had his heart set on the emergency room. He liked the action and the adrenaline rush. But in 1991, after completing his residency in family medicine at the University of Rochester, he tried something different: becoming the physician at Chase Memorial Nursing Home in New Berlin, New York. He discovered that he enjoyed working with the elderly, getting to know them, hearing their stories. He also discovered that nursing homes were seriously flawed—even the best-performing facilities. At Chase, the equipment was up-to-date, the staff was dedicated, and the inspection record was spotless. Yet the residents were miserable. "What appalled me was how lonely and bored they were," Thomas says. "It was painfully obvious to me that they were dying in front of my eyes."

He concluded that nursing-home residents suffer from three plagues: loneliness, helplessness, and boredom. They feel lonely because they've been uprooted from their family, friends, and even their pets. They feel helpless because they've lost control of their lives; for the most part, they eat, sleep, get dressed, and bathe according to the institution's schedule. Finally, they feel bored because the few activities that are available to them, such as watching television, aren't meaningful or fulfilling. "Care for the elderly is not simply about health care or medicine or technology," Thomas says. "It's about creating the right environment and caring relationships that sustain an older adult in his last years."

While working at Chase, Thomas received a $200,000 grant to improve life for the facility's residents. The experiment gave rise to Eden Alternative. Bringing animals into nursing homes was not a new idea, but in the past, they were usually brought in for visits. They didn't live on the premises, as Thomas prefers. That way, the animals become companions, and the residents grow attached to them. As one of the 10 Eden principles says, "Loving companionship is the antidote to loneliness."

If the elders—Thomas finds the term more dignified—are able, they lend a hand in grooming or feeding the animals, watering plants, or reading with children. These activities not only allow residents to engage in everyday physical therapy, but they also satisfy another fundamental human need, one that often gets neglected: giving care, as opposed to only receiving it.

At Eden facilities, residents and staff are partners. Whenever possible, the two groups work together, voting on what type of pet to add or what type of decorations to put up. Staff members understand that what they call the workplace is a far more intimate and personal place to residents: It's home. And that understanding shapes decisions. Eden removes hierarchical or autocratic management. Like the residents, the certified nurse assistants, who make up the bulk of the staff, have more control over their schedules and help make decisions about how to divvy up work. "What you find is that as the managers do to the staff, the staff does to the elders," says Thomas. "So if you treat the staff well, the elders will benefit."

That's the case in the Toomsboro Nursing Center, a 62-bed facility in rural Georgia. Since adopting the Eden model, the staff has become more responsive and more unified, and the care has become more compassionate and individualized, says Jane Lough, an administrator at the center. Instead of giving orders, Lough tells the certified nurse assistants, "You know this resident. Tell me what you think she needs." By working in teams—the Conquerers, Earth Angels, Outrageous Girlfriends,

and Untouchables—employees began seeing beyond their roles as cook, laundry aide, nurse, and housekeeper. They realized that every staff member provides care in one way or another. As the stickers that they wear declare, "I'm a world-maker." "That's one of Dr. Thomas's terms," says Lough. "In a nursing home, very little of the outside world comes in, except for the staff. They are the residents' world, and they have the opportunity to make it a special place."

Eden does not reverse the aging process, of course, but studies, including one done by the Texas Long Term Care Institute in San Marcos, Texas, indicate that the residents' overall health does improve: They had fewer infections and required less medication. Meanwhile, the staff absenteeism went down and retention went up—a significant improvement in an industry that is notorious for high turnover.

"Relationships are the foundation of good health care," Thomas says. "This is nothing new. But it's not something that the industry has made a priority." In fact, some institutions actively discourage relationships between staff and residents. "When I started out, I was told, 'You don't share yourself with residents, because it hurts too much when they die,'" says Lough. "That's definitely not the attitude here."

Voices in the Garden (Part II) *Kathleen Perra, director of nursing, St. Luke's Home, New Hartford, New York: "Every day last summer, we had school-age day care here. There were kids screaming down the hall, cats jumping on tables. It was bedlam, but it was great. You want those unpredictable things happening for the residents. Of course, health-care workers favor predictability. We work around schedules. I'd say the biggest change with the Eden program is for the staff."*

Method: Warmth, Suction, Frost

Nursing homes that are designed like gardens provide an apt metaphor for Bill Thomas's program, because, like a garden, Eden Alternative doesn't occur naturally. It requires preparation, hard work, and continuous scrutiny as it evolves. Otherwise, if the changes are taken for granted or neglected, Eden eventually shrivels up and dies.

Since founding their organization, Bill and Jude Thomas have become change experts out of necessity. Merely tweaking facilities wasn't effective. Creating an Eden involves a complete transformation. "Some homes think that Eden and the operation of the facility are two separate things," he says. "But Eden is all over. It affects everything you do."

Says director of nursing Kathleen Perra: "Every day last summer, we had school-age day care here. There were kids screaming down the hall, cats jumping on tables. It was bedlam, but it was great"

The duration and success of the change process depends on what Bill Thomas calls the "warmth" of the organization. A warm culture is open to change, because employees have trust and generosity for one another, whereas a cold culture is characterized by pessimism and cynicism. After conducting a survey to determine an organization's temperature, the Thomases or one of 5,000 Eden associates nationwide begin "warming the soil." In some cases, managers hold a potluck dinner at someone's house, where they can't discuss work. Employees also perform good deeds, or mitzvahs, for their colleagues and the residents without expecting anything in return. "You open people's minds by opening their hearts," Thomas says.

Before virtually every step—before adding pets, before switching to self-scheduling—the staff votes. If the outcome isn't unanimous, the group continues the education process. "You can't force change on anybody," says Thomas. "Consensus is the only way. You have to get the entire staff to see the advantages for themselves and become excited about what you're going to do. We call it creating 'suction.'"

Thomas also expects setbacks, or "frost," as he puts it. It's a natural part of change. "I tell the leaders to expect that what they're changing will be smashed to bits, and when that happens, they have to be ready to pick up the pieces and move forward," says Thomas. "People are going to get scared. They're going to make mistakes." Every year, about 5% of Eden homes drop the program. But Thomas doesn't give up hope for them. He prefers to think that they're experiencing a long frost.

Voices in the Garden (Part III) *Ron Rothstein, president and COO, Levindale Hebrew Geriatric Center and Hospital, Baltimore, Maryland: "You don't cure the three plagues overnight. Some of our residents have been here a while, and they've become depressed. It takes time to bring out the best in them. I'm a type A personality—a 'gotta get it done today' type. But culture change is slow. And subtle. You don't necessarily see the relationships between people every day."*

Momentum: Progressives vs. Stalwarts

Eden Alternative's headquarters isn't located in an actual garden. But almost. It's on a lush farm in the rolling hills of upstate New York, 60 miles southeast of Syracuse. On 220 acres that had been abandoned for 50 years, Bill and Jude Thomas brought Summer Hill Farm to life, building a house, barn, retreat center, and 14-room lodge. It's here that you fully appreciate how much of a Renaissance man Thomas is. In the fields behind his house, he uses draft horses to pull the machinery that cuts and rakes the hay. Come wintertime, he takes the family on a horse-drawn-carriage ride into the snowy woods to tap maple sap in order to produce Summer Hill Syrup.

In a very real sense, Summer Hill is the Thomases' personal Eden, a home with dogs and children and individuals who need long-term medical care. Hannah and Haleigh Thomas, 5 and 7, suffer from a rare neurological disorder that prevents them from being able to see, speak, and walk. During a break in the Eden training, Jude checks on them and their nurse and dotes on the dark-haired girls in the double stroller. "When people ask if the Eden program can make a difference in someone who's in a nursing home, I tell them that it can, because I see how Hannah and Haleigh respond to loving care," says Jude. "I honestly believe they're alive because of Eden."

When her husband isn't at Summer Hill, he's spreading the word to nursing-home administrators, regulators, insurance companies, policy makers, and industry associations. He gives about 40 talks a year. Thomas is an optimist—"It can be different," his business card says—but he's also a realist. He knows that he can't fix the country's nursing homes on his own. He relies on Eden associates to promote the program, share success stories, and conduct training sessions in their communities.

Part of changing an industry is about choosing wisely where to focus your energy. In long-term care, as in any field, the stalwarts vastly outnumber the progressives. In general, Thomas says, the progressives have ideas and enthusiasm but lack real authority or management skills, and the stalwarts have authority and experience but resist changes in the status quo. Thomas doesn't turn down invitations to address the latter, but he doesn't court them either. "The reason I'm not racing to Edenize 17,000 nursing homes across the country is because I know that I'll never win over the stalwarts," he says. "I'm focusing on the progressives, because they're interested in changing things."

Ultimately, Eden Alternative is a repair for a broken industry. The replacement, says Thomas, is his Greenhouse Project. It involves houses that are built for small groups of elders and that have a dedicated staff. They are actual homes, instead of an institution that calls itself a home. St. Luke's Home, where Thomas used to be the medical director, expects to break ground on the first greenhouses within the next couple of years. After that, he says, the next logical stage is an Eden Village, where the greenhouses and the elders are part of a larger community.

But why stop there? he wonders. Why not apply these principles to other institutions, such as schools and prisons? Thomas jokes about starting a group called "Institutions Anonymous." Maybe he's only half joking. "Don't get me started," he says.

CHUCK SALTER (csalter@fastcompany.com) *is a Fast Company senior writer based in Baltimore. Learn more about Eden Alternative on the Web (www.edenalt.com), or contact* **BILL THOMAS** *by email (thomaswh@edenalt.com).*

A Home for the Rest of Your Life

Continuing-care communities promise independence now and all the help you need later on.

JANE BENNETT CLARK

Four days. That's how long Lucy and Dick Thomson had to make the decision of a lifetime: Stay in Saginaw, Mich., where they had met before World War II, or pull up stakes and move to a cottage that they had never seen in a new development that was swimming in mud. The couple had placed a small deposit on a cottage at the unfinished site in Lake Forest, Ill., at the urging of their son, who lives nearby. But they were taken aback when the call came that the cottage was available. The message: Grab it now or lose your place in line. That was six years ago.

Today, the Thomsons smile at the memory as they show off their two-bedroom cottage, a sunny space decorated in pale green, yellow and cream. The couple, both 84, enjoy good health and a full calendar at Lake Forest Place, a continuing-care retirement community run by the Presbyterian Homes, in Evanston, Ill. Should their health fail, they are assured of getting help, either in their home or elsewhere on campus. Says Lucy, "it was the best decision we've made in our whole life."

Lake Forest Place is one of 2,100 continuing-care communities across the country that offer independent living, in either cottages or apartments, along with various levels of care. Unlike assisted-living facilities, which can ask you to leave when your money runs out or you need skilled nursing, these communities promise to keep you for life, usually in exchange for an upfront six-figure deposit and monthly fees. Most offer amenities such as fitness clubs, restaurant-style meals and a busy social schedule. Says Linda Fodrini-Johnson, a geriatric-care manager with an office in San Francisco, "It's a nice choice for the healthy senior who wants to be socially engaged."

Continuing-care communities also present a conundrum: To qualify, you must be reasonably healthy—healthy enough that you could still stay in your own home. In fact, most retirees remain in their homes or go directly to assisted living at about age 80 or older. Those who do enter a life-care community typically wait until they are at least 75.

But moving to the right place at the right time can prolong your vitality, says Karen Love, founder of the Consumer Consortium on Assisted Living. The communities are "wonderful environments because they're supportive," she says. "Typically, the food is excellent. There's transportation. If I want a buddy to go shopping with, there are tons of people to pick from." You could actually live longer and healthier in such settings, says Larry Minnix, president of the American Association of Homes and Services for the Aging. "They give the services that people need when they need them, in a place they can call home," Minnix says.

The Thomsons had no immediate plans to leave Saginaw six years ago, but they did have compelling reasons to move someday. All four of their parents had ended their days in grim nursing homes, and the couple's four children had already moved away. "We were wondering what our parents were going to do," says Richard Jr., known as Tom. When Lake Forest Place sprang up near his home outside of Chicago, the family saw an opening. Says Dick, a pilot who parachuted out of his aircraft after it was hit over Hungary during World War II, "It was time to hit the silk."

Go in With Your Eyes Open

It's easy to see why the Thomsons are pleased with their decision. The sea of mud is long gone, and their cottage, which backs to a beautifully landscaped area, boasts a full kitchen, a laundry room and a garage. In the Town Center, the community's main building across the road, the paneling, arched windows and overstuffed chairs easily compete with the ambiance of any country club. Residents can work out in the fitness club or take a dip in one of the community's several pools.

But Dick steers clear of the parts of the complex that offer nursing care or help with eating and dressing. "When it comes to assisted living, I'm in denial," he admits. And he's not alone, says Laurie Duncan, a CPA who owns Choices for Aging, a geriatric-care management company in Arlington, Va. "People like to look at the apartments, the dining facilities—but when you suggest a visit to the health facilities, they say, 'No thanks.'"

As understandable as the ostrich approach might be, anyone looking to secure a comfortable future should "make sure they tour every bit of a community, including the assisted-living and nursing-home areas," says Nicole Muller of Brecht Associates, a firm that specializes in senior housing. Odors, poor housekeeping or residents who look parked are obvious red flags. "The atmosphere should feel comfortable to the person looking at it, not scary."

Lake Forest Place can rightly boast of its caregiving: It's accredited by the Commission on Accreditation of Rehabilitation Facilities. (To find out if a facility has earned the commission's okay, go to www.carf.org.) State inspection reports, required for assisted-living and nursing-home units, provide another glimpse into quality control—if you can decipher them. Geriatric-care managers offer insight into such reports, as well as the skinny on local retirement communities. To find one in your area, call the National Association of Professional Geriatric Care Managers, at 520-881-8008, or go to www.caremanager.org.

Whatever the measuring stick, facilities that come up short, says Duncan, usually share the same problem: poor staffing. "You can have a beautiful lobby, but if you don't have the staff, you're not going to give good care," she says. "If you're paying minimum wage and don't have good training—that's where the rubber meets the road."

The bottom line is that good caregiving requires plenty of willing arms, Duncan says. "In the nursing units, if you have one aide for every nine residents, each resident is getting much less than one hour of one-on-one care during a shift. If one aide is out, then are residents going to get showered or moved? On the assisted-living end, people who need help getting in and out of bed or a chair won't get help if there's only one aide for 15 residents."

Assuming the care and staff are top-notch, you'll need to explore how much help can be brought into your apartment before the community moves you from one level to another, especially when dementia is involved. Grouping cognitively impaired residents isn't necessarily bad, says Gail Kohn, of Linking Partners, a long-term-care consulting firm. But be sure to ask whether and how it is done.

Some states dictate the circumstances in which you will be moved from an assisted-living to a nursing unit; in others, the managers of the community—preferably with the input of family members—make the call. Either way, ask how many nursing beds have been set aside for residents, says Chris Cooper, a registered financial adviser in Toledo who specializes in geriatrics. In a large community, "if there are only 12 beds, they could be full when you need them."

The path between independent living and the nursing unit doesn't have to be one-way. At Lake Forest Place, for instance, stroke victims and surgery patients can practice getting in and out of a full-scale car or climb stairs in the rehab center, giving them a leg up on recovery. The Erickson Retirement Communi-

ties, based in Baltimore, go a step further: They have doctors and other health-care providers on their campuses. "That's a big innovation," Minnix says.

A New Beginning

Just how do two people trade the house where they have lived for 45 years—and the town where they met, married and raised four kids—for a community of total strangers? Piece of cake, says Lucy Thomson. "We've met tons of people. We invite them over for a drink, then go to the town center for dinner. When you go, you have to mingle and it's boy-girl-boy-girl. Everyone has been reading something different. You exchange ideas."

Her son Tom, who heads the microbiology laboratory at Evanston Northwestern Health Care, happily concurs. "We thought it would be hard for our parents to pull up roots from the town where our family had been for generations, but it just worked," he says. "In Saginaw, they knew everyone and had done everything. This has been a social rebirth."

The Thomsons connected in their new setting in part because the residents of life-care communities tend to be likeminded, says Fodrini-Johnson. "These are bright people who are used to doing the research and finding the answers to complex problems." Dick, who spent his career manufacturing automotive parts, agrees with that assessment. "The whole campus is composed of top professionals."

Still, each community has its own flavor. For instance, the Kendal Communities—most of whose small campuses are located near liberal-arts colleges—attract residents who want to take classes or participate in campus functions. The Erickson communities draw members who like a wide range of activities. Religion, politics and socioeconomic status each play a role in the matchmaking process, says Kohn.

But little things like dining-room seating arrangements can be an important indication of how thoughtfully a community brings you into the mix. At the Erickson communities, for instance, residents are led to tables by a hostess rather than left to hunt for a seat. "You never sit alone," says Trudy Couch, who lives in Riderwood Village, in Silver Spring, Md. Couch spent several nights in the guest suites at Riderwood to get a feel for the place before moving in. "I noticed how friendly the staff members were."

Although the Thomsons first visited Lake Forest Place as a mudhole, any uncertainty about their move has vanished. Lucy attends yoga class or walks the trail beyond her house in the morning. Dick has taken a spot on the finance committee. They meet friends for dinner in the dining room three or four times a week. Says Lucy, "We've never been happier."

Nursing Homes: Business as Usual

Two decades after the passage of a federal law to clean up the nation's nursing homes, bad care persists and good homes are still hard to find.

In 1987, Congress passed a landmark law meant to improve nursing home care for the elderly. But our investigation reveals that poor care is still all too common, especially at nursing homes run by for-profit chains, now the dominant force in the industry.

CONSUMER REPORTS' analysis found that not-for-profit homes generally provide better care than for-profit homes, and that independently run nursing homes appear to provide better care than those that are owned by chains. In a separate study, we found that many states are lax in penalizing bad homes.

For this report, we analyzed the three most recent state inspection reports for some 16,000 nursing homes across the U.S. We also examined staffing levels and so-called quality indicators, such as how many residents develop pressure sores when they have no risk factors for them.

The Consumer Reports Nursing Home Quality Monitor, formerly the Nursing Home Watch List, is available free at www.ConsumerReports.org/nursinghomes. It lists facilities in each state that rank in the best or worst 10 percent on at least two of our three dimensions of quality. By examining the kinds of homes that tend to cluster at either end of the continuum, we can make some judgments about how likely a facility is to provide proper care.

This year's list, financed by a grant from The Commonwealth Fund, a philanthropic organization, is the fifth we've published since 2000. We've seen little evidence that the quality of care has improved since then. Indeed, 186 of the homes cited for poor care on this list have also appeared on earlier lists of poor-quality homes.

Consider the White Blossom Care Center, part of a for-profit chain in San Jose, Calif. From the outside, it looks like many of the nursing homes that dot the California landscape: wings of residents' rooms and a parking lot full of cars. Inside we saw nothing that would arouse unease. Residents nodded off in wheelchairs, and aides chatted at nurses' stations as an occasional visitor walked through the halls.

White Blossom, though, is no ordinary nursing home. It's one of 12 that have been on each of our lists of poorly performing homes since 2000. Its state inspection, conducted last August and current when our reporter visited in December, raised troubling questions about the care it delivers.

Page after page of the unusually long document detailed failures to follow doctors' orders, perform a pain assessment, mon-

---

CR Quick Take

Our investigation found that the state agencies responsible for overseeing nursing home care have often failed to correct problems. But consumers can increase their odds of choosing a good nursing home if they narrow their search to certain types. Our findings:

- Not-for-profit homes are more likely to provide good care than for-profits, based on our analysis of inspection surveys, staffing, and quality indicators.
- The same analysis shows that independently run homes are more likely to provide good care than chains.
- Through its influence in politics, the industry has whittled down the protections of the 1987 federal law.

---

dishes and utensils. The 43-page report told of a stroke victim with swallowing problems who was left unsupervised with mushy material in her mouth. And it mentioned a medication error that could have been fatal. The survey also reported on the facility's plans to correct the deficiencies that were cited.

The survey, which by federal law must be "readily accessible" in every nursing home, was not visible in the lobby when our reporter arrived. Only after she insisted on seeing it did the home's administrator produce it. A staff member at the front desk said the report wasn't initially available because it was being used by someone else at the time. Steven Earle, White Blossom's administrator, wouldn't comment on specific deficiencies but said that they had been corrected.

In the three most recent state surveys we analyzed, 657 homes across the country were cited for failing to make their inspection results readily accessible.

Skimping on Care?

While our investigation suggests that you or a family member might receive better care at a not-for-profit, independently owned facility, they make up a small portion of the industry. Since the establishment of Medicaid, the state and federal program for the poor and the elderly, in the 1960s, for-profit homes have come to dominate the field.

"In some chains we see facilities that will consistently do poorly," says Paul Dreyer, director of licensing and certification in the Massachusetts Department of Public Health. "Sometimes it hasn't been the chain's priority to make facilities the best they can be. The focus is maximizing some kind of return to investors."

Bruce Yarwood, president and CEO of the American Health Care Association (AHCA), which represents primarily for-profit homes, says that poor homes are a "chronic, tough issue." He notes that many nursing home executives have trouble escaping Wall Street's quarterly earnings pressure. But, he says, "For every bad story there are probably 50 good ones."

Nursing home researchers say that the most serious problems sometimes show up in small, for-profit chains within a state. In New York, for example, Healthcare Associates, wholly owned by Anthony Salerno, jointly administers a network of 12 separately incorporated facilities. Salerno is the largest shareholder in all the facilities. Three of the homes have been on our quality-monitor list.

Earlier this year Eliot Spitzer, New York's attorney general, sued one of the three homes, the Jennifer Matthew Nursing and Rehabilitation Center in Rochester, alleging abuse and neglect. Investigators used a hidden camera to show that call bells were placed out of residents' reach and that patients would go unturned and unwashed for hours. That facility was a four-time repeater on our lists. The legal case is ongoing; a lawyer for the center did not respond to requests for comment.

One reason the independently owned, not-for-profit facilities might do a better job is that they tend to have more staff, which experts agree is crucial to good care. We found that on average, not-for-profits provided almost an hour of additional nursing care each day per resident, compared with for-profit facilities. They also provided nearly twice as much care from registered nurses.

In 2002, a study conducted for the federal Centers for Medicare & Medicaid Services (CMS) noted that without a daily average of 2.8 hours of care from nurse aides and 1.3 hours from licensed nurses, residents were more likely to experience poor outcomes—pressure sores and urinary incontinence, for example. "Most nursing homes are staffed significantly below that," says John Schnelle, director of the Borun Center, a joint venture of UCLA and the Jewish Home for Aging that does research on long-term care.

The CMS, however, has not recommended or adopted minimum staffing standards, a point of contention for nursing home advocates, who are pushing for them. Marvin Feuerberg, a technical director at the CMS, says officials even watered down the 2002 study's executive summary when it was given to Congress.

Instead, current rules say that staffing must be sufficient to meet the needs of nursing home residents, a standard so vague that it makes penalizing nursing homes that skimp on care almost impossible. Rules do require homes to have 8 hours of registered nursing and 24 hours of licensed nursing coverage per day. But the standard applies to all homes, no matter how many residents they have. So a nursing home with 200 residents can use the same-size staff as one with 20.

Inadequate staffing puts residents at risk. Glen Barnhill, 46, of Nashville, lived in Tennessee nursing homes for several years after he suffered a gunshot wound to the head. Barnhill, a quadriplegic who needs a ventilator to breathe, says he would sometimes go into respiratory distress while waiting for a call light to be answered. "I'd be in bed gasping and fighting for air, not knowing when the nurse would come," he says.

The AHCA says that minimum staffing rules cannot be an unfunded mandate on the part of the government. "If you're required to have x amount and certain types of staff, you need reimbursement," says Sandra Fitzler, the group's senior director of clinical operations. More money from Medicaid, which pays for more than half of all nursing home stays, would improve staffing, the industry says.

But money is not always the problem. We examined Medicaid reimbursement for nursing homes in 2002, the last year for which we had complete data. We found no evidence that the average state Medicaid payment to nursing homes had a significant impact on the percentage of homes identified as poor performers.

Playing Politics

Nursing homes are not major donors to national political campaigns, but they wield considerable clout in state capitals, where their $500, $1,000, and $3,000 contributions count with gubernatorial, state legislative, and judicial candidates.

In Arkansas, for example, the industry was a top contributor to state candidates in 2004, according to Followthemoney.org, a nonpartisan database of campaign contributions. The Arkansas Health Care Association, which represents for-profit nursing homes, gave almost $100,000 that year to candidates in the state.

The trade association also maintains an office near the Arkansas Capitol in Little Rock, where legislators can stop in and enjoy a free lunch three times a week during legislative sessions.

"They contribute a large amount of money to people's campaigns" and the politicians become beholden, says state Sen. Mary Anne Salmon, a Democrat. She adds, "Nursing homes have stopped some very good legislation that would have made things better for the elderly."

Messages from legislators, subtle and not so subtle, filter down to regulators, who have learned that nursing homes will challenge them if they press too hard. Grachia Freeman, a former nursing home inspector in Arkansas, says that supervisors "would not let me write deficiencies I wanted to write" for a facility she was inspecting. Now a nurse at a VA hospital in North Little Rock, she adds, "They were angry with me for investigating and told me not to complete the survey." We made several efforts to interview regulators in the long-term-care unit of the Arkansas Department of Health and Human Services but were repeatedly rebuffed.

This pressure "gives facilities the confidence to push back in so many ways, like appealing citations and sanctions because they know that state legislators tend to be very protective of homes in their districts," says Iris Freeman, principal consultant with Advocacy Strategy, a Minneapolis firm that works with community groups on behalf of the elderly and disabled.

Shopsmart
How You Can Find Good Nursing Home Care

Choosing a humane, well-run nursing home can be one of the most important decisions you'll make in life. Unfortunately, it can also be one of the most rushed. Even when good information is available, you may have little time to digest it, especially if a hospital discharge planner says your relative must be out in 24 hours. He or she will often suggest a particular nursing home in the area, but you may not know whether the home is your best choice or a very bad one.

If you find yourself in this situation, first know that you can use your appeal rights under Medicare to extend the hospital stay for two days. That will buy you additional time. Then follow these steps:

Get the names of local facilities. The Eldercare Locator (800-677-1116) will refer you to your local agency on aging. It, in turn, can supply you with a list of nursing homes and contact information for the local ombudsman, a government official whose job is to investigate nursing home complaints and advocate for residents and their families.

Consult our Quality Monitor. (www.Consumer Reports.org/nursinghomes). It will help you cross potentially bad homes off your list. Avoid facilities that have appeared on our list repeatedly and those that performed poorly on two of our three dimensions of quality. If a nursing home near you is on our "good" list, put it on your list of possibilities. Also check state penalty information on our site. If a nursing home has received a state fine, even a small one, consider that a warning.

Check the ownership. A resident's chances of receiving good care are better at an independent not-for-profit facility than at a for-profit chain. You should ask whether the facility is about to (or has) changed owners. One that's on the auction block might have problems, just as one with a new owner might be getting better. Be aware that if the facility is part of a large corporation that has split itself into smaller, limited-liability companies, you may have little recourse against the home if things go badly for your family member.

Check with the local ombudsman. He or she should be able to tell you about homes in your area. We say "should" because many ombudsmen have encountered pressure from the industry and are now very careful about what they say. Comments such as "You may want to look further" or an unenthusiastic "They're OK" could be warning signals.

Don't depend on the federal Web site. The Centers for Medicare & Medicaid Services maintains a Nursing Home Compare site at *www.medicare.gov*. But our comparison of the information on that site and the state inspection reports on which it is based show that you'll probably get an incomplete and possibly misleading picture of any home that you have under consideration.

Visit the homes. Once you've narrowed your search, make unannounced visits. Connie Smith of Little Rock, Ark., visited five homes, several repeatedly, before selecting the Greenhurst Nursing Center in Charleston, Ark., for her son Jordan, 23, who as a child became a quadriplegic due to a BB gun accident. She's pleased with the personal attention he has received. When Jordan turned 21, the nursing home administrator put a drop of beer on his lips to mark his coming of age.

Read each home's Form 2567. That is the facility's state inspection survey, which should be "readily accessible." If it's not and you have difficulty obtaining it, consider that a warning that the facility may be hiding damaging information. A lengthy survey with lots of violations indicates problems. The administrator might tell you they've been fixed, which may or may not be true. But even a deficiency-free survey is no guarantee of good care. It may merely mean that the inspectors were not looking very hard.

Visit the homes again. Drop in between 9:30 and 10 a.m., for example, to see how many people are still in bed. Homes with too few staff members don't get people out of bed until late in the day, if at all. Also visit at dinnertime. If 75 percent of the residents are eating in their rooms, that's not a good sign. Most people prefer to be out of bed and to eat in the dining room. Ask the nurse aides how many residents they each care for. The smaller the number, the better.

Ask about top-level turnover. If the administrator and the director of nursing have worked at a facility for several years, that's a positive sign. Frequent changes in those positions indicate instability, which could translate into poor care.

Talk to the administrator. Try to get a sense of his or her philosophy of care and how well it's communicated to staff members. Good care begins with the facility's leadership.

Easing Off of Enforcement

Although the number of deficiency citations written by state inspectors has increased 7.6 percent since 2003, according to the CMS, inspectors appear to be watering them down. Each one carries a letter code, from A through L, indicating the scope and severity of the violation. Citations labeled G through L denote actual harm or the potential for death. Codes I through L indicate that the harm was widespread, affecting many people.

State inspectors are now writing fewer deficiencies with codes that denote actual harm, such as avoidable pressure sores and medication errors. "We are going back to a less stringent and simpler enforcement," says a federal analyst familiar with nursing home inspection data at the CMS. "Everything is becoming a D level. Nursing facilities are going to challenge anything above a D level if it carries a mandatory penalty, can be used in a tort case, or will be publicly disclosed."

In 2000, 40 percent of all deficiencies carried a D designation. By 2005, the number had risen to 54 percent. The reason, says the analyst, is pressure from nursing homes on under-staffed state agencies that find it hard to muster the resources to defend their citations in court.

The most common remedy for violations is a "plan of correction." The nursing home acknowledges there is a problem and promises to fix it within a specified period. Often the problem is corrected but soon resurfaces, a phenomenon regulators call yo-yo compliance.

Token Fines or None at All

The 1987 nursing home reform law provided for monetary penalties that could be imposed by states and the federal government. But that hasn't meant that fines are collected. In fact, last year the federal Office of the Inspector General found that the CMS did not take all the required steps to collect 94 percent of past-due penalties.

Some states are doing no better. Even when inspectors find that homes are providing poor care, regulators may be slow to impose fines, if they levy them at all.

In 2003 and 2005, CONSUMER REPORTS examined whether states were levying fines against our sample of poorly performing homes. We found that the ones that could impose fines were not always using that authority. Our earlier study found that in states with the power to impose fines, only 55 percent of the facilities in our sample that could have received one actually did. In our most recent analysis, we found that states fined just 50 percent of such homes.

Eight of the 12 five-time repeaters on this year's list of poorly performing homes had not received state fines between 1999 and 2004. The others received minimal penalties. California regulators, for instance, fined White Blossom a total of $10,800 during the six years it was on our lists. The largest fine it received in any one year was $3,600.

When fines are assessed, they tend to be low, sometimes absurdly so. Consider the slap on the wrist given the Willow Tree Nursing Center in Oakland, Calif. In 2001, according to state records, a 38-year-old paraplegic with poor cognitive ability left the home on a pass. When he did not return until 2 a.m., the home's administrator ordered a nurse not to let him back in. Regulators cited the facility for failing to keep a resident free from mental abuse and assessed a fine of $700. The state, however, collected only $455 and closed the case. Seventeen months later, the state again cited Willow Tree, for failing to report an allegation of abuse within 24 hours. This time, a nurse who allegedly put a pillow over a resident's face, said, "I'm going to smother you," and then walked out of the room laughing after the patient pushed it off. The state collected $600.

States can reduce an already meager fine by 35 percent if the nursing home agrees not to appeal. The median fine in 1999 for the homes we looked at was $4,800; in 2004 it had dropped to $3,000. Less than 2 percent of the homes received a fine greater than $100,000.

"The system hasn't been hard enough on those who view penalties as the cost of doing business," says David Hoffman, a former federal prosecutor in Philadelphia who has sued many nursing homes and now consults with the industry about improving the quality of its care.

Shutting Down a Home

The CMS can disqualify a home from the Medicare and Medicaid programs, cutting off federal funds. But that remedy, the most drastic in the agency's arsenal, is used less frequently than in the past. In 1998, the number of terminations peaked at 51; in 2005 there were only 8.

States can also try to shut down what they judge to be poorly performing facilities. In 2005, Indiana regulators investigated a complaint that a student nurse aide at the Hanover Nursing Center in Hanover had beaten a resident in the face, an immediate-jeopardy violation. That inspection resulted in a 62-page report detailing numerous violations.

Regulators placed a 45-day ban on admitting new residents to the home but lifted it after further inspection. In February, Hanover's license expired, and state officials refused to grant a new one. The facility is appealing the loss of its license and a federal fine of $117,500 for the immediate-jeopardy violation. Meanwhile, it continues to operate.

Declaration of Independents

Home is where you want to live forever. Here's how.

BARBARA BASLER

Suzanne Stark, 79, lives in a book-lined apartment in central Boston's lovely Beacon Hill neighborhood. Independent and active, the author and freelance writer nevertheless acknowledges there are times when problems arise and she needs help. Like when her beloved cat Zenobia became suddenly, violently ill, and Stark couldn't get her into a carrier to take her to the veterinarian.

"I tried everything, and then I called Beacon Hill Village," she says. "I said, 'I know this is weird, but can you send someone to help me get this cat in the carrier?' And they did."

Beacon Hill Village is a revolutionary, all-encompassing concierge service created by residents who want to grow old in the homes they have lived in for years. Now, they can do that, confident that even as they age they can deal with almost any contingency, large or small, without relying on relatives or friends. To preserve their independence, they can turn to the village, as the nonprofit association is known, which helps its 320 members find virtually any service they need—from 24-hour nursing care to help with a wayward cat, often at a discounted fee.

Their innovation is so appealing that a national expert on aging at the Massachusetts Institute of Technology asserts it could well change the way Americans—and the rest of the world—grow old. "The assisted living and the die-with-a-golf-club-in-your-hand communities had better take notice," says Joseph Coughlin, director of the MIT AgeLab, a think tank on aging.

This fresh concept is already attracting attention far beyond the quaint cobblestone walkways of Beacon Hill. In the three years since it started, the village has received more than 200 inquiries—from places as diverse as Manhattan and Las Vegas.

The group's grassroots creators are now writing a how-to manual so others can replicate the village in their own neighborhoods. And MIT is working on a plan of the concept that could be used around the world.

"With Beacon Hill Village you have life, you don't have retirement," Coughlin says. The village not only links members to carefully vetted personal trainers, caterers, house cleaners, plumbers and computer advisers, it also offers them a number of free benefits such as weekly car service to the grocery. Other free benefits include monthly lectures by notable Bostonians, exercise classes and special health clinics—all activities that take place in neighborhood churches, schools and a community center.

The village hasn't yet had a request it couldn't help fill, says Judy Willett, the social worker hired to direct the association and its two other full-time employees. "We even had a member in the hospital call and ask us to find someone to pick up her betting slips at the track. And we did," she says.

"We wanted everything you'd find in a retirement community or assisted living—but we wanted these services in our own homes," explains Susan McWhinney-Morse, 72, the president of Beacon Hill Village, who was one of the 12 residents who helped create it. "We didn't want to leave the neighborhood we love."

Village founder and member J. Atwood "Woody" Ives, 69, says, "Even the places they call active retirement communities tend to be depressing. They're so artificial—everybody there is old." But, he says, by staying in his own neighborhood, "I see college students, couples, young families, old people. There is a great mix here, and I think that adds to the quality of life."

Any neighborhood resident age 50 or older can join the village. Its members include retirees in their 90s as well as working people in their 50s and 60s. "The younger ones join because they like the convenience of our services or they need help caring for a parent who lives with them," Willett says. "They want to support Beacon Hill Village, make sure it will be there as they age."

Membership costs $550 a year per person, $750 a year per couple and $100 a year for lower-income residents, who also get a $250 credit toward services. And the village has people who charge as little as $15 an hour for odd jobs.

The woman the village sent to help Suzanne Stark with Zenobia spent all afternoon with them—driving Stark and her cat to the vet, waiting, then driving them to the animal hospital and finally home. "That saved Zenobia's life," Stark says. The cost of the service: $35.

In many cases remaining at home and using the village's à la carte services is much cheaper than assisted living, Willett says. If, however, someone becomes ill enough to need 24-hour care or other expensive services, the total costs probably will equal those of a nursing home, "but with one big difference: You are in your own home."

Village employees not only provide information and referrals, they telephone members to check that each job was completed satisfactorily. Although members are entitled to highly personalized attention, the tiny staff—operating out of a one-room neighborhood office—has never been overwhelmed be-

How to Build Your Own Village

HUDDLE Form a core group of about a dozen high-profile neighbors with diverse skills and backgrounds.

COUNT YOUR CHICKENS Research your community—the number of residents over age 50, their average income, etc. Beacon Hill Village used census information to determine if there are enough people to support the venture.

KNOW YOUR CUSTOMERS Commission a survey to find out what services people want and what they will pay for them.

LINE UP PLAYERS Contact key local businesses and health providers—from local hospitals and home care agencies to repair services—to gauge their interest in working with your group.

DO THE MATH Draw up a business plan, estimating membership income and service costs. Beacon Hill Village used Harvard MBA alumni. Local universities or colleges may offer similar free consultation.

PASS THE HAT Raise seed money. 30 percent of your estimated budget. Much of Beacon Hill Village's start-up money came from contributions by neighborhood residents who believed in the idea.

GET A CHIEF Hire a director who will be the face and voice of your enterprise as you continue to recruit members and service providers.

cause only about a third of the members call the village frequently. Another third use it now and then, while the remainder draw mainly on its social offerings—lectures, weekly lunches in a local restaurant and day trips to places like the Newport Jazz Festival.

"The social aspect is the secret sauce here," says MIT's Coughlin. "Just bringing services to your door doesn't ensure a good life. People, especially older people living alone, need to be engaged, they need reasons to go out, to be a part of a community. And the village works to give them that."

The core group of 12 residents laid the groundwork for the project with meticulous research, drawing up a business plan, vetting and recruiting a number of businesses and health providers, all of them eager to have a reliable stream of customers. Two key concerns joined their effort early and helped anchor it—Harvard Medical School's Massachusetts General Hospital and HouseWorks, a Boston home services company.

The gifted amateur organizers, however, were canny enough to realize they needed help. By donating their own money and raising contributions from others in the neighborhood who believed in the idea, they hired professionals to help market the village concept to residents. They also approached several foundations for money for the subsidized memberships.

The village still relies on foundations and support from board members and the community, but membership is growing by about eight new members a month.

"Membership fees pay for about 50 percent of our expenses, and within a year we think that will rise to 60 percent," Willett says.

The leafy streets of Beacon Hill are lined with 19th-century townhouses where people such as Henry James and Louisa May Alcott once lived. Today's residents live in a dense mix of fine homes, imposing apartment buildings, condos and even subsidized housing for older people, but they still tend to be well heeled and well educated. Can their aging solution really be transplanted to other, very different communities?

Yes, says Coughlin, because innovations "always start at the top, rather than the middle or the bottom. Of all the ideas we've seen here at the AgeLab, this one has got a better chance of going mainstream than many others."

Establishing this city-bred idea in the suburbs and beyond may actually be easier "because the cost of living, the cost of services is much less expensive there than here," says Sue Bridge, 66, one of the founders who, with help from alumni volunteers from Harvard University's School of Business, wrote the village's business plan.

Coughlin points out that "some of the best-knit communities in America are not in the city but in the country, in rural agricultural areas where institutions of faith often organize services and contacts for people."

Transportation in the suburbs or exurban areas could be an issue, but he does not see it as an insurmountable problem. "You have to think creatively," he says. "Missoula, Montana, for example, uses its airport shuttles in the off-peak hours to ferry older residents where they want to go and to take families to visit relatives in nursing homes."

"What we need," Coughlin says, "are folks with the passion to work these things out." Those people may be in a neighborhood association or they may be entrepreneurs "who see an explosion of disposable income and a demand for services that needs to be met."

One of the biggest obstacles to this effort to change the way people age has been the residents themselves. Village research shows that of the 13,000 people in the Beacon Hill area, 14 percent are age 60 or older, and some of these people were the most resistant.

"We couldn't believe all of the people we approached about joining who told us, 'That's a great idea, but I'm not ready yet,' " says board member Ives. "These were people in their 80s and 90s. People just hate to admit they need any kind of help."

Instead, "too many deal with aging by cutting back on where they go and when, what they do, who they see," says Bridge. "Their lives become more and more constricted. When they join the village, suddenly life opens up again."

One resident who initially resisted the village is now a booster. "They treat me like a queen," says Dorothy Weinstein, 97, who recently signed up for a village trip to New Hampshire to see the fall leaves. "They've been a saving grace."

She uses the village grocery service and calls the office when she needs an escort to her clinic appointments. The village even has volunteers who accompany her on neighborhood walks.

A resident of Beacon Hill for 53 years, still living in the house where she and her late husband raised their sons, Weinstein wouldn't think of moving.

"Where would I be as content as I am here?" she asks. "I look out my window at the park. I see people passing. I talk to old neighbors I know. This is the way I want things."

UNIT 8

Social Policies, Programs, and Services for Older Americans

Unit Selections

Key Points to Consider

- Why do most older persons not see the new Medicare prescription drug card as really solving the problem of high cost drugs?

- Why do many people believe the U.S. government should legalize the practice of importing drugs from foreign countries?

- Why does Thomas Bethell believe that privatization of the Social Security fund would hurt older women?

- Why does Pamela Herd believe that privatization of Social Security or Medicare would be most harmful to poor older persons?

- What are the different ways that the financial solvency of the Social Security program could be achieved without privatization?

- What are the advantages and disadvantages of a single payer system of universal health coverage?

- What does William Greider propose as a new retirement program to replace all those that are now having financial difficulties of being terminated?

Student Website

www.mhcls.com/online

Internet References

Further information regarding these websites may be found in this book's preface or online.

Administration on Aging
   http://www.aoa.dhhs.gov

American Federation for Aging Research
   http://www.afar.org/

American Geriatrics Society
   http://www.americangeriatrics.org

Community Transportation Association of America
   http://www.ctaa.org

Consumer Reports State Inspection Surveys
   http://www.ConsumerReports.org

Medicare Consumer Information From the Health Care Finance Association
   http://cms.hhs.gov/default.asp?fromhcfadotgov=true

National Institutes of Health
   http://www.nih.gov

The United States Senate: Special Committee on Aging
   http://www.senate.gov/~aging/

It is a political reality that older Americans will be able to obtain needed assistance from governmental programs only if they are perceived as politically powerful. Political involvement can range from holding and expressing political opinions, voting in elections, participating in voluntary associations to help elect a candidate or party, and holding political office.

Research indicates that older people are just as likely as any other age group to hold political opinions, are more likely than younger people to vote in an election, are about equally divided between Democrats and Republicans, and are more likely than young people to hold political office. Older people, however, have shown little inclination to vote as a bloc on issues affecting their welfare despite encouragement by senior activists, such as Maggie Kuhn and the leaders of the Gray Panthers, to do so.

Gerontologists have observed that a major factor contributing to the increased push for government services for the elderly has been the publicity on their plight generated by such groups as the National Council of Senior Citizens and the American Association of Retired Persons (AARP). The desire of adult children to shift the financial burden of aged parents from themselves onto the government has further contributed to the demand for services for the elderly. The resulting widespread support for such programs has almost guaranteed their passage in Congress.

Now, for the first time, there are groups emerging that oppose increases in spending for services for older Americans. Requesting generational equity, some politically active groups argue that the federal government is spending so much on older Americans that it is depriving younger age groups of needed services.

The articles in this section raise a number of problems and issues that result from an ever-larger number and percentage of the population living to age 65 and older. In "Have Seniors Been Dealt a Bad Hand? Medicare's Drug Discount Cards," the article points out how much money older people would have by ordering drugs online from Canadian pharmacies rather than using

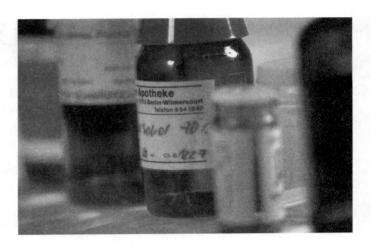

the new Medicare drug prescription card program. In "Social Security's 70th Anniversary: Surviving 20 Years of Reform," the author points out the success of the Social Security program and why he believes it will be financially solvent for well into the future. In "Universalism Without the Targeting: Privatizing the Old-Age Welfare State," Pamela Herd points out how privatization would threaten the current redistribution of monies and services that Social Security and Medicare provide to maintain an adequate standard of living for the very poor.

Patricia Barry in "Coverage For All," reviews Massachusetts and Vermont's universal health care coverage programs and points out that these may well be the direction that health care coverage in the United States is headed in the near future. William Greider in "Riding Into the Sunset" gives the economic problems of the current retirement funds and proposes a mandatory and universal saving system that he believes would be more durable than the current programs.

Have Seniors Been Dealt a Bad Hand?

Medicare's Drug Discount Cards

When Medicare's drug discount cards were unveiled in May, 74-year-old Evelyn Levin considered enrolling in a plan. An interim measure until Medicare's full drug benefit begins in 2006, these cards would, in the words of the Bush administration, "give seniors the power to save on prescription drugs" and "demand the best prices." The only tangible benefit of the 2003 Medicare law seniors will see before November's elections, the White House and other supporters of the law are anxious to see the cards succeed.

The question is: Are seniors grateful for the cards or just confused and frustrated?

Evelyn and her husband, Seth, 70, together take six prescription medicines daily. For the past several years, this Manhattan couple has purchased their drugs online from a Canadian pharmacy. A web-savvy senior, Evelyn figured she would visit Medicare's website to research the cards. It was there she ran into her first problem. "I couldn't get through to the site because too many people were trying to access it at the same time and it was overloaded."

Medicare officials estimated 7 million hits to the website were made the first week the cards became available. Medicare's toll-free hotline, an option for seniors without Internet access, was also busy, logging 1.7 million calls in the first week, 10 times more than usual.

Choosing from the more than 70 Medicare-approved cards has generated widespread confusion among many seniors and their families. "When I was finally able to get through to the website I found it very, very confusing," Evelyn remarked. Aside from the sheer number of choices, the cards do not lend themselves to simple comparisons. Each card offers different discounts, different drugs and different participating pharmacies.

"It took a lot of research and reading to get the information I needed to make the right choices for us," Evelyn said. "And after all that, I was furious by what I found. The card companies can change their discounts every week, but we would be locked into a card for a year! There may be a 15 percent discount one week and none the next. It's just not worth it."

Evelyn's complaints echo those commonly expressed by other seniors and advocates. As drug prices and discounts continue to fluctuate, confused seniors are struggling to determine which card will work best with their personal circumstances. A Harvard University study revealed average drug card savings would range around 17% off retail prices. However, those savings pale in

Tips for Choosing a Medicare Drug Discount Card

Do Your Homework

Research all your options. Visit Medicare's website at www.medicare.gov or call 1-800-MEDICARE and have available a list of your drugs. You will not find one card that offers discounts on all your medications, so choose a plan that offers the greatest discounts on your most expensive drugs. Compare the benefits of the various plans to all your current discounts and decide whether you should even enroll in a plan.

Beware of Discount Card Scams

Medicare-approved drug cards will not be sold by any telemarketer or door-to-door salesman. Do not give any personal information, including your Social Security number or credit card information, to someone over the phone. Legitimate drug card sponsors will be stamped with an official logo and are listed on Medicare's website www.medicare. gov/assistanceprograms or you can confirm their legitimacy by calling 1-800-MEDICARE.

Low-Income Seniors Get Credit

If you do not have any drug coverage and earn $12,569 annually (or $16,862 for a couple), sign up for the card. Low income beneficiaries receive an annual $600 credit on the card and will not have to pay an annual fee; although they will have co-pays of 5% to 10% for each prescription. Visit Medicare's website at www.medicare.gov or call 1-800-MEDICARE to sign up.

comparison to the 40% discounts Levin finds in Canada. "I have an ulcer and for 100 pills it's $190 in Canada, compared to $360 in the United States—it's almost half the price," Evelyn explained. "Buying from Canada always saves me money and buying online couldn't be more simple. It's a no-brainer. For middle-class people like us, it ensures there's money for other things like food." Evelyn and Seth Levin are not the only ones to discover

Comparing Your Prescription Drug Discount Options

Ask prospective card sponsors these questions before joining a drug discount program

Cost of Drugs

1. **How much will each drug I take cost under the program?**
2. **What other costs will I have?**
   - Is there a monthly premium
   - Is there an annual enrollment fee?
   - Is there a deductible?
   - Is there a co-pay?
3. **Are the costs of the program worth it?**
4. **How will I be able to find out about changes to the list of discounted drugs?**

Access to Discounts

1. **Will I be able to use the pharmacies I normally use?**
2. **Are discounts available by mail order?**

If you are in a Medicare Private Plan (HMO or PPO)

1. **How does the HMO's drug coverage coordinate with the program?**

Service Area

1. **Does the program work outside my state?**
2. **What happens if I travel outside my area?**

that the cards do not yield the same savings as retiree health benefits, state drug assistance programs, or Canadian purchases.

As of June 1, the first day card discounts went into effect, only 2.8 million of Medicare's 35 million eligible beneficiaries had signed up for a card. Most, however, were automatically enrolled into the cards because they belong to a Medicare-managed care plan. Only about 400,000 actually chose to sign up. Medicare officials are hoping that 7.3 million beneficiaries will eventually sign up for a card.

There is little dispute, however, that the 7.2 million low-income beneficiaries who have no drug coverage and are eligible for the $600 credit should sign up for a card. The government will spend $4.6 million on outreach programs in urban and rural areas to enroll low-income seniors and persons with disabilities, according to the Department of Health and Human Services. At least six states—Maine, Massachusetts, Michigan, New Jersey, Connecticut and New York—intend to automatically enroll low-income seniors who are already in state drug assistance programs into a Medicare-approved card plan. Some states have decided against automatic enrollment because the state drug program is already more generous than the discount cards.

As seniors try to make sense of the new Medicare reality, the cards portend the greater complexity that lies ahead. "The 2006 drug benefit promises even more daunting complexity," predicts Robert Hayes, president of the Medicare Rights Center, an independent organization that provides counseling services. "The administration and Congress should create what the American people want and need: a prescription drug program that treats everyone equal, negotiates fair drug prices and provides reliable and comprehensive coverage."

Despite Medicare's offerings, Evelyn and Seth Levin are likely to continue doing what they've been doing all along: getting their drugs outside the U.S. "I'm not one to march or go to rallies," Evelyn said, "but I will march in protest if the government stops allowing seniors to buy their drugs from Canada. Once again, we are at the mercy of big business and the administration. We must all speak out against those who would make it difficult, and in some cases impossible, to pay for our needed medications."

Social Security's 70th Anniversary: Surviving 20 Years of Reform

L. RANDALL WRAY

Social Security turned 70 on August 14, [2005], although no national celebration marked the occasion.[1] Rather, our top policymakers in Washington continue to suggest that the system is "unsustainable." While our nation's most successful social program, and among its longest lived, has allowed generations of Americans to live with dignity in retirement, many think it is time to retire Social Security itself. They claim it is necessary to shift more responsibility to individuals and to scale back the promises made to the coming waves of retiring baby boomers.

Even the nonpartisan Social Security Administration has been enlisted in the effort to lower expectations, posting on its website the following caution to today's 26-year-old: "Unless changes are made, when you reach age 62 in 2041, benefits for all retirees could be cut by 26 percent and could continue to be reduced every year thereafter. If you lived to be 100 years old in 2079 (which will be more common by then), your scheduled benefits could be reduced by 32 percent from today's scheduled levels." Private accounts, lower benefits, and—perhaps—higher taxes are the prescribed remedy for "unfunded" trillions of commitments we have made to tomorrow's seniors. In this note, I provide a brief assessment of the curious transformation of America's most popular and efficient safety net into a program that is widely regarded as requiring thorough reform.

There is no question that Social Security has been under attack by well-organized and well-funded opponents for the past two decades. As my colleague Max Skidmore has documented, the enemies of the program have been there from the beginning, but they have had little success until recently (Skidmore 1999). Originally, the program was criticized on the basis that it was socialistic. However, the framers of the Social Security Act anticipated such claims and consequently formulated the program as if it were an insurance plan, with payroll taxes that could be counted as "contributions" and "benefit payments" that bore some relation to the contributions. Americans came to believe that they earned benefits because they "paid into" the program. And because the program was never means tested, it enjoyed wide support. Hence, rather than socialistic welfare, the program has been viewed as little different from a pension plan. For several de-

cades, this misconception effectively quashed criticism, so the program was expanded, rather than cut (Wray 2001).

However, beginning in the 1980s, the critics seized on an apparent weakness. Slower economic growth after 1970, lower birth rates, longer life spans, and especially the coming retirement of a wave of baby boomers all supposedly threatened the long-run financial viability of Social Security. The enemies of the program formulated a two-pronged attack. First, they began a campaign to convince younger people that because of shaky finances they would never collect benefits equal to what they paid into the program (Skidmore 1999). This became an increasingly easy sell for younger, high-income workers because the redistributive aspects of the program provide fairly low "money's worth" returns for the "pension" provided by Social Security. (Note that the debate mostly ignored all the "non-pension" aspects of the program, such as disability and survivors' benefits, which make it a good deal for just about all Americans.) Second, the Greenspan Commission was formed in 1983 to resolve the long-run financial problems with "reforms" that included large payroll tax increases and a gradual rise of the normal age of retirement (Papadimitriou and Wray 1999a). These changes reinforced the claim that Social Security was a bad deal for younger workers, who were already seeing take-home pay fall during a period in which labor was under attack by the Reagan administration.

After the Greenspan Commission had "solved" the financial problems, the Social Security Administration adopted increasingly pessimistic assumptions for its long-run forecasts—as documented by Skidmore (2001) and by actuary David Langer (2000). Not surprisingly, a "looming financial crisis" reappeared, and hysteria about reforming Social Security was revived. Taxes would have to be raised, benefits would have to be cut, and, more importantly, the return on Trust Fund assets would have to be increased. As the stock market performed well throughout most of the 1980s and then picked up the pace in the 1990s, the enemies saw a chance to privatize the program while playing the role of savior. At the same time, the "friends" of Social Security, mostly Democrats and Big Labor, also saw a chance to exploit popular fears. They would play along with the enemies, pretending there really was a financial problem, so that *they* could save Social Security and thereby win votes. Polls consistently show that voters trust Democrats more on Social Security; hence, given a choice between Republican schemes to "save" the program through privatization or Democratic plans to "save" it by placing the Trust Funds off limits, the voters would choose the Democrats.

I have been writing about Social Security since the late 1980s, and in 1990, I published a critique of *Can America Afford to Grow Old?* a book by Henry Aaron, Michael Bosworth, and Gary Burtless that argued that the only way to take care of baby boomers would be to immediately increase national saving (Wray 1990, 1990–91; Aaron et al. 1989; Aaron 1990–91). This could be done, according to the authors, by running budget surpluses, adding to national savings, and increasing the size of the Trust Fund. Hence, this book could be seen as a road map for the evolving Democratic party position during the Clinton years. However, I argued at the time that a larger Trust Fund could not in any way provide for future retirees, nor would it add to national savings. Rather, the Trust Fund represents a leakage that lowers aggregate demand; all else being equal, this lowers economic growth and thus makes it more difficult to take care of future retirees. Aaron wrote a response to my piece, arguing that he had thought that such "vulgar Keynesianism" was "blessedly extinct" (Aaron 1990–91). According to Aaron, running budget surpluses to add to the Trust Fund would indeed increase saving and lower interest rates, thus stimulating investment and economic growth, making it easier to take care of retirees.

As we now know, the Clinton budget did turn sharply toward surplus, and those surpluses were projected at the time to continue for at least a generation. A number of economists advocated "saving" this surplus for future retirees. As laid out in the plan by Aaron, et al., President Clinton proposed to take a portion of each year's surplus and add it to the Trust Fund (Wray 1999a, 1999b). Essentially, this would allow double counting of the surplus run by Social Security, since most of the budget surpluses accrued during the Clinton years were due to payroll taxes that far exceeded program benefits. During the 2000 presidential race, Al Gore used Social Security "lockboxes" as a primary campaign issue, confusing an internal bookkeeping operation (as Social Security's assets in the Trust Fund equal the Treasury's liabilities to Social Security, this is a case of the government owing itself) with availability of "finance" for the government as a whole. A wide variety of economists (including Aaron) embarrassed themselves by claiming that this was "good economics," going so far as to sign a petition in support of the plan (Wray 1999b).

I was told by economic advisors to top Democrats and big unions that they realized lockboxes were nonsense but believed it was politically pragmatic to endorse irregular accounting as a means to "save" the program. I responded that there was no need to run budget surpluses in order to credit Social Security's Trust Fund; the government can immediately credit the Trust Fund with trillions of dollars of assets, offset by the Treasury's commitment to make timely benefit payments when and as necessary (Wray 1999b). Most importantly, I worried about the long-term damage that would be done to the program by creating a false crisis and then resolving it with a preposterous gimmick. Of course, the Democrats' strategy did backfire: Gore lost the election, the Clinton budget surpluses brought down the economy and morphed into huge deficits "as far as the eye can see," and President Bush took on Social Security "reform" as a major goal of his administration. Ironically, the Republicans now quote President Clinton whenever Democrats try to deny that the program faces a crisis, leaving Dems in the untenable position of either admitting they were lying in the 1990s or that they are lying now (Wray 2005).

During the Clinton years I wrote a series of pieces critical of alternative plans to "save" Social Security, including those proposed by Democrats as well as those advanced by Republicans (Wray 1999a, 1999b; Papadimitriou and Wray 1999a, 1999b). After reading one of these critiques (Papadimitriou and Wray 1999b), Charles P. Blahous, policy director for Senator Judd Gregg (R-NH), engaged me in a series of e-mail exchanges. He accepted my critiques of the Clinton plan, but was bothered by my critique of the Gregg-Breaux proposal (which, briefly, included partial privatization, a government-subsidized savings plan, and a combination of benefit cuts and tax hikes; Blahous had apparently played some role in formulating the plan, and many of its features were included in later reform proposals).He also insisted that there really was a Social Security crisis and that the only feasible solution would be to privatize. He raised a number of issues that appeared at the time to be rather bizarre: that the crisis would begin as soon as tax revenue fell below benefit payments (that is, long before the Armageddon date cited by many economists as the year in which the Trust Fund is expected to be depleted); that faster economic growth would make the problem *worse*; that under current law, benefits would have to be cut by more than a quarter as soon as the Trust Fund was depleted; and that Social Security was a terrible deal for blacks and for women. More interestingly, when President Bush appointed his Reform Commission to study the problem, none other than Blahous was picked as executive director.[2] Blahous's hand could be seen all over the various reports issued by the Commission, with many of the same arguments that he had made previously in e-mails to me. The Commission claimed that Social Security was "broken" and required a "complete overhaul"; it bemoaned the bad deal cut for women and minorities; it engaged in a sleight of hand by comparing its "reforms" against "current law benefits" that were actually a quarter below those promised in the current benefit formula (none of the proposed reforms came close to providing the legislated benefits); it claimed that the present value of Social Security's shortfall was $3.2 trillion; and it proposed partial privatization and benefit cuts as the solution (Wray 2001).[3] What appeared then to be bizarre claims are now commonplace.

However, terrorism and security issues forced Social Security to the back burner during the first Bush term. After reelection, Bush felt he had a mandate to return to privatization of Social Security. At first, supporters of privatization claimed that it would resolve the "financial crisis"; eventually, the President admitted that the private accounts would worsen the program's finances (Wray 2005). Finally, he returned to the Commission's suggestion to drop wage indexing of future benefits (at least for all but the lowest-income workers) and hinted that he would consider elimination of the cap on wages subject to taxation (Wray 2005). If successful, these changes would substantially erode the support of middle- and upper-income earners, who would face huge cuts to benefits and higher taxes. Partial privatization would almost certainly lead to lower retirement payments for many lower-income workers (with management fees eating up the returns on their small accounts). Further, as many middle- and upper-income workers would opt for the privatization alternative, the amount of benefits received directly from Social Security by them would fall toward insignificance (Krugman 2005). Over the long haul, the nonprivatized portion of Social Security would be converted to a "welfare" program, important only to low-income people. This could be the last straw for what has long been America's most successful and popular government program.

The truth is that Social Security does not, and indeed *cannot*, face any financial crisis. It is a federal government program and as such cannot become insolvent. Social Security benefits are paid in the same way that the federal government makes expenditures for all of its other programs: by cutting a Treasury check or, increasingly, by directly crediting a bank account. Social Security is an unusual program only in that we pretend the payroll taxes "pay for" benefits; in reality, trying to maintain a balance between these flows is purely a politically inspired accounting procedure. Any federal government spending must be accounted for, but it cannot be *financially* constrained by specific or even general tax revenues. Further, the Trust Fund does not and cannot provide finance for Social Security. So long as the full faith and credit of the U.S. government stands behind the promised benefits, they can and will be paid, whether the Trust Fund has a positive or negative balance. Many proponents of the current system who understand this economic reality still want to accumulate a Trust Fund on the argument that it provides political protection. Perhaps the Trust Fund provided cover at one time, but it no longer serves even that purpose. It is precisely because there is a Trust Fund that the privatizers are making headway: if there were no Trust Fund, there would be nothing to privatize. Indeed, some of the privatizers see the trillion and a half dollars in the Trust Fund as a potential boost to flagging equity markets. Further, the eventual "exhaustion" of the Trust Fund plays a critical role in all of the schemes to increase returns on assets through privatization. Hence, the irregular accounting only hinders development of a clear understanding of the issues involved.

Social Security provides a substantial measure of security for aged persons, survivors, and disabled persons—and their dependents. It has never missed a payment, nor will it ever do so, as long as the full faith and credit of the U.S. government lies behind the program. Reform might be desired, and might even be necessary, but not because of any mythical looming financial crisis. Our nation is undergoing slow but important demographic changes that probably warrant informed discussion of the future shape of Social Security. While the baby boomers receive all the attention, other demographic and economic changes may be more important, including a greater proportion of female-headed households, higher immigration and the rising proportion of "minority" populations (already a majority in several states), and increasing economic inequality. Combined with the disappearance of employer-provided defined benefit pension plans and reduced employment security, these trends actually might strengthen the arguments for more generous and secure publicly provided safety nets—*not* for benefit cuts and privatization. However, none of these challenges rises to the level of a programmatic crisis; we will have years and even decades to make adjustments to Social Security should we decide they are necessary. In the meantime, happy 70th birthday, Social Security, with many happy returns.

Notes

1. Interestingly, the only reference to the anniversary available on the Social Security Administration's website is an *Orlando Sentinel* editorial by Jo Anne B. Barnhart, commissioner of Social Security, who notes that while the program has paid "approximately $8.4 trillion in benefits to nearly 200 million people," and while the benefits for "our parents, grandparents, and great-grandparents . . . are secure and will be paid . . . the same cannot be said for my teenage son and his friends" (Barnhart 2005).

2. Before that appointment, Blahous served as executive director of the business-sponsored Alliance for Worker Retirement Security from June 2000 through February 2001. He joined the National Economic Council on February 26, 2001, and now serves as special assistant to the president for economic policy.

3. See Diamond and Orszag (2002a) for a careful analysis of the Commission's reports. Blahous tried to defend the claims made for the various "reforms" in a memo characterized by *New York Times* columnist Paul Krugman as "hysterical. The number of non sequiturs and misrepresentations Mr. Blahous manages to squeeze into just a few pages may set a record" (Krugman 2002). See Blahous's response (2002) and Diamond and Orszag's rejoinder (2002b).

References

Aaron, Henry J. 1990–91. "Comment: Can the Social Security Trust Fund Contribute to Savings?" *Journal of Post Keynesian Economics* 13:2: 171.

Aaron, Henry J., Barry P. Bosworth, and Gary Burtless. 1989. *Can America Afford to Grow Old?* Washington, D.C.: Brookings Institution.

Barnhart, Jo Anne B. 2005. "Social Security Boss: Send Signal of Strength." *Orlando Sentinel,* August 11. www.ssa.gov/article081105.htm

Blahous, Charles P. 2002. "Problems with the Diamond/Orszag Paper on the Proposals of the President's Commission to Strengthen Social Security." June 18. Available from Peter A. Diamond, MIT, or Peter R. Orszag, Brookings Institution.

Diamond, Peter A., and Peter R. Orszag. 2002a. "An Assessment of the Proposals of the President's Commission to Strengthen Social Security." Washington, D.C.: The Brookings Institution. www.brookings.edu/views/papers/orszag/20020618.htm

———. 2002b. "A Response to the Executive Director of the President's Commission to Strengthen Social Security." Washington, D.C.: Center on Budget and Policy Priorities. www.cbpp.org/6-25-02socsec.pdf

Krugman, Paul. 2002. "Fear of All Sums." *New York Times*, June 21. www.pkarchive.org/column/062102.html

———. 2005. "A Gut Punch to the Middle." *New York Times*, May 2.

Langer, David. 2000. "Cooking Social Security's Deficit." *Christian Science Monitor,* January 4.

Papadimitriou, Dimitri B., and L. Randall Wray. 1999a. *Does Social Security Need Saving? Providing for Retirees throughout the Twenty-first Century.* Public Policy Brief No. 55. Annandale-on-Hudson, N.Y.: The Levy Economics Institute.

———. 1999b. "More Pain, No Gain: The Breaux Plan Slashes Social Security Benefits Unnecessarily." Policy Note 1999/8. Annandale-on-Hudson, N.Y.: The Levy Economics Institute.

Skidmore, Max J. 1999. *Social Security and Its Enemies: The Case for America's Most Efficient Insurance Program.* Boulder, Colorado: Westview Press.

———. 2001. "What Happened to the Social Security Surplus? An Examination of the Trustees' Projections." Paper presented at "The Social Security 'Crisis': Critical Analysis and Solutions" conference at the University of Missouri–Kansas City.

Wray, L. Randall. 1990. "A Review of *Can Americans Afford to Grow Old?: Paying for Social Security*, by Aaron, Bosworth, and Burtless." *Journal of Economic Issues* 24:4: 1175–1179.

———. 1990–91. "Can the Social Security Trust Fund Contribute to Savings?" *Journal of Post Keynesian Economics* 13:2: 155–170.

———. 1999a. "The Emperor Has No Clothes: President Clinton's Proposed Social Security Reform." Policy Note 1999/2. Annandale-on-Hudson, N.Y.: The Levy Economics Institute.

———. 1999b. "Surplus Mania: A Reality Check." Policy Note 1999/3. Annandale-on-Hudson, N.Y.: The Levy Economics Institute.

———. 2001. "Killing Social Security Softly with Faux Kindness: The Draft Report by the President's Commission on Social Security Reform." Policy Note 2001/6. Annandaleon-Hudson, N.Y.: The Levy Economics Institute.

———. 2005. "Manufacturing a Crisis: The Neocon Attack on Social Security." Policy Note 2005/2. Annandale-on-Hudson, N.Y.: The Levy Economics Institute.

Senior Scholar **L. RANDALL WRAY** is a professor at the University of Missouri–Kansas City and director of research at the Center for Full Employment and Price Stability.

The Levy Economics Institute is publishing this research with the conviction that it is a constructive and positive contribution to the discussion on relevant policy issues. Neither the Institute's Board of Governors nor its advisers necessarily endorse any proposal made by the author.

Universalism Without the Targeting

Privatizing the Old-Age Welfare State

Decades of conservative attempts to scale back Social Security and Medicare, by limiting the program's universality through means testing and drastic benefit cuts, have failed. Thus, after numerous unsuccessful attempts at dismantling the U.S.'s universal old-age welfare state, or even meaningfully restraining its growth, conservative critics have developed a new approach. They are wrapping promarket "privatization" policy proposals in the popular universal framework of Social Security and Medicare. What is fundamentally different about privatization is that it embraces (or at least acquiesces to) key aspects of universalism, including broad-based eligibility and benefits that "maintain accustomed standards of living," which leave universal programs with rock-hard public support. Proponents argue privatization will "save" these programs. What distinguishes this approach from past retrenchment efforts is that promarket privatization policies, while supporting key universal tenets, will retrench Social Security's and Medicare's redistributive facets. Instead of limiting the most popular features of universalism, privatization proposals limit the redistributive elements of our large social insurance programs.

Pamela Herd, PhD[1]

Social Security and Medicare are the United States' most popular social welfare policies. Despite decades of conservative attempts to scale them back, our universal old-age welfare state remains the bedrock of American social policy. Attempts to limit the programs' universality through means testing and drastic benefit cuts have failed. Moreover, Social Security and Medicare have almost exclusively expanded their breadth and depth since their inceptions.

Thus, after numerous unsuccessful attempts at dismantling the U.S.'s universal old-age welfare state, or even meaningfully restraining its growth, conservative critics have developed a new approach. They are wrapping promarket "privatization" policy proposals in the popular universal framework of Social Security and Medicare. As President Bush argues, he wants to institute individual accounts to save Social Security. What is fundamentally different about privatization as a reform goal is that it embraces (or at least acquiesces to) key aspects of universalism, including broad-based eligibility and benefits that "maintain accustomed standards of living," which leave universal programs with rock-hard public support (Korpi, 1983; Korpi & Palme, 1998).

Privatizing Social Security and Medicare would not change universal eligibility, unlike means testing reforms or proposals to make contributions to both programs voluntary. And in regards to benefits, a common refrain from privatization proponents runs along these lines: "Such an enormous financial gap (referring to Medicare and Social Security's current fiscal problems) cannot be closed by raising taxes and cutting benefits, which would greatly harm working people and retirees. The only solution is to reform the system by taking advantage of the efficiencies, incentives, competition, and productivity of the private sector" (Ferraro, 1998). Basically, privatizing will address the program's fiscal problems with a limited, and in some cases, positive impact on benefits. The validity of these claims are addressed in this article. Nonetheless, true or not, the key claim with this new reform approach is the promise to maintain key features of universal policies, particularly broad-based eligibility and generous benefits, which keeps middle-class Americans happy and the program popular.

But while privatization proponents promise a generous and robust old-age welfare state, privatization will retrench the redistributive aspects of both Social Security and Medicare. Ironically, past less popular retrenchment efforts, including means testing and even benefit cuts, did not directly challenge the redistributive nature of these programs.

The Political Strength of Universal Programs

Throughout the world, universal programs, like Social Security and Medicare, are consistently the most popular social welfare policies. Basically, when all citizens contribute to and benefit

---

[1]LBJ School of Public Affairs, University of Texas, Austin.

from a social policy it engenders enormous amounts of public support and loyalty for those policies. The evidence for this is overwhelming (Korpi & Palme, 1998). Any cuts or retrenchment to these programs must pass the muster of middle-class voters who benefit from them, and politicians are loathe to risk negative reactions from such a large voting block.

Any approach that would have significantly and negatively impacted the Social Security benefits of middle-class Americans, thereby undermining the program's universal principles, has gained no traction. Conservative politicians in the United States have faced voters' wrath in the past when they have attempted to do just that. Republican nominee Barry Goldwater's suggestion that participation in Social Security be made "voluntary" became a symbol of his "radical conservativism" (Derthick, 1979, p. 187) and contributed to his landslide loss to Lyndon Johnson in the 1964 election. Throughout the 1980s and into the 1990s proposals to means test Social Security benefits fell on deaf ears. Reagan was attacked in the 1980s for proposals to reduce Social Security benefits. Examples like these led to Social Security's nickname as the "Third Rail" of politics. Thus, during the past 50 years, most changes to Social Security have expanded the number of beneficiaries and the size of those benefits.

Medicare, created in 1965 compared to Social Security's inception in 1935, has a similar, albeit a much shorter, political history. Most changes to the program have expanded, as opposed to retrenched, benefits. The most recent of which was the inclusion of a prescription drug benefit. And programmatic reforms that would undermine its universal principles have been met with significant resistance. One of the prime examples of this is the 1988 Medicare Catastrophic Coverage Act, which while expanding benefits, would have instituted significantly higher charges for higher income beneficiaries. The Act was unpopular with seniors, and it was repealed in 1989 (Rice, Desmond, & Gabel, 1990).

What connects all these past reform efforts is that they did not explicitly challenge Social Security's and Medicare's redistributive features. Instead, they tried to limit the programs' universality through means testing or significantly limit the depth of that universality by advocating large benefit cuts. Means testing, in theory, is actually more redistributive. And benefit cuts, though they would be hardest for the poorest, would not alter the programs' redistributive structures. Of course, though, the long-term concern with means testing or dramatic benefit cuts is that they would *eventually* destroy our most successful redistributive social policies by undermining the programs' popularity among the general public; means testing and drastically cutting benefits would hamper middle-class benefits and thus their support for the old-age welfare state.

This is not to say, however, that small benefit cuts, means testing, and decreasing eligibility ages have not happened or that they are no longer being proposed. Universalism has been "stretched" (Kingson, 1994). Social Security's eligibility age rose from 65 to 67, and higher income beneficiaries now have their benefits taxed. In the next few years, high-income Medicare beneficiaries will pay higher premiums, and changes in 1997 entailed that beneficiaries would pay more

for their benefits. Further, proposals to privatize have been accompanied by proposals to reduce benefits to offset Social Security's long-term fiscal problems. But these potential benefit cuts are a separate policy issue from privatization. Moreover, advocates argue that necessary benefits cuts due to Social Security's fiscal problems will be smaller because of privatization.

Ultimately, what makes privatization different from past retrenchment efforts is that it embraces key aspects of universalism to generate public support for reforms while attacking these programs' redistributive features that have for so long been protected within the programs' popular universal frameworks. That said, I am not arguing that privatization will have no negative impact on universality. The extent to which universal programs inspire social solidarity and mutual obligation would likely be harmed by a reform that fosters the individualistic, rather than collective, aspects of Social Security. Moreover, privatization would likely weaken important insurance aspects of the program, particularly disability and spousal and survivor benefits. That said, Social Security has always fostered an individualistic spirit by clearly linking individual retirement worker benefits, and to a lesser extent disability benefits, with individual earnings. In the end, most privatization proponents claim privatization will maintain the aspects of universalism that keep programs popular—broad-based eligibility and generous benefits.

The Growing Popularity of Privatization

Unlike past retrenchment efforts, the idea of privatization is gaining traction among the public. Support for privatizing Social Security varies from 50% to 70% depending on the question wording, though the support is far greater among younger than older Americans. Contrastingly, public support for past retrenchment efforts is far weaker. The percentage of individuals approving means testing Social Security benefits comes in at about 40%, while reducing benefits comes in at 35% (Public Agenda, 2004). Even in the most recent polls where support for President Bush's partial privatization plan has fallen, the majority of Americans (56%) support diverting a portion of their payroll tax into an individual account, whereas support for means testing benefit cuts is much lower (Social Polling Report, 2005).

Support for privatizing Medicare is even more striking. To fix Medicare's fiscal problems, almost 8 in 10 Americans support allowing seniors to choose among many private health plans with a fixed monetary contribution from the government (Employee Benefit Research Institute [EBRI], 2001). Comparatively, 54% support increasing Medicare premiums for those with incomes above $50,000, while 27% favor increasing the age of eligibility (EBRI).

The following two sections, which explore Social Security and Medicare separately, answer these two questions. First, why is privatization more popular than past reform or retrenchment efforts? Specifically, how is this reform agenda being sold? Second, how does this reform agenda line up with the conservative agenda and what are the impacts of this on the redistributive elements of Social Security and Medicare?

Social Security

Most Social Security privatization proposals entail shifting about 2%–4% of the 12.4% payroll tax (split between employers and employees) into individual accounts that Americans would invest in the stock market. That 2%–4% would now be a contribution to an individual account. The key reason for the popularity of these reform proposals, compared to past reform approaches, is that they do not undermine the principles of universalism that have kept the program popular. These reforms promise the maintenance of relatively generous benefits and universal eligibility. In fact, proponents argue that privatizing Social Security will "save" it from bankruptcy and limit the need for large benefit cuts to fix its fiscal problems (President's Commission to Strengthen Social Security, 2001).

While I will examine these claims momentarily, what is critical to point out is that a major reason why privatization has been a relatively popular reform idea is because politicians and policy advocates no longer talk about eliminating or downsizing the program. Instead, privatization is framed as a way to save Social Security. Yet, this is a reform that can still meet a common conservative principle: limited government intervention. Specifically, privatization would give individuals more control over their payroll taxes, and the government would have a lesser ability to redistribute. Privatizations falls in line with past retrenchment efforts, means testing and benefit cuts, because it shifts individual contributions back toward individuals who would bear the risks and rewards of controlling these resources.

Part of the public support for privatization is because proponents argue it will help save a bankrupt social policy. But is it really bankrupt? Many have shown how the "crisis" is severely overstated (Quadagno, 1996). The Social Security trustees estimate that the program's 75-year shortfall could be fixed by a 1.9% increase in payroll tax (shared between employers and employees), which hasn't been raised since 1983, while the Congressional Budget Office (CBO, 2004a) estimates a 1% increase. Another way to lend some proportion to the issue is that while President Bush has specifically argued Social Security is financially unsustainable in its current form, the money spent on the recent tax cut would have completely offset the 75-year shortfall. Finally, the projections that show a deficit are based on all kinds of assumptions about fertility, mortality, immigration, and the economy. For those in their 20s, the analogous forecast is predicting what their children, who are not born yet, will be doing in retirement. (Herd & Kingson, 2005)

Further, would privatization "save" Social Security? The argument to prefund the system is theoretically appealing. There would be no fiscal problem if each individual was funding their own retirement. But when theory hits the ground, the possibility that creating individual accounts will financially save Social Security is not even a remote certainty (Diamond & Orszag, 2002). First and foremost it would cost around 2 trillion dollars to switch the system over. Current beneficiaries need their benefits as future individual account holders shift their payroll taxes towards those accounts. Thus, there is a need for additional revenue.

And though proponents argue privatization would increase peoples' benefit, this claim is questionable. The privatization proposal that came from the President's Commission to Strengthen Social Security made benefit comparisons between the current and proposed system based on current projected benefit levels reduced by 30% to account for the shortfall (Diamond & Orszag, 2002). Then, using this baseline, they claimed privatization would increase Social Security benefits when, in fact, benefits would be substantially reduced to address the shortfall. Aside from the shortfall issue, administrative costs and the ability of individuals to invest wisely call into question whether individual accounts can produce the strong return proponents of privatization hope for (CBO, 2004a).

How Privatizing Undermines Redistribution

The effort to privatize Social Security has its roots in neoliberalism, which argues against most government intervention. The basic theory is that income is best left in the hands of individuals, as opposed to the government. The notion of redistribution, shifting resources from wealthier to poorer Americans, runs contrary to this sentiment. And this is precisely why opponents of government intervention dislike Social Security. While it is questionable that privatizing Social Security will "save" it, there is little doubt it will have a significant and negative impact on the program's progressiveness. So how does creating individual accounts, or privatizing Social Security, undermine the program's progressiveness? Privatization limits the program's ability to redistribute.

While Social Security's universal structure has engendered wide public support among middle class Americans, it has also been enormously successful at protecting some of the poorest Americans. In 1970, before the largest expansion of Social Security benefits with the automatic cost of living increases, about 1 in 4 elderly persons lived below the poverty line. In 2003, just 1 in 10 elderly persons lived below the poverty line (Census Bureau, 2004). Comparatively, the poverty rate for children rose and remained stagnant for working-age adults.

Social Security protects poor Americans because, as Theda Skocpol (1991) argues, it "targets within universalism." Poor Americans benefit from the re-distributive benefit formula. Simply, low-income workers have a higher percentage of their lifetime earnings replaced by their benefits than do high-income workers. It is these beneficiaries who are most vulnerable to poverty. Not including Social Security benefits in individuals' incomes raises the poverty rate from 10% to almost 50% (Porter, Larin, & Primus, 1999).

Targeting, however, is done under the cover of universalism. Unlike means tested programs, like the eliminated Aid to Families with Dependent Children (AFDC), which are constantly retrenched because they lack broad support, universal programs like Social Security maintain popular support because everyone contributes to and benefits from the program.

The shift toward individual accounts would restrain Social Security's ability to redistribute resources. The high-income replacement rates that low-income workers receive may be threatened by privatization. Quite simply, the more payroll taxes are diverted to individual accounts, the less the government will be able to redistribute those resources. Of course, women, Blacks, and Hispanics would be particularly hard hit given their relatively low earnings. Compared to the White man's dollar, women still earn just 70 cents, Black women earn just 63 cents, Hispanic women earn 53 cents, and Black and Hispanic men earn 60 cents (National Committee on Pay Equity, 2004).

One of the most enlightening studies of privatization was done in the county of Galveston, Texas (Wilson, 1999). On January 1, 1982, the county opted out of Social Security and developed a privatized system. The study found that those with higher earnings had higher benefits under this plan than they would have under the Social Security system. Contrastingly, low earners had lower benefits under the plan than they would have under Social Security. Their initial benefit was about 4% lower. But because Social Security institutes cost of living increases to offset inflation, the difference grows over time. So after 15 years, their benefit would be 63% of what it would have been under Social Security. More moderate earners would have a higher initial benefit, but after 15 years their benefit would be 91% of their original benefit and after 20 years it would be just 78%. Contrastingly, the highest earners would have an initial benefit 177% of their Social Security benefit. After 20 years it would be equivalent to what their Social Security would have been. Overall, they would have obtained a substantial gain through a private contribution system.

There are numerous reasons other than restricting redistribution as to why disadvantaged groups do not fare well. There is concern about peoples' ability to make good investment decisions (Williamson & Rix, 1999). Others point out the relatively high administrative costs for small accounts (CBO, 2004b). Women, who live 7 years longer than men on average, will not gain as much from individual benefits more directly linked with overall contributions; Social Security does not penalize women for their longer life spans (Williamson & Rix). And of course the smaller one's income in retirement the less able one is to absorb large changes in income that would likely occur if it was heavily tied to the stock market (Herd & Kingson, 2005).

A final salient concern is how those benefiting from the insurance portion of the program, particularly disabled workers and survivors, would fare given money would be shifted out of the insurance portion of the program and into private accounts. The basic insurance benefit would thus be around one third lower for survivors and disabled beneficiaries (Diamond & Orszag, 2002). Survivors, however, could inherit whatever savings had built up in the deceased worker's account, which would be highly dependent on the age he or she died at. The size of disabled workers' accounts would be highly dependent on the age at which they became disabled. Generally, the individual account, particularly for disabled workers, would not have accrued enough value, leading to lower benefits overall than under the current system.

Medicare

Currently, older Medicare beneficiaries pay the same premiums, deductibles, and co-payments to their primary health insurance provider: the federal government. A small percentage of beneficiaries are covered by HMOs. But regardless of whether beneficiaries participate in fee-for-service or an HMO, individuals are guaranteed a set of covered services (benefits) regardless of cost. It is a defined benefit. Moreover, all those individuals are placed in the same "pool" to determine the cost of premiums. The most common privatization proposal for Medicare would basically entail providing older Americans with a voucher with which they would buy their health insurance coverage from a host of private insurance providers, who would offer an array of different plans with varying copayments and services, in addition to traditional Medicare. In essence, the system would shift toward a defined contribution approach, where a contribution, as opposed to a certain level of benefits, is guaranteed. Unlike in the current system (a defined benefit) where the government contributes more toward sicker and generally poorer beneficiaries, everyone would receive the exact same monetary voucher benefit (a defined contribution). How this amount is determined will depend upon policy details. A pure defined contribution would pay, for example, $500 toward a premium. Another variation, however, premium support, would set the amount at a percentage, say 90%, of the average premium amount. Another key difference is that older Americans would no longer be in the same insurance pool. The result is that premiums and benefits would vary widely.

The reason privatizing Medicare is a more popular reform than limiting eligibility through significant means testing or raising the program's eligibility age is because, similar to privatizing Social Security, privatizing Medicare is being sold as the way to save this universal program. Some privatization proponents argue it would protect Medicare from fiscal ruin and improve its benefits without requiring increases to the eligibility age, benefit cuts, or significant means testing (Bush, 2004). Other proponents, however, are more pragmatic and acknowledge benefits cuts will be necessary (Pauly, 2004). While I will examine these claims momentarily, it is critical to note that privatization is being sold in such a way that does not challenge the basic aspects of universalism that make Medicare popular. Everyone contributes and everyone would continue benefiting; the size of the beneficiary pool would not be decreased due to an increased age of eligibility or significant means testing. What would change is the extent to which Medicare subsidizes the sickest, and generally the poorest, beneficiaries.

Much like the claims made by proponents of privatizing Social Security, there is no evidence that privatizing Medicare will improve its fiscal problems. Medicare's dilemma is far more serious than Social Security's. Currently, Medicare comprises 2.7% of gross domestic product (GDP). By 2030 it will comprise 7% of GDP (MedPAC, 2004). But what is often ignored is that Medicare's fiscal problems are rooted in the larger problems of the U.S. health care system. Overall, health care spending is expected to rise from 15.3% of GDP to 25% of GDP from 2004 to 2030 (MedPAC). The only country in the industrialized world without the government as the primary health insurer for its citizens and residents is also consistently the most expensive system in the world.

Proposals to privatize would severely limit the government's role as the primary health insurer to all older Americans and expand the private sector's role. But Medicare has been far more effective at controlling health care costs than the private sector has been (Boccuti & Moon, 2003). From 1972 to 2002, average annual cost increases have been 9.6% in Medicare compared to 11.1% in the private sector. There are two reasons for the government's success at holding prices down. First, the large pool of beneficiaries (almost all older Americans) makes it easy to negotiate low prices with health care providers and suppliers. Second, it has much lower administrative costs: 3% compared to the private sector's 12.8% (Davis, 2004).

The goal of privatizing Medicare is to reduce the government's current role as the primary health insurer for almost older Americans. Proponents argue that older Americans should be able to "decide what kind of health plans they want, the kinds of benefits packages they want, the medical treatments and procedures they want, and the premiums, co-payments, deductibles, and coinsurance they are willing to pay" (Lemieux, 2003; Moffit, 2004). More choice will lead to more competition and further reduce prices. Ultimately, proponents argue that the increased competition that results from privatizing Medicare is a way to "save" and improve Medicare without resorting to benefit cuts or tax increases.

But there is no evidence that increased competition will reduce costs (Moon & Herd, 2002; Rice & Desmond, 2002). First, the larger number of companies, and consequently different health plans, involved will increase administrative costs. Second, for competition to reduce costs, elderly people would have to switch plans on an almost yearly basis, but there is significant evidence that older adults will not switch plans (Buchmueller, 2000). Third, it will be very difficult for seniors to sort out which plans will give them the most for their money. It is difficult to compare plan benefits and costs because plans vary so widely within and between health insurance companies.

How Privatization Will Undermine Redistribution Within Medicare

How does Medicare redistribute? The redistributive nature of Medicare is less obvious than Social Security's. But the key progressive feature of Medicare is that, regardless of how sick or poor, individuals are guaranteed access to the same basic coverage at the same costs as wealthier and healthier individuals. This is most certainly not the case for younger Americans who may not be able to access health insurance or often have to pay considerably more for it depending on their employment status, health status, and where they live.

The key to understanding Medicare's success is understanding what older people's health insurance dilemmas were before Medicare. Before Medicare was enacted in 1965 about three quarters of older Americans had inadequate health insurance coverage, and half had no coverage whatsoever (Century Foundation, 2001). Wealthier older Americans were the only ones able to afford health insurance. Moreover, buying health insurance as individuals in the market left them with few protections. The sickest older Americans could be charged exorbitant premiums making the coverage unaffordable. Now all older Americans are guaranteed affordable health insurance. Their Medicare premiums are not effected by how sick they are or where they live. And most polls show approval ratings for the program at almost 90% among the elderly people who rely on it (Public Agenda, 2004).

Again, the long-term goal of privatization supporters is to dramatically reduce the role of Medicare fee-for-service or rather limit the government's current role as the primary health insurance provider for older Americans. Though the government does contract out Medicare's administrative responsibility to private companies, ultimately the government determines what services beneficiaries receive and how much they have to pay. Under a defined contribution approach, the government plan—Medicare fee-for-service—would just be one of hundreds of primary health insurance plans with varying premiums and services covered.

The problem for poorer and sicker beneficiaries is that these changes are likely to increase their health care costs. Multiple insurance pools make it much harder to spread and redistribute the costs of health care from the sickest and poorest beneficiaries to the healthiest and wealthiest. In the current system, everyone is in the same insurance pool so costs are spread evenly; the more pools, the harder to evenly spread costs. The problem is that HMOs are skilled at attracting the healthiest individuals who bring the highest profits. Studies show that sicker individuals end up concentrated in certain plans when people have multiple options. With a defined contribution approach, the sickest and most expensive beneficiaries would be concentrated in fee-for-service Medicare. Sick and expensive beneficiaries concentrated in one plan drives up costs, leaving these vulnerable beneficiaries with extraordinarily high premiums, deductibles, and copayments (Moon & Herd, 2002; Rice & Desmond, 2002).

Unlike with Social Security, partial privatization of Medicare has already begun. And these experiments demonstrate the problems with privatization for sicker and poorer Americans. The main example is the participation of HMOs in Medicare. Millions of older Americans have participated in an HMO as opposed to traditional Medicare fee-for-service. Beneficiary premiums remained the same, but for years those elders in HMOs, who are the healthiest and wealthiest, received better benefits than the average participant in Medicare fee-for-service. The government was overpaying the HMOs. But as soon as the reimbursements were corrected, HMOs began dropping Medicare coverage. In 1998, 17% of beneficiaries participated in an HMO; by 2004 that had fallen to 11% (Kaiser Family Foundation, 2004a). In 2002, Congress significantly increased reimbursements to HMOs to further encourage their participation. Currently, the government pays an extra $552 per enrollee in Medicare HMOs as compared to fee-for-service, even though the sickest and poorest beneficiaries are in Medicare fee-for-service (Cooper, Nicholas, & Biles, 2004).

The second piece of privatization in Medicare is the new prescription drug bill, whereby private insurers, as opposed to the government, will provide coverage (Kaiser Family Foundation, 2004b). The benefit premium will vary depending on where beneficiaries live and what kind of plan they choose. Beneficiaries already in HMOs will simply receive their coverage through them. Beneficiaries who want to remain in Medicare fee-for-service (who are sicker and poorer beneficiaries) will have to buy an additional policy from a private insurer, which is on top of whatever Medigap coverage they currently have. There is concern that Medicare fee-for-service participants will have to pay more for less coverage due to the stand-alone nature of the coverage. The overall incentive is to push more individuals into HMOs and away from fee-for-service Medicare.

Conclusion

Neither privatizing Social Security nor privatizing Medicare explicitly threatens two basic universal principles that keep these programs popular: broad-based eligibility and relatively generous benefits for the middle class. While additional policy changes to deal with these programs' fiscal problems could threaten either of these principles, proponents argue that privatization will help offset the impact of any benefit cuts. This is likely a key explanation as to why these reforms have received far more public support than past attempts at retrenching Social Security and Medicare. Instead of attacking Social Security and Medicare as draining and wasteful programs that should be limited, proponents argue privatization will "save" these programs.

What privatization does clearly limit is the redistribution that occurs within these programs. The magnitude of the impact on redistribution, however, will depend on policy details. A few recent proposals for Medicare and Social Security have tried to limit the impact of reform on poor beneficiaries (see Pauly, 2004). That said, the basic premise of these proposals is to more tightly link individual contributions with individual benefits, which reduces the potential for redistribution. Given Social Security's and Medicare's success at securing the incomes and protecting the health of elderly Americans, we need to pay close attention to the ramifications of privatization on the beneficiaries who need these programs the most.

References

Boccuti, C., & Moon, M. (2003). Comparing Medicare and private insurers. *Health Affairs, 22,* 230–237.

Buchmueller, T. C. (2000). The health plan choice of retirees under managed competition. *Health Services Research, 35,* 949–957.

Bush, G. W. (2004). *Framework to modernize and improve Medicare fact sheet.* Retrieved September 15, 2004, from http://www.whitehouse.gov/news/releases/2003/03/20030304-l.html

Census Bureau. (2004). *Income, poverty, and health insurance coverage in the United States: 2003.* Retrieved September 10, 2004, from http://www.census.gov/prod/2004pubs/p60-226.pdf

Century Foundation. (2001). *Medicare reform.* Retrieved September 10, 2004, from http://www.medicarewatch.org

Congressional Budget Office. (2004a). *The outlook for Social Security.* Retrieved January 15, 2005, from http://www.cbo.gov/showdoc.cfm?index=5530&sequence=0

Congressional Budget Office. (2004b). *Administrative costs of private accounts in Social Security.* Retrieved January 15, 2005, from http://www.cbo.gov/showdoc.cfm?index=5277&sequence=0

Cooper, N., Nicholas, L., & Biles, B. (2004). *The cost of privatization.* New York: Commonwealth Fund.

Davis, K. (2004). Making health care affordable for all Americans. Testimony before the Senate Committee on Health, Education, Labor, and Pensions, January 28, 2004. Retrieved January 15, 2005, from http://www.cmwf.org/usr_doc/davis_senatehelptestimony_714.pdf

Derthick, M. (1979). *Policymaking for Social Security.* Washington, DC: Brookings Institution.

Diamond, P., & Orszag, P. (2002). *Reducing benefits and subsidizing individual accounts.* New York: The Century Fund.

Employee Benefit Research Institute (EBRI). (2001). *Medicare awareness, satisfaction, confidence, and reform.* Retrieved September 10, 2004, from http://www.ebri.org/facts/0701fact.pdf

Ferrara, P. (1998). *The next step for Medicare reform.* Policy analysis no. 305. Washington, DC: CATO Institute.

Herd, P., & Kingson, E. (2005). Selling Social Security. In R. Hudson (Ed.), *The future of age-based public policy* (pp. 183–204). Baltimore, MD: Johns Hopkins University Press.

Kaiser Family Foundation. (2004a). *Medicare fact sheet: Medicare Advantage, March 2004.* Retrieved January 15, 2005, from http://www.kff.org

Kaiser Family Foundation. (2004b). *Summaries of the Medicare Modernization Act of 2003.* New York: Author.

Kingson, E. (1994). Testing the boundaries of universality. *The Gerontologist, 34,* 736–742.

Korpi, W. (1983). *The Democratic class struggle.* London: Routledge.

Korpi, W., & Palme, J. (1998). The paradox of redistribution and strategies of equality. *American Sociological Review, 63,* 661-687.

Lemieux, J. (2003). *Explaining premium support.* Retrieved September 1, 2004, from http://www.centrists.org

MedPac. (2004). *A data book: Health care spending and the Medicare program.* Medicare Payment Advisory Commission. Retrieved September 1, 2004, from http://www.medpac.gov/publications/congressional_reports/Jun04DataBookSec6.pdf

Moffit, R. (2004). What federal workers are doing today that you can't. Webmemo #604. Washington, DC: The Heritage Foundation.

Moon, M., & Herd, P. (2002). *A place at the table.* New York: The Century Foundation.

National Committee on Pay Equity. (2004). Fact sheet on gender pay gap. Retrieved September 3, 2004, from http://www.pay-equity.org/info.html

Pauly, M. (2004). Means testing in Medicare. *Health Affairs, web exclusive,* W4 (549).

Porter, K., Larin, K., & Primus, W. (1999). *Social security and poverty among the elderly.* Washington, DC: Center on Budget and Policy Priorities.

President's Commission to Strengthen Social Security. (2001). *Strengthening Social Security and creating personal wealth for all Americans.* Retrieved September 4, 2004, from http://www.css.gov

Public Agenda. (2004). *Opinion polling on Medicare.* Retrieved Month, day, year, from http://www.publicagenda.org/issues/major_proposals_detail.cfm?issue_type=ss&e list=l

Quadagno, J. (1996). Social Security and the myth of the entitlement crisis. *The Gerontologist, 36,* 391–399.

Rice, T., & Desmond, K. (2002). *An analysis of reforming Medicare through a premium support plan.* New York: Henry J. Kaiser Foundation.

Rice, T., Desmond, K., & Gabel, J. (1990). The Medicare Catastrophic Coverage Act. *Health Affairs, 9,* 75–87.

Skocpol, T. (1991). Targeting within universalism. In C. Jencks & P. E. Peterson (Eds.), *The urban underclass*, (pp. 411–436). Washington, DC: The Brookings Institution.

Polling Report. (2005). Title of report. Retrieved April 3, 2005, from http://www.pollingreport.com

Williamson, J., & Rix, S. (1999). Social Security reform: Implications for women. Boston College, Boston, MA. Retrieved September 1, 2004, from http://www.bc.edu/centers/crr/papers/wp_1999-07.pdf

Wilson, T. (1999). Opting out: The Galveston plan and Social Security. PRC WP 99–22, Wharton School, University of Pennsylvania, Philadelphia.

Address correspondence to **PAMELA HERD**, LBJ School of Public Affairs, University of Texas, Austin, PO Box Y, Austin, TX 78713-8925. E-mail: pherd@mail.utexas.*edu*

From *The Gerontologist,* Vol. 45, no. 3, pp. 292-298. Copyright © o. 3 by The Gerontological Society of America. Reprinted by permission of the publisher.

Coverage for All

Two states have enacted universal health care plans.
Are they leaders or simply anomalies?

PATRICIA BARRY

After years of mounting evidence that the U.S. health care system has become dysfunctional—with nearly 46 million uninsured, costs escalating and some of America's largest employers cutting back on benefits—something unexpected happened this spring: two states enacted laws intended to create near-universal health coverage for their residents, starting next year.

What riveted the attention of health policy experts was that both these measures, though very different, had strong bipartisan support. In both Massachusetts and Vermont, they were passed by Democratic-controlled legislatures and signed into law by Republican governors. Only two lawmakers in Massachusetts voted against that state's bill, with its landmark—and highly controversial—requirements that all residents purchase health insurance and most employers contribute or face penalties.

Across the nation, the "first reaction to Massachusetts was marveling at the political accomplishments—how they were able to craft a compromise between a Republican governor and two Democratic leaders with very different ideas," says Paul Ginsburg, president of Washington's Center for Studying Health System Change. "And that's going to inspire other states to try."

For over a decade, since the Clinton health reform proposals tanked, Washington, riven by opposing ideologies, has remained in near-paralysis over the rising tide of uninsured and underinsured Americans. The right wing promotes more private insurance options, mainly high-deductible health savings accounts. The left wing favors a national "single-payer" system, run by the federal government.

Most Americans, however, want universal health coverage—whether private or public or mixed—that they can afford, according to recent opinion polls. The bipartisan Citizens' Health Care Working Group set up by Congress reported last month that of 23,000 people contacted, "over 90 percent ... believed it should be public policy that all Americans have affordable coverage." The group has called on Congress to guarantee such coverage by 2012.

So, will the Massachusetts and Vermont initiatives point the way for other states or even the nation? And, for consumers, just how universal, affordable and dependable is the coverage they're planning?

Massachusetts

No state has ever attempted to require all residents to buy health coverage. Under the new law, people in Massachusetts who are uninsured must buy coverage by July 1, 2007, and all businesses with more than 10 employees that do not provide insurance must pay a "fair share" contribution of up to $295 per year to the state for each worker.

That concept of "shared responsibility" was a major political key to the law's passage, experts say. Companies that already provide health insurance welcomed the opportunity to level the competitive playing field with those that do not. Even so, Gov. Mitt Romney, in signing the law, vetoed the $295 assessment on employers—a veto the legislature overrode.

Individuals who do not comply will lose their personal tax exemption in 2007 and after that will face fines of 50 percent of the monthly cost of health insurance for each month without it. But there is a caveat. They will not be compelled to buy insurance if they can't find affordable coverage. The state has not yet defined what "affordable" will mean. And it does not intend to set levels of premiums, deductibles and copayments.

The state has become the first to adopt an idea promoted by the Heritage Foundation, a conservative Washington think tank. The law sets up a clearinghouse—called the Connector—intended to link uninsured individuals and companies having fewer than 50 employees to a choice of "affordable" health plans designed by private insurers and regulated by the state.

The Connector aims to offer these two groups the advantages that many people in large employer-sponsored groups now enjoy—deeper discounts, premiums paid out of pretax dollars and an opportunity to change plans every year.

And it offers them a further unique advantage. Their coverage will be portable. If they change full-time jobs, or are part-time or temporary employees working several jobs, their coverage remains in place.

This is a fundamentally different approach to solving the problem of the uninsured, says Edmund Haislmaier, a Heritage Foundation expert who helped formulate the Massachusetts law. "If you make the insurance stick to the people instead of to the job, you'd probably solve at least half this problem with no new money."

The law also offers subsidized coverage (no deductibles, premiums on a sliding scale) to residents with incomes up to 300 percent of the federal poverty level (about $29,000 for an individual, $40,000 for a couple, $60,000 for a family of four). And it aims to make health coverage more affordable for young adults.

The law has plenty of detractors from both ends of the political spectrum. AFL-CIO President John Sweeney called the mandate for people to have insurance an "unconscionable" step that will "bankrupt many middle-class families." Michael Tanner, director of health studies at the libertarian Cato Institute, said that it presages "a slow but steady spiral downward toward a government-run national health care system."

For Massachusetts residents, the devil will be in the details. Just how much people who are not eligible for subsidies will have to pay in premiums, deductibles and copays under the private plans provided through the Connector is not yet known, though early estimates place monthly premiums at about $300 for an individual and $600 for a couple.

Comprehensive employer-sponsored health policies for a family in Massachusetts currently run about $12,000 to $14,000 a year. How will insurers offer new options for less?

Some believe it can't be done. The choice could be between costly plans that offer good benefits and inexpensive plans that cut benefits or have very high deductibles, says David Himmelstein, M.D., associate professor of medicine at Harvard Medical School and co-founder of a physicians group that promotes a national single-payer health system. The law, he says, "will force you to purchase either something you can't afford or something you can afford but which will be nearly useless in the actual coverage it offers."

Supporters also acknowledge the challenges. "We're very aware of the issues around cost sharing," says John McDonough, executive director of MA HealthCare for All, a grassroots group that helped get the law passed. "It will take a huge amount of implementation by [all] stakeholders to make sure that this is done well and done right" over the next few months. But he adds: "They're fully committed to doing that."

Vermont

Unlike the "stick" of mandated coverage proposed by Massachusetts, Vermont's new law is more of a "carrot" that lawmakers hope will achieve the same goal—near-universal health care coverage in the state by 2010.

Vermont will provide a new voluntary, standardized plan—called Catamount Health—for uninsured residents. It will be offered by private insurers, and its benefits and charges will be similar to those in the average BlueCross BlueShield plan in Vermont. Unlike Massachusetts', the Vermont plan has defined costs. Enrollees will pay $10 for office visits; 20 percent coin-

Highlights of the Massachusetts law ...

- All residents required to have health insurance by July 1, 2007.
- All employers required to offer insurance or contribute up to $295 a year for each uninsured employee.
- Fines for residents and businesses not complying—except individuals unable to find "affordable" policies, or businesses with 10 or fewer employees.
- The Connector links individuals and companies with under 50 employees to a choice of "affordable" private health plans paid for out of pretax dollars.
- Health insurance obtained through the Connector is portable when enrollee changes jobs.
- Subsidized premiums on a sliding scale for enrollees with incomes of up to 300 percent of the federal poverty level.

... and the Vermont law

- Catamount Health plan for uninsured residents starts Oct. 1, 2007.
- Businesses with more than eight employees pay up to $365 a year for every uninsured employee.
- Plan offers portable coverage through private insurers and defined benefits and costs, including annual caps on out-of-pocket spending.
- Subsidized premiums on a sliding scale for enrollees with incomes of up to 300 percent of the federal poverty level.
- Incentives for enrollees with chronic conditions who participate in a disease management program; payments for doctors who promote preventive care and healthy living.

surance for medical services; tiered copays of $10, $30 or $50 for prescription drugs; and a $250 annual deductible for an individual or $500 for a family for in-network services (double those amounts for out-of-network). Another big benefit: Out-of-pocket expenses will be capped at $800 a year for an individual and $1,600 for a family using in-network services (almost double for out-of-network).

Premiums have yet to be determined but are likely to be around $340 a month for an individual. People with incomes below 300 percent of the federal poverty level would be eligible for premium subsidies.

Plan supporters are confident it will attract uninsured Vermonters without the need for a mandate because its benefits are more comprehensive than the only other plans that many can now afford. "Most folks tell us they do not want to be in a high-deductible health saving account where they're paying maybe $5,000 out of pocket before they reach some kind of catastrophic benefit," says Greg Marchildon, state director for AARP Vermont, which helped drive the new legislation. "They basically describe it as paying to be uninsured."

Employers are not required to provide health insurance, but those with more than eight employees must help fund Catamount Health by paying a dollar a day for every uninsured worker.

The other centerpiece of the Vermont law is a landmark program offering special care with financial incentives—such as waived deductibles and free services and testing—to people with chronic illness.

Vermont is the first state to formally recognize that about 80 percent of health care dollars are consumed by people with chronic conditions (such as diabetes, high blood pressure, heart disease and obesity) and that many cannot afford the screening and services that prevent expensive complications.

In terms of holding down costs as well as improving general health, "the last thing you want for those patients is high copays, deductibles or anything that will deter them from ongoing routine medical management," says Kenneth Thorpe, chairman of the health policy department at Emory University in Atlanta and the main architect of the Vermont legislation.

"If this is done well—and experts in Vermont believe it will become the gold standard for how you manage chronic disease," AARP's Marchildon adds, "we think that over time we're going to save tens of millions of dollars."

Will Other States Copy?

Other states will be closely watching Massachusetts and Vermont over the next year to see if they can implement their laws or if they'll run into roadblocks.

Analysts point to a number of reasons why other states may not rush to replicate those laws in their entirety. Both states, for example, have far smaller uninsured populations than the national average, tight regulations on health insurers already in place and, above all, sufficient financing (mainly from federal dollars) to fund the programs for at least a few years.

"But individual components of the reforms—yes, I think you will see states replicating them," says Laura Tobler, a health policy analyst at the National Conference of State Legislatures. She cites as examples Massachusetts' compulsory insurance and its Connector program and Vermont's chronic care program.

Yet experts on each law say the whole state system must be changed to achieve universal coverage. Haislmaier of the Heritage Foundation says the unique approach in Massachusetts is "to reform the market, not the products, to create a single unified mechanism that gets rid of these distinctions between [insurance for] individuals and small groups and large groups."

In Vermont's case, says Emory's Thorpe, reform "can't just be about costs or the uninsured. You've got to convince people who [already] have health insurance that they are going to get more affordable and better-quality health care with less administrative hassle than they have today."

Financing also relies on an integrated system. As more residents get coverage, the funds the two states now use to pay the hospital bills of the uninsured will be shifted to subsidies that help more low-income enrollees get coverage.

Many experts say Massachusetts and Vermont set aside ideologies to forge a compromise, and that this could well spur a renewed debate on national health coverage in the 2008 election.

"The whole history of national health [reform] has been of people overreaching and getting nothing," says Ginsburg of the Center for Studying Health System Change. "A lot of people have interpreted the term 'universal' as meaning single-payer, and that's a source of confusion. To me, universal just means that everybody's covered, no matter what the mechanism."

Riding Into the Sunset

The Geezer Threat

WILLIAM GREIDER

In 1900 Americans on average lived for only 49 years and most working people died still on the job. For those who lived long enough, the average "retirement" age was 85. By 1935, when Social Security was enacted, life expectancy had risen to 61 years. Now it is 77 years—nearly a generation more—and still rising. Children born today have a fifty-fifty chance of living to 100. This inheritance from the last century—the great gift of longer life—surely represents one of the country's most meaningful accomplishments.

Yet the achievement has been transformed into a monumental problem by contemporary politics and narrow-minded accounting. "The nation faces a severe economic threat from the aging of its population combined with escalating health costs," a *Washington Post* editorial warned. Others put it more harshly. "Greedy geezers" are robbing from the young, bankrupting the government. Painful solutions must be taken to avoid financial ruin. Or so we are told.

A much happier conviction is expressed by Robert Fogel, a Nobel Prize-winning economist at the University of Chicago and a septuagenarian himself. America, he reminds us, is a very wealthy nation. The expanding longevity is not a financial burden but an enormous and underdeveloped asset. If US per capita income continues to grow at a rate of 1.5 percent a year, the country will have plenty of money to finance comfortable retirements and high-quality healthcare for all citizens, including those at the bottom of the wage ladder. When politicians talk about raising the Social Security retirement age to 70 in order to "save" the system, they are headed backward and against the tide of human aspirations. The average retirement age, Fogel observes, has been falling in recent decades by personal choice and is now around 63. Given proper financing arrangements, he expects the retirement age will eventually fall to as low as 55—allowing everyone to enjoy more leisure years and to explore the many dimensions of "spiritual development" or "self-realization," as John Dewey called it.

"What then is the virtue of increasing spending on retirement and health rather than goods?" Fogel asked in his latest book, *The Fourth Great Awakening and the Future of Egalitarianism* (2000). "It is the virtue of providing consumers in rich countries with what they want most." What people want is time—more time to enjoy life and learning, to focus on the virtuous aspects of one's nature, to pursue social projects free of economic necessity, to engage their curiosity and self-knowledge or their political values. The great inequity in modern life, as Fogel provocatively puts it, is the "maldistribution of spiritual resources," that is, the economic insecurity that prevents people from exploring life's larger questions. Everyone could attain a fair share of liberating security, he asserts, if government undertook strategic interventions in their behalf.

Fogel's perspective is generally ignored by other economists, but sociologists and psychologists recognize his point in the changing behavior of retirees. The elderly are redefining leisure, finding "fun" in myriad activities that lend deeper meaning to their lives. An informal shadow university has grown up around the nation in which older people are both the students and the teachers. They do "volunteer vacationing" and "foster grandparenting." They rehab old houses for the needy, serve as self-appointed environmental watchdogs or act as ombudsmen for neglected groups like indigent children or nursing-home patients. They dig into political issues with an informed tenacity that often withers politicians. In civic engagement, they are becoming counselors, critics, caregivers and mentors equipped with special advantages—the time and freedom to act, the knowledge and understanding gained only from the experience of living.

When the "largest generation" reaches retirement a few years from now, the baby boomers will doubtless alter the contours of society again, perhaps more profoundly than in their youth. Theodore Roszak, the historian who chronicled *The Making of a Counter Culture* thirty-six years ago, thinks boomers taking up caregiving and mentoring roles will inspire another wave of humanistic social values (perhaps expressed more maturely this time around). "More than merely surviving we will find ourselves gifted with the wits, the political savvy and the sheer weight of numbers to become a major force for change," Roszak wrote in *America the Wise* (1998). "With us, history shifts its rhythm. It draws back from the frenzied pursuit of marketing novelties and technological turnover and assumes the measured pace of humane and sustainable values. We may live to see wisdom become a distinct possibility and compassion the reigning social ethic." The "retired," he predicts, will seek to become reintegrated with the working society and claim a larger role in its affairs. Some elderly may reclaim the ancient role of respected "elders" who keep alive society's deeper truths and remind succeeding generations of their obligations to the nation's longer term. None of these possibilities are likely to unfold, however, if the promise of economic security for retirement is eviscerated in the meantime.

Fogel's optimism sounds eccentric amid the gloom and doom of the Social Security debate and the more threatening deterioration under way in private pensions and personal savings. Fogel skips over the snarled facts of current politics. He thinks big-picture and long-term. He won the Nobel Prize by producing unorthodox economic history that traced the deeper shifts in demographics and living conditions across generations, even centuries. His thinking is especially provocative because the conclusions collide with both left and right assumptions. Fogel is a secular Democrat, yet he extols the conservative evangelical awakening as a valuable social force. He sounds alternately conservative and liberal on economic issues, yet he thinks government should engineer a vast redistribution of financial wealth, from top to bottom, to insure equitable pensions for all.

Fogel's solution is a new national pension system alongside Social Security—a universal "provident fund" that requires all workers to save a significant portion of their wage incomes every year to provide for their future. He proposes a savings rate of 14.7 percent (though taking Social Security benefits and taxes into account, a lower rate would suffice for a start). The contributions would be mandatory but set aside as true personal savings, not as a government tax. The accumulating nest eggs would belong to the individual workers and become a portable pension that goes with them if they change jobs, but the wealth would be invested for them through a broadly diversified pension fund. Employers would no longer be in charge (though they could still contribute to worker savings to attract employees). The government or independent private institutions would manage the money, investing conservatively in stocks, bonds and other income-generating assets while allowing workers only limited, generalized choices on their investment preferences.

Fogel's vision of expanding leisure and greater human fulfillment is actually receding at the moment. The time for big ideas is now.

The concept resembles the forced savings plans adopted in some Asian and Latin American countries, but Fogel's favorite prototype is American: TIAA-CREF, the pension system that exists for nearly all college professors (a nonprofit institution founded in 1917 by Andrew Carnegie). Another model could be the government's own Thrift Savings Plan, which manages savings wealth for federal employees. Lifelong healthcare, Fogel adds, could be guaranteed for all by setting aside another 9.8 per-

cent from current incomes. "If you take the typical academic, we all have TIAA-CREF," he explains. "The universities require of us that we invest anywhere from 12.5 to 17.5 percent of our salaries in a pension fund—mandatory—but it's all in my name. I can leave it to whomever I want. It has entered my sense of well-being for many years. The fund has earned about 10 percent a year since the 1960s, so retirement is not a burden to the university."

Obviously, people with low or even moderate incomes could not afford such savings rates, and even diligent savings from their low wages would not be enough to pay for either retirement or healthcare. Fogel has a straightforward solution: Tax the affluent to pay for the needy. A tax rate of 2 or 3 percent, applied progressively to families in the top half of income distribution, could finance the "provident fund" for those who can't pay for themselves. "This is a problem, not of inadequate national resources, but of inequity," he observes.

Fogel's big thinking—a system of compulsory savings, with the federal government taking charge—sounds way too radical for this right-wing era, and probably even most Democrats would shy away from the concept. But keep Fogel's solution in mind as we examine the sorry condition of retirement security. The current political debate is not even focused on the right "crisis," much less on genuine solutions. It is not Social Security that's financially threatened but healthcare and the other two pillars of retirement security—employer-run pension plans and the private savings of families. Many millions of baby boomers realize as they approach the "golden years" that they can't afford to retire at all, much less retire early. They will keep working because they lack the wherewithal to stop. Retiring for them would mean a drastic fall in their standard of living. Fogel's vision of expanding leisure and greater human fulfillment is actually receding at the moment. The time for big ideas is now.

Grasshoppers and Ants

When George W. Bush launched Social Security reform with his promise of new personalized savings accounts for everyone, he did not seem to grasp that most Americans already have such accounts. During the past generation tax-exempt 401(k) and IRA accounts—the individualized "defined contribution" approach—became the principal pension plan for working people, displacing the traditional company pension provided by employers who assume the risks and promise a "defined benefit" to workers at retirement. The do-it-yourself version of pensions is a flop, as many Americans have painfully learned. When older employees look at their monthly balance statements, they are more likely to experience fear than Bush's romanticized thrill of individual risk-taking.

Picking stocks for themselves has left many employees, perhaps as many as 40-45 percent, without an adequate nest egg for retirement. When Bush explains further that he intends to divert trillions from Social Security to finance his "ownership society," it makes people even more nervous. Social Security pays very modest average benefits—roughly equivalent to the federal minimum wage— but it is the last safety net. For nearly half of the private-sector workforce, it is the only safety net. The far more threatening problem is elsewhere—shrinking pensions, collapsed personal savings and soaring costs for health insurance.

The bleak reality is reflected in those 401(k) account balances. Of the 48 million families who hold one or more of the accounts, the median value of their savings is $27,000 (which means half of all families have less than $27,000). Among older workers on the brink of retiring (55 to 64 years old) who have personal accounts, the median value is $55,000. That's only enough to buy an annuity that would pay $398 a month, far short of middle-class living standards. What's strange and disturbing about their low accumulations is that these older workers have been investing during the best of times—the "super bull market" of soaring stock prices that lasted nearly twenty years. The Congressional Research Service summarized the sobering results: Median pension savings "would not by themselves provide an income in retirement that most people in the United States would find to be adequate."

This grand experiment was launched nearly twenty-five years ago by Ronald Reagan, but with very little public debate because the pension changes were obscured by more immediate controversies—Reagan's regressive tax cuts and massive budget deficits. His Treasury under secretary explained the reasoning: "The evidence of the past suggests that people do not behave like grasshoppers. They are much more like ants." For lots of reasons, most Americans turned out not to be like the proverbial ants, storing food for winter. People either misjudged their future need for savings or couldn't afford to put much aside or bet wrong in the stock market and got wiped out. But corporate managements turned out to be the true grasshoppers, living for the moment and ignoring the future. Companies took advantage of the 401(k) innovation to escape their traditional responsibility to employees. They dumped old defined-benefit pension plans and adopted the new version, which requires much smaller employer contributions and thereby reduces labor costs dramatically. Good for the bottom line, bad for the country's future.

"The whole thinking was: Let's relieve the employers of this burden and empower individuals," explains Karen Ferguson, longtime director of the Pension Rights Center in Washington. "The problem is, it has failed—and failed miserably—and no one wants to say that."

Pension protection is actually shrinking, despite the proliferation of 401(k) accounts and the alleged prosperity of the 1980s and '90s. In the private sector, fewer employees participate in pension plans of any kind now than twenty years ago, down from 51 percent to 46 percent (the defined-benefit company pensions that once covered 53 percent now protect only 34 percent). The value of pension wealth, meanwhile, fell by 17 percent for workers in the middle and below, mainly because their voluntary savings were weak or nonexistent, yet soared for those at the top—"an upsurge in pension wealth inequality," economist Edward Wolff of New York University observed.

In sum, pensions became less valuable. And fewer families have one. That helps explain why Bush's plan encountered popular resistance. In these circumstances, whacking Social Security benefits or raising the retirement age does not sound like "reform." But neither political party has yet summoned the nerve to acknowledge the implications of the failed experiment or to propose serious solutions.

The most threatening problem is not Social Security; it is shrinking pensions, collapsed personal savings and soaring health costs.

The circumstances look even more ominous—the very opposite of Professor Fogel's sunny vision—because personal savings also collapsed during the long, slow-motion weakening of pensions. Given the stagnating wages for hourly workers and easier access to credit, families typically managed to stay afloat by working more jobs and by borrowing more. Saving for the future was not an available option for many. In 1982 personal savings peaked at $480 billion, then began an epic decline. Last year the national total in personal savings was only $103 billion—down nearly 80 percent from twenty-five years ago. As Eugene Steuerle of the Urban Institute points out, the federal government now spends more money on tax subsidies to encourage the individual forms of pension savings—$115 billion last year—than Americans actually save.

The one potential bright spot in this story might be real estate—the family wealth that accumulates gradually through home ownership and the rising market value of houses. Given the current housing boom and runaway prices in the hotter urban markets, many families might salvage retirement plans by selling their homes and moving to less expensive dwellings. The trouble is, families have been living off that wealth—borrowing, almost dollar for dollar, against the rising price of their homes through equity-credit lines or refinanced mortgages. From 1999 through 2003, the value of family homes rose by a spectacular $3.3 trillion, but families' actual equity in those properties changed little because mortgage borrowing rose nearly as fast.

Thus, people financed routine consumption by borrowing against their long-term assets—that's real grasshopper behavior. And the situation could turn very ugly if the housing bubble pops and home prices fall. People will find themselves stuck paying off a mountain of debt on homes that are suddenly worth less than the mortgages. They will not only need to keep working; they might also be filing for bankruptcy.

'Just as wealth and income are being redistributed to the wealthy, so is leisure.' —economist Teresa Ghilarducci

How could this have happened in such a wealthy nation—especially during an era when stock prices were rising explosively? The basic explanations are familiar: rising inequality and reactionary economic policies, launched first by Reagan, then elaborated by Bush II and resisted only faintheartedly by Democrats. The corporate "social contract" was discarded; regressive tax-cutting rewarded capital and the well-to-do; numerous other measures fractured the broad middle class. The wages of hourly workers—80 percent of the private-sector workforce—have been essentially unchanged in terms of real purchasing power for three decades (no one in politics wants to talk about that, either). The political system continues to defer to the needs of corporations despite the torrent of financial scandals and extreme greed displayed by egomaniacal CEOs. All these factors contributed to the erosion of retirement security. Economist Teresa Ghilarducci, a pension authority at Notre Dame, remarks, "Just as wealth and income are being redistributed to the wealthy, so is leisure."

In fact, Ghilarducci argues, allowing the pension system to deteriorate serves a long-term interest of business: avoiding future labor shortages when the baby-boom generation moves into retirement. "All this retirement policy is really a labor policy," she asserts. "It's motivated by these experts who say, Hey, wait, we're going to need to do what we can to encourage people to work longer. A whole range of economists and elite opinion makers is talking about a labor shortage where, God forbid, wages would increase. That's what they're worried about—making sure there isn't a corporate profit squeeze, that skill shortages and upward wage pressures are checked."

This development is already lengthening working lives, she finds. The average retirement age, rather than gradually declining toward 55, as Fogel foresees, has turned around in the past few years and is slowly increasing. "I'm not against older people working if they want to," Ghilarducci says. "I'm against policies that force them back into the workforce because they've lost their pensions or their healthcare costs have gone up."

O ne need not question the sincerity of the right's ideological convictions to see that their policy initiatives are also designed to benefit important political patrons. With the transition to 401(k) accounts, corporate employers were major winners. Ghilarducci's examination of 700 companies over nearly two decades found that their annual pension contributions dropped by one third—from $2,140 to $1,404 per employee—as they shifted from defined-benefit pensions to the less expensive defined-contribution model. Not surprisingly, the traditional company pension began to disappear or shrink as large industrial companies hacked away at the uncompetitive costs. The number of younger workers with the traditional form of pension is much smaller and falling fast.

Wall Street banks and brokerages were big winners too, since they began competing for the millions of new "investors" with their individual stock accounts. This enormous influx of customers helped fuel the long stock-market boom and encouraged the exaggerated promises made by both corporations and financial firms. The overall economy was probably damaged too, because mutual funds competed for customers by going after rapid, short-term gains rather than focusing on the long-term investments financed by patient capital. When the stock-market illusions burst in 2000, the meltdown evaporated lots of retirement accounts too, especially for those innocent risk-takers who had bet their savings on NASDAQ's high-flying tech stocks.

The most damning fact about the 401(k) experiment is that it has failed to fulfill the original purpose: boosting savings for ordinary Americans. Academic studies have confirmed that the personal accounts produced "very little net savings" or "statistically insignificant" gains. While every worker could participate in theory, the practical reality is that only the more affluent families could afford to take full advantage of the 401(k) tax break—sheltering their annual 401(k) contributions from income taxes. But typically they did so simply by moving money from other conventional savings accounts into the tax-exempt kind.

More affluent Americans thus reduced their income taxes, but their net savings did not actually increase. For two decades, the federal government has been heavily subsidizing "savings" by the people who needed no inducement because they were already saving. Think of it as welfare for the virtuously well-to-do. A rational government would phase out such a misconceived program. Bush is instead proposing to make the contradictions worse by adding still other tax-exempt savings vehicles designed to benefit the affluent.

The old system of defined-benefit pensions had many strengths by comparison, but it was never a solution to the national problem either. Even at their peak, the traditional corporate pensions left out half of the workforce. Larger companies, especially in unionized industrial sectors, provided strong benefits for their employees, responding to labor's bargaining demands and to attract well-qualified people. But the millions of very small firms, where more Americans work, almost never offered pensions. The burden either seemed too costly or too complicated to administer. Generally, their workers are the folks who depend solely on Social Security.

The corporate pensions are also not portable (a problem the individual accounts were supposed to solve). And pension law gives corporate managers ample latitude to game their pension funds to enhance the company's bottom line. Stories of elderly retirees stranded by their old employers are now commonplace: broken promises on healthcare and other benefits that go unpunished. Instead of accumulating larger surpluses during the good times, the corporations often did the opposite, leaving their pension funds severely underfunded for the bad times, when shortfalls couldn't be overcome. Employees have no representatives to speak for them in the decision-making. If a corporate pension fund goes belly up, its liabilities are dumped on the government's insurance agency, which is getting strapped itself.

A logical and achievable solution exists to correct this mess. Government should create a new hybrid pension that combines the best aspects of defined-benefit and defined-contribution versions—one that requires all workers to save for the future and no longer relies on the "good will" of employers. Given modern employment patterns, workers do need a portable pension that stays with them, job to job. But their voluntary savings are simply too small and erratic—too vulnerable to manipulation by financial brokers—to produce secure results in the stock-market casino. Either they get lured into wild gambles or they park their savings in mutual funds that gouge them with inflated fees and commissions while catering to the corporations that are the funds' largest customers (this conflict of interest between large and small customers is endemic to the US financial system; guess who loses). The employees' money will produce far more reliable accumulations if it is invested for them by professionals at a major independent pension fund that works only for them.

The fundamental truth (well understood among experts) is that individualized accounts can never match the investment returns of a large common fund, broadly diversified and soundly managed, because the pension fund is able to average its results over a very long time span, thirty years or more. A few wise guys might beat the casino odds, but the broad herd of small investors will always be captive to the random luck of bad timing and their own ignorance. The right wing's celebration of individual risk-taking in financial markets is like inviting sheep to the slaughter.

The super bull market is over. Its gorgeous returns will not return for many years, maybe many decades. But a very large, diversified pension fund—managed solely in the interests of its contributors—provides the vehicle for "shared luck." It can smooth out the ups and downs among all participants, young and old, lucky and unlucky. It can invest for long-term economic development rather than chase stock-market fads. Good returns for retirees, good results for the economy.

These are the very qualities Professor Fogel envisions. They describe trustworthy pension systems, like TIAA-CREF, which reliably serves many thousands of individual employees (teachers and professors) who are scattered across many different employers (schools and universities). The present reform debate is not thinking this way. Collective action is out of fashion, especially if the government is involved. Significant reform would require institution-building. The transition would pose many technical difficulties. "There are obstacles, but I don't think that's the problem," Ghilarducci says. "The obstacle is imagination."

Pro-Life Pension Reform

The Pension Rights Center just conducted a year-long "conversation on coverage" that pulled together experts from business and labor, the insurance industry, Wall Street finance, academia, AARP and other interested sectors. The workshop sessions produced a long list of worthy ideas for patching up the broken system, but that was the problem: The proposals basically involved incremental tinkering with the status quo, not universal, mandatory solutions. To get all these diverse interests to join the conversation, Karen Ferguson confides, the center had to stipulate that "mandatory" would not be discussed.

"The bottom line is that the companies always have the upper hand, even though they've gotten huge subsidies and tax benefits," she explains. "The system is voluntary, so companies can always opt out." Indeed, the politics of pension reform is usually a discussion about what new favors and concessions should be granted to employers to get them to do the "right thing" for their employees. This political logic led to the current failure. "Voluntary" is a loser, as the past twenty years amply demonstrated, be-

cause it gives companies controlling leverage over what is possible. And even well-intentioned executives will always have to choose between the company's self-interest and its employees (guess who usually loses). Only the government has the reach and power to design and oversee a pension system that truly serves all. During the past generation, most corporations discarded their obligations under the old social contract. It seems only fair they should forfeit political control too.

A universal savings system that covers everyone because it is mandatory could prove to be as durable (and popular) as Social Security.

Plausible plans in addition to Fogel's do exist that offer genuine solutions. A universal savings system that covers everyone because it is mandatory could prove to be as durable (and popular) as Social Security. It balances equity by subsidizing the savings of lower-income workers. It creates authentic individual ownership and incentives to save more for the future, consume less in the present. It operates free of Wall Street profiteers and under government supervision, adhering to well-established principles of sound investing. Employers could be discouraged from further abandoning their obligations by penalties in the tax code. Many other nations, large and small and far less wealthy, have created such systems. Americans would need to craft their own distinctive version.

One promising example, designed by economist Christian Weller for the Economic Policy Institute, proposes a modest savings rate of 3 percent of wages, but combined with the existing Social Security benefits, it would approach the level of retirement security envisioned by Fogel. The government would contribute substantial savings for low earners and also match additional contributions made by the workers or their employers. Weller estimates this would cost around $48 billion a year—less than half the federal tax subsidy now devoted to all pension plans. Weller's design is robustly equitable, scaled to help the bottom rungs most and top income earners least. Combined with Social Security, low earners (wages of $24,000 or less) would enjoy a pension that replaces 83 percent of their peak working wages. Average earners would get 60 percent replacement, high earners only 48 percent. This makes sense, because higher-income families have much greater opportunity to augment pensions with other sources of income and savings. The working poor do not.

Essentially, Weller has updated and expanded a mandatory savings plan that was proposed nearly twenty-five years ago—a last gasp from the Carter Administration. Reagan's election and laissez-faire politics snuffed the idea. While still modest in scale, Weller's design represents a meaningful start toward Fogel's larger vision of a 15 percent savings rate. Since the Social Security tax now collects 12.6 percent of wages jointly from workers and employers, it is not plausible at this point to add another 15 percent to labor costs for pension savings. However, as the new pension system matures and public confidence is established, a gradual transition can be pursued that adds little by little to the personal savings rate, offset by equivalent reductions in the payroll tax for Social Security—thus yielding greater savings and lower taxes. Both government systems would continue in place, one as the fundamental safety net of social insurance, the other as the universal, expanding pillar for comfortable retirement.

Ghilarducci thinks much of the accumulating wealth could be stored and invested by large private pension funds, organized by unions or other groups for workers at multiple employers (much like TIAA-CREF's role for universities). A successful existing model is the unified pension systems for the building and construction trades. Co-managed by unions and companies, they encourage industry and labor to collaborate on joint training and other productivity-enhancing endeavors that can raise the quality of work and wages.

While most politicians don't dare embrace a "mandatory" solution—not yet, anyway—it is not self-evident that ordinary Americans would reject one, if properly educated about the alternatives. Most people are conflicted. They know they need to save more—retirement is a very meaningful investment for them—but it's very hard to accomplish, given the competing pressures. They like the concept of personal accounts but are also aware of their vulnerability as amateur investors. In her conversations with union presidents, Ghilarducci finds they are more in favor of an "add on" national pension than raising the payroll tax for Social Security. "You can sell workers if their name is on it," she concludes. "If you had a system that says you must contribute 3 percent of wages to your mandatory savings account, you would actually have two-thirds of the workers grateful that they are being forced to save. You wouldn't get that if they were forced to pay another 3 percent in taxes into Social Security."

The retirement question—choices of mandatory or voluntary, universal or incremental—embodies a classic dilemma often facing liberal politics. Do reformers pursue the larger, more provocative approach that invites greater resistance but would fundamentally solve the problem? Or do they opt for smaller, safer measures that have a better chance of adoption and will demonstrate good intentions, if not a genuine remedy for society? For several decades, it seems obvious, most Democrats have chosen the side of caution: thinking small, offering symbolic gestures, avoiding fights over fundamental solutions. One can see where this strategy has gotten the party. The gestures are no longer taken seriously, since they don't lead anywhere. The public no longer associates Democrats with big ideas or principled commitments to authentic reform. We await incautious politicians with the courage to pursue their unfashionable convictions.

Index

Index

Test Your Knowledge Form

We encourage you to photocopy and use this page as a tool to assess how the articles in *Annual Editions* expand on the information in your textbook. By reflecting on the articles you will gain enhanced text information. You can also access this useful form on a product's book support Web site at *http://www.mhcls.com/online/*.

NAME: DATE:

_____

TITLE AND NUMBER OF ARTICLE:

_____

BRIEFLY STATE THE MAIN IDEA OF THIS ARTICLE:

_____

LIST THREE IMPORTANT FACTS THAT THE AUTHOR USES TO SUPPORT THE MAIN IDEA:

_____

WHAT INFORMATION OR IDEAS DISCUSSED IN THIS ARTICLE ARE ALSO DISCUSSED IN YOUR TEXTBOOK OR OTHER READINGS THAT YOU HAVE DONE? LIST THE TEXTBOOK CHAPTERS AND PAGE NUMBERS:

_____

LIST ANY EXAMPLES OF BIAS OR FAULTY REASONING THAT YOU FOUND IN THE ARTICLE:

_____

LIST ANY NEW TERMS/CONCEPTS THAT WERE DISCUSSED IN THE ARTICLE, AND WRITE A SHORT DEFINITION:

We Want Your Advice

ANNUAL EDITIONS revisions depend on two major opinion sources: one is our Advisory Board, listed in the front of this volume, which works with us in scanning the thousands of articles published in the public press each year; the other is you—the person actually using the book. Please help us and the users of the next edition by completing the prepaid article rating form on this page and returning it to us. Thank you for your help!

ANNUAL EDITIONS: Aging 07/08

ARTICLE RATING FORM

Here is an opportunity for you to have direct input into the next revision of this volume.
We would like you to rate each of the articles listed below, using the following scale:

1. **Excellent: should definitely be retained**
2. **Above average: should probably be retained**
3. **Below average: should probably be deleted**
4. **Poor: should definitely be deleted**

Your ratings will play a vital part in the next revision.
Please mail this prepaid form to us as soon as possible.
Thanks for your help!

RATING	ARTICLE	RATING	ARTICLE
	1. Elderly Americans		21. How to Survive the First Year
	2. The Economic Conundrum of an Aging Population		22. The Big Squeeze
	3. Living Longer		23. Old. Smart. Productive.
	4. Puzzle of the Century		24. The Broken Promise
	5. The Demographic Drivers of Aging		25. Work/Retirement Choices and Lifestyle Patterns of Older Americans
	6. Will You Live to Be 100?		26. More Hospice Patients Forgoing Sustenance
	7. The 2005 White House Conference on Aging		27. The Grieving Process
	8. Women's Sexuality as They Age: The More Things Change, the More They Stay the Same		28. Start the Conversation
	9. As Good As It Gets		29. Mind Frames Towards Dying and Factors Motivating Their Adoption by Terminally Ill Elders
	10. Cohabitation Among Older Adults: A National Portrait		30. (Not) the Same Old Story
	11. We Can Control How We Age		31. A Home for the Rest of Your Life
	12. Society Fears the Aging Process		32. Nursing Homes: Business As Usual
	13. Ageism in America		33. Declaration of Independents
	14. The Secret Lives of Single Women		34. Have Seniors Been Dealt a Bad Hand? Medicare's Drug Discount Cards
	15. The Under-Reported Impact of Age Discrimination and Its Threat to Business Vitality		35. Social Security's 70th Anniversary: Surviving 20 Years of Reform
	16. Primary Care for Elderly People: Why Do Doctors Find It So Hard?		36. Universalism Without the Targeting: Privatizing the Old-Age Welfare State
	17. Breakthrough		37. Coverage For All
	18. Marital History and the Burden of Cardiovascular Disease in Midlife		38. Riding Into the Sunset
	19. The Disappearing Mind		
	20. The Extent and Frequency of Abuse in the Lives of Older Women and Their Relationship With Health Outcomes		

(Continued on next page)

BUSINESS REPLY MAIL
FIRST CLASS MAIL PERMIT NO. 551 DUBUQUE IA

POSTAGE WILL BE PAID BY ADDRESEE

McGraw-Hill Contemporary Learning Series
2460 KERPER BLVD
DUBUQUE, IA 52001-9902

NO POSTAGE
NECESSARY
IF MAILED
IN THE
UNITED STATES

ABOUT YOU

Name

Date

Are you a teacher? ❑   A student? ❑
Your school's name

Department

Address   City   State   Zip

School telephone #

YOUR COMMENTS ARE IMPORTANT TO US!

Please fill in the following information:
For which course did you use this book?

Did you use a text with this ANNUAL EDITION?   ❑ yes ❑ no
What was the title of the text?

What are your general reactions to the *Annual Editions* concept?

Have you read any pertinent articles recently that you think should be included in the next edition? Explain.

Are there any articles that you feel should be replaced in the next edition? Why?

Are there any World Wide Web sites that you feel should be included in the next edition? Please annotate.

May we contact you for editorial input?   ❑ yes ❑ no
May we quote your comments? ❑ yes ❑ no